Upper Gastrointestinal Bleeding

Editor

IAN M. GRALNEK

GASTROENTEROLOGY
CLINICS OF NORTH AMERICA

www.gastro.theclinics.com

Consulting Editor
GARY W. FALK

December 2014 • Volume 43 • Number 4

ELSEVIER

1600 John F. Kennedy Boulevard ● Suite 1800 ● Philadelphia, Pennsylvania, 19103-2899
http://www.theclinics.com

GASTROENTEROLOGY CLINICS OF NORTH AMERICA Volume 43, Number 4
December 2014 ISSN 0889-8553, ISBN-13: 978-0-323-32650-6

Editor: Kerry Holland
Developmental Editor: Susan Showalter

Gastroenterology Clinics of North America (ISSN 0889-8553) is published quarterly by Elsevier Inc., 360 Park Avenue South, New York, NY 10010-1710. Months of issue are March, June, September, and December. Business and Editorial Offices: 1600 John F. Kennedy Blvd., Suite 1800, Philadelphia, PA 19103-2899. Customer Service Office: 6277 Sea Harbor Drive, Orlando, FL 32887-4800. Periodicals postage paid at New York, NY and additional mailing offices. Subscription prices are $320.00 per year (US individuals), $160.00 per year (US students), $530.00 per year (US institutions), $350.00 per year (Canadian individuals), $651.00 per year (Canadian institutions), $445.00 per year (international individuals), $220.00 per year (international students), and $651.00 per year (international institutions). Foreign air speed delivery is included in all *Clinics* subscription prices. All prices are subject to change without notice. **POSTMASTER:** Send address changes to *Gastroenterology Clinics of North America*, Elsevier Health Sciences Division, Subscription Customer Service, 3251 Riverport Lane, Maryland Heights, MO 63043. Telephone: 1-800-654-2452 (U.S. and Canada); 314-447-8871 (outside U.S. and Canada). Fax: 314-447-8029. E-mail: journalscustomerservice-usa@elsevier.com (for print support); journalsonlinesupport-usa@elsevier.com (for online support).

Reprints. For copies of 100 or more, of articles in this publication, please contact the Commercial Reprints Department, Elsevier Inc., 360 Part Avenue South, New York, New York 10010-1710. Tel. 212-633-3874, Fax: 212-633-3820, E-mail: reprints@elsevier.com.

Gastroenterology Clinics of North America is also published in Italian by II Pensiero Scientifico Editore, Rome, Italy; and in Portuguese by Interlivros Edicoes Ltda., Rua Commandante Coelho 1085, 21250 Cordovil, Rio de Janeiro, Brazil.

Gastroenterology Clinics of North America is covered in *MEDLINE/PubMed (Index Medicus), Excerpta Medica, Current Contents/Clinical Medicine, Science Citation Index, ISI/BIOMED,* and *BIOSIS*.

Contributors

CONSULTING EDITOR

GARY W. FALK, MD, MS
Professor of Medicine, Division of Gastroenterology, Hospital of the University of Pennsylvania, University of Pennsylvania Perelman School of Medicine, Philadelphia, Pennsylvania

EDITOR

IAN M. GRALNEK, MD, MSHS, FASGE
Chief, Hospital-Wide Ambulatory Care Services, Head, GI Outcomes Unit and Senior Physician Department of Gastroenterology, Rappaport Faculty of Medicine, Rambam Health Care Campus, Technion-Israel Institute of Technology, Haifa, Israel

AUTHORS

ABDULLAH M.S. AL-OSAIMI, MD, FACP, FACG, AGAF
Medical Director of Liver Transplantation, Chief, Division of Hepatology; Associate Professor of Medicine and Surgery, Department of Medicine, Temple University Health System, Temple University School of Medicine, Philadelphia, Pennsylvania

SUMEET K. ASRANI, MD, MSc
Baylor University Medical Center, Dallas, Texas

ANNA BAIGES, MD
Barcelona Hepatic Hemodynamic Laboratory, Liver Unit, Hospital Clinic, Institut d'Investigacions Biomèdiques August Pi-Sunyer (IDIBAPS), Ciber de Enfermedades Hepáticas y Digestivas (CIBEREHD), Barcelona, Spain

ALAN BARKUN, MD, MSc
Divisions of Gastroenterology and Clinical Epidemiology, McGill University Health Center, McGill University, Montréal, Canada

KENNETH F. BINMOELLER, MD
Interventional Endoscopy Services, California Pacific Medical Center, San Francisco, California

ANDRÉS CÁRDENAS, MD, MMSc, AGAF
GI/Endoscopy Unit, Hospital Clinic, Institut d'Investigacions Biomèdiques August Pi-Sunyer (IDIBAPS), Ciber de Enfermedades Hepáticas y Digestivas (CIBEREHD), Barcelona, Spain

YEN-I CHEN, MD
Division of Gastroenterology, McGill University Health Center, McGill University, Montréal, Canada

PHILIP WAI YAN CHIU, MD, FRCSEd
Professor, Department of Surgery, Institute of Digestive Disease, Prince of Wales Hospital, The Chinese University of Hong Kong, Hong Kong, China

JUAN CARLOS GARCIA-PAGAN, MD, PhD
Barcelona Hepatic Hemodynamic Laboratory, Liver Unit, Hospital Clinic, Institut d'Investigacions Biomèdiques August Pi-Sunyer (IDIBAPS), Ciber de Enfermedades Hepáticas y Digestivas (CIBEREHD), Barcelona, Spain

VIRGINIA HERNANDEZ-GEA, MD, PhD
Barcelona Hepatic Hemodynamic Laboratory, Liver Unit, Hospital Clinic, Institut d'Investigacions Biomèdiques August Pi-Sunyer (IDIBAPS), Ciber de Enfermedades Hepáticas y Digestivas (CIBEREHD), Barcelona, Spain

I. LISANNE HOLSTER, MD, PhD
Department of Gastroenterology and Hepatology, Erasmus MC University Medical Centre, Rotterdam, The Netherlands

JAWAD A. ILYAS, MD, MS
Gastroenterology and Hepatology, Department of Medicine, Baylor College of Medicine, Houston, Texas

PATRICK S. KAMATH, MD
Division of Gastroenterology and Hepatology, Mayo Clinic College of Medicine, Rochester, Minnesota

FASIHA KANWAL, MD, MSHS
Gastroenterology and Hepatology, Department of Medicine, Baylor College of Medicine; Center for Innovations in Quality, Effectiveness, and Safety (IQuESt), Michael E. DeBakey Veterans Affairs Medical Center, Houston, Texas

JOSHUA C. KLEIN, BS
Research Fellow, Department of Emergency Medicine, George Washington University, Washington, DC

ERNST J. KUIPERS, MD, PhD
Department of Gastroenterology and Hepatology, Erasmus MC University Medical Centre, Rotterdam, The Netherlands

SUMIT KUMAR, MD, MRCP
Abington Memorial Hospital, Abington, Pennsylvania

JAMES YUN WONG LAU, MD, FRCSEd
Department of Surgery, Institute of Digestive Disease, Prince of Wales Hospital, The Chinese University of Hong Kong, Hong Kong, China

MICHAEL J. LEVY, MD
Professor of Medicine, Division of Gastroenterology and Hepatology, Mayo Clinic, Rochester, Minnesota

YIDAN LU, MD
Division of Gastroenterology, McGill University Health Center, McGill University, Montréal, Canada

ANDREW C. MELTZER, MD, MS
Assistant Professor, Department of Emergency Medicine, George Washington University, Washington, DC

SUJAL M. NANAVATI, MD
Associate Clinical Professor, Interventional Radiology, Department of Radiology and Biomedical Imaging, University of California, San Francisco, California

KAMRAN QURESHI, MD
Division of Hepatology, Assistant Professor of Medicine, Department of Medicine, Temple University Health System, Temple University School of Medicine, Philadelphia, Pennsylvania

GIANLUCA ROTONDANO, MD, FASGE, FACG
Division of Gastroenterology and Digestive Endoscopy, Hospital Maresca, Azienda Sanitaria Locale Napoli 3 Sud, Torre del Greco, Italy

ARUN J. SANYAL, MBBS, MD
Professor of Internal Medicine, Pharmacology and Molecular Pathology, Division of Gastroenterology, Department of Internal Medicine, Virginia Commonwealth University School of Medicine, Richmond, Virginia

SANJAYA K. SATAPATHY, MBBS, MD, DM
Division of Surgery, Methodist University Hospital Transplant Institute, University of Tennessee Health Sciences Center, Memphis, Tennessee

ERIC T.T.L. TJWA, MD, PhD
Department of Gastroenterology and Hepatology, Erasmus MC University Medical Centre, Rotterdam, The Netherlands

FRANK WEILERT, MD
Waikato Hospital, Hamilton, New Zealand

LOUIS M. WONG KEE SONG, MD
Associate Professor of Medicine, Division of Gastroenterology and Hepatology, Mayo Clinic, Rochester, Minnesota

Contents

Foreword: Upper GI Bleeding   xiii

Gary W. Falk

Preface: Upper GI Bleeding   xv

Ian M. Gralnek

Epidemiology and Diagnosis of Acute Nonvariceal Upper Gastrointestinal Bleeding   643

Gianluca Rotondano

Acute upper gastrointestinal bleeding (UGIB) is a common gastroentero-
logical emergency. A vast majority of these bleeds have nonvariceal
causes, in particular gastroduodenal peptic ulcers. Nonsteroidal antiinflammatory drugs, low-dose aspirin use, and *Helicobacter pylori* infection
are the main risk factors for UGIB. Current epidemiologic data suggest that
patients most affected are older with medical comorbidit. Widespread use
of potentially gastroerosive medications underscores the importance of
adopting gastroprotective pharamacologic strategies. Endoscopy is the
mainstay for diagnosis and treatment of acute UGIB. It should be performed within 24 hours of presentation by skilled operators in adequately
equipped settings, using a multidisciplinary team approach.

**Upper Gastrointestinal Bleeding: Patient Presentation, Risk Stratification,
and Early Management**   665

Andrew C. Meltzer and Joshua C. Klein

The established quality indicators for early management of upper gastrointestinal (GI) hemorrhage are based on rapid diagnosis, risk stratification,
and early management. Effective preendoscopic treatment may improve
survivability of critically ill patients and improve resource allocation for all
patients. Accurate risk stratification helps determine the need for hospital
admission, hemodynamic monitoring, blood transfusion, and endoscopic
hemostasis before esophagogastroduodenoscopy (EGD) via indirect measures such as laboratory studies, physiologic data, and comorbidities.
Early management before the definitive EGD is essential to improving
outcomes for patients with upper GI bleeding.

Endoscopic Management of Acute Peptic Ulcer Bleeding   677

Yidan Lu, Yen-I Chen, and Alan Barkun

This review discusses the indications, technical aspects, and comparative
effectiveness of the endoscopic treatment of upper gastrointestinal
bleeding caused by peptic ulcer. Pre-endoscopic considerations, such
as the use of prokinetics and timing of endoscopy, are reviewed. In addition, this article examines aspects of postendoscopic care such as the
effectiveness, dosing, and duration of postendoscopic proton-pump inhibitors, *Helicobacter pylori* testing, and benefits of treatment in terms of
preventing rebleeding; and the use of nonsteroidal anti-inflammatory drugs,
antiplatelet agents, and oral anticoagulants, including direct thrombin and
Xa inhibitors, following acute peptic ulcer bleeding.

Endoscopic Management of Nonvariceal, Nonulcer Upper Gastrointestinal Bleeding   707

Eric T.T.L. Tjwa, I. Lisanne Holster, and Ernst J. Kuipers

Upper gastrointestinal bleeding (UGIB) is the most common emergency condition in gastroenterology. Although peptic ulcer and esophagogastric varices are the predominant causes, other conditions account for up to 50% of UGIBs. These conditions, among others, include angiodysplasia, Dieulafoy and Mallory-Weiss lesions, gastric antral vascular ectasia, and Cameron lesions. Upper GI cancer as well as lesions of the biliary tract and pancreas may also result in severe UGIB. This article provides an overview of the endoscopic management of these lesions, including the role of novel therapeutic modalities such as hemostatic powder and over-the-scope-clips.

Emerging Endoscopic Therapies for Nonvariceal Upper Gastrointestinal Bleeding   721

Louis M. Wong Kee Song and Michael J. Levy

 Videos of hemostasis of an actively bleeding gastric Dieulafoy lesion, hemostasis of an actively bleeding duodenal ulcer, carbon dioxide–based cryotherapy of diffuse gastric antral vascular ectasia, radiofrequency ablation of gastric antral vascular ectasia, animation of the OverStitch endoscopic suturing device, and OverStitch suture closure of endoscopic submucosal dissection defect accompany this article

Several new devices and innovative adaptations of existing modalities have emerged as primary, adjunctive, or rescue therapy in endoscopic hemostasis of gastrointestinal hemorrhage. These techniques include over-the-scope clip devices, hemostatic sprays, cryotherapy, radiofrequency ablation, endoscopic suturing, and endoscopic ultrasound–guided angiotherapy. This review highlights the technical aspects and clinical applications of these devices in the context of nonvariceal upper gastrointestinal bleeding.

What if Endoscopic Hemostasis Fails?: Alternative Treatment Strategies: Interventional Radiology   739

Sujal M. Nanavati

Since the 1960s, interventional radiology has played a role in the management of gastrointestinal bleeding. What began primarily as a diagnostic modality has evolved into much more of a therapeutic tool. And although the frequency of gastrointestinal bleeding has diminished thanks to management by pharmacologic and endoscopic methods, the need for additional invasive interventions still exists. Transcatheter angiography and intervention is a fundamental step in the algorithm for the treatment of gastrointestinal bleeding.

What If Endoscopic Hemostasis Fails?: Alternative Treatment Strategies: Surgery   753

Philip Wai Yan Chiu and James Yun Wong Lau

Management of bleeding peptic ulcers is increasingly challenging in an aging population. Endoscopic therapy reduces the need for emergency surgery in bleeding peptic ulcers. Initial endoscopic control offers an opportunity for selecting high-risk ulcers for potential early preemptive surgery. However, such an approach has not been supported by evidence in the literature. Endoscopic retreatment can be an option to control ulcer rebleeding and reduce complications. The success of endoscopic retreatment largely depends on the severity of rebleeding and ulcer characteristics. Large chronic ulcers with urgent bleeding are less likely to respond to endoscopic retreatment. Expeditious surgery is advised.

Epidemiology, Diagnosis and Early Patient Management of Esophagogastric Hemorrhage   765

Sumit Kumar, Sumeet K. Asrani, and Patrick S. Kamath

Acute variceal bleeding (AVB) is a potentially life-threatening complication of cirrhosis and portal hypertension. Combination therapy with vasoactive drugs and endoscopic variceal ligation is the first-line treatment in the management of AVB after adequate hemodynamic resuscitation. Short-term antibiotic prophylaxis, early resuscitation, early use of lactulose for prevention of hepatic encephalopathy, targeting of conservative goals for blood transfusion, and application of early transjugular intrahepatic portosystemic shunts in patients with AVB have further improved the prognosis of AVB. This article discusses the epidemiology, diagnosis, and nonendoscopic management of AVB.

Primary Prophylaxis of Variceal Bleeding   783

Jawad A. Ilyas and Fasiha Kanwal

Gastroesophageal varices are present in almost half of patients with cirrhosis at the time of initial diagnosis. Variceal bleeding occurs in 25% to 35% of patients with cirrhosis. Effective and timely care can prevent variceal bleeding (primary prophylaxis). For example, clinical studies demonstrate that both beta-blockers and endoscopic variceal ligation are effective in preventing a first episode of variceal bleeding. The major challenge is to screen patients in a timely manner and institute a form of therapy that has the highest chance of success in terms of patient compliance and effectiveness.

Endoscopic Hemostasis in Acute Esophageal Variceal Bleeding   795

Andrés Cárdenas, Anna Baiges, Virginia Hernandez-Gea, and Juan Carlos Garcia-Pagan

Acute variceal bleeding (AVB) is a milestone event for patients with portal hypertension. Esophageal varices bleed because of an increase in portal pressure that causes the variceal wall to rupture. AVB in a patient with cirrhosis and portal hypertension is associated with significant morbidity and mortality. The initial management of these patients includes proper resuscitation, antibiotic prophylaxis, pharmacologic therapy with vasoconstrictors, and endoscopic therapy. Intravascular fluid management, timing of endoscopy, and endoscopic technique are key in managing these patients. This article reviews the current endoscopic hemostatic strategies for patients with AVB.

Endoscopic Management of Gastric Variceal Bleeding   807

Frank Weilert and Kenneth F. Binmoeller

> Expert knowledge of endoscopic management of gastric varices is essential, as these occur in 20% of patients with portal hypertension. Bleeding is relatively uncommon, but carries significant mortality when this occurs. Inability to directly target intravascular injections and the potential complication related to glue embolization has resulted in the development of novel techniques. Direct visualization of the varix lumen using endoscopic ultrasound (EUS) allows targeted therapy of feeder vessels with real-time imaging. EUS-guided combination therapy with endovascular coiling and cyanoacrylate injections promise to provide reduced complication rates, increased obliteration of varices, and reduced long-term rebleeding rates.

Nonendoscopic Management Strategies for Acute Esophagogastric Variceal Bleeding   819

Sanjaya K. Satapathy and Arun J. Sanyal

> Acute variceal bleeding is a potentially life-threatening complication of portal hypertension. Management consists of emergent hemostasis, therapy directed at hemodynamic resuscitation, protection of the airway, and prevention and treatment of complications including prophylactic use of antibiotics. Endoscopic treatment remains the mainstay in the management of acute variceal bleeding in combination with pharmacotherapy aimed at reducing portal pressure. This article intends to highlight only the current nonendoscopic treatment approaches for control of acute variceal bleeding.

Approach to the Management of Portal Hypertensive Gastropathy and Gastric Antral Vascular Ectasia   835

Kamran Qureshi and Abdullah M.S. Al-Osaimi

> Gastric antral vascular ectasia (GAVE) and portal hypertensive gastropathy (PHG) are important causes of chronic gastrointestinal bleeding. These gastric mucosal lesions are mostly diagnosed on upper endoscopy and can be distinguished based on their appearance or location in the stomach. In some situations, especially in patients with liver cirrhosis and portal hypertension, a diffuse pattern and involvement of gastric mucosa are seen with both GAVE and severe PHG. The diagnosis in such cases is hard to determine on visual inspection, and thus, biopsy and histologic evaluation can be used to help differentiate GAVE from PHG.

Index   849

GASTROENTEROLOGY
CLINICS OF NORTH AMERICA

FORTHCOMING ISSUES

March 2015
Gastroparesis
Henry P. Parkman and
Pankaj Jay Pasricha, *Editors*

June 2015
Barrett's Esophagus
Prasad G. Iyer and
Navtej Buttar, *Editors*

September 2015
H. Pylori Therapies
David Y. Graham and
Akiko Shiotani, *Editors*

RECENT ISSUES

September 2014
Biologics in Inflammatory Bowel Disease
Edward V. Loftus, *Editor*

June 2014
Eosinophilic Esophagitis
Ikuo Hirano, *Editor*

March 2014
Gastroesophageal Reflux Disease
Joel E. Richter, *Editor*

RELATED INTEREST

Gastrointestinal Endoscopy Clinics of North America,
October 2011 (Vol. 21, Issue 4)
Upper Gastrointestinal Bleeding
Col. Roy K.H. Wong, *Editor*

Foreword
Upper GI Bleeding

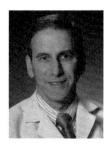

Gary W. Falk, MD, MS
Consulting Editor

One of the most common problems encountered by gastroenterologists throughout the world is upper gastrointestinal (GI) bleeding. Furthermore, upper GI bleeding represents a true emergency with risk for mortality with each episode. The approach to upper GI bleeding has evolved over the years to involve a combination of pharmacologic, endoscopic, radiologic, and surgical approaches. However, GI bleeding most definitely does not follow a "one-size-fits-all" approach. To address the current state-of-the-art, Dr Ian Gralnek, a well-recognized authority in upper GI bleeding, has assembled internationally recognized experts in the field. This update on a host of important issues in both variceal and nonvariceal upper GI bleeding is both timely and practical. I hope you enjoy this issue of *Gastroenterology Clinics of North America*.

Gary W. Falk, MD, MS
Division of Gastroenterology
University of Pennsylvania Perelman School of Medicine
9 Penn Tower
One Convention Avenue
Philadelphia, PA 19104, USA

E-mail address:
gary.falk@uphs.upenn.edu

Gastroenterol Clin N Am 43 (2014) xiii
http://dx.doi.org/10.1016/j.gtc.2014.09.002
0889-8553/14/$ – see front matter © 2014 Elsevier Inc. All rights reserved.

gastro.theclinics.com

Preface

Upper GI Bleeding

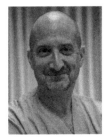

Ian M. Gralnek, MD, MSHS, FASGE
Editor

Acute gastrointestinal bleeding (GI) is one of the most common clinical problems in gastroenterology and all too frequently rousts many a gastroenterologist from their slumber when on call. The most common type of acute GI bleeding is *upper* GI bleeding. However, not all upper GI bleeding is alike...acute upper GI bleeding is divided into nonvariceal and variceal causes. This issue of *Gastroenterology Clinics of North America* is all about acute upper GI bleeding and is divided, not surprisingly, into two distinct sections: section I is devoted to nonvariceal upper GI bleeding and section II is devoted to variceal upper GI bleeding.

Acute nonvariceal upper GI bleeding may originate from the esophagus, stomach, or duodenum, essentially anywhere proximal to the Ligament of Treitz. In Section I, Dr Gianluca Rotondano, Hospital Maresca, Torre del Greco, Italy, begins with a review of the epidemiology and diagnosis of acute nonvariceal upper GI bleeding. We then turn to patient presentation, risk stratification, and how to initially medically manage these bleeding patients. I am pleased to have one of our emergency medicine colleagues, Dr Andrew Meltzer, Department of Emergency Medicine, George Washington University, contribute this important article and provide a unique viewpoint from the emergency department where most of these patients initially present. As we all know, endoscopic hemostasis is the accepted standard of care for patients with acute nonvariceal upper GI bleeding. Moreover, peptic ulcer bleeding is the most common nonvariceal cause of acute upper GI bleeding; thus, Drs Yidan Lu, Yen-I Chen, and Alan Barkun from McGill University, Montreal, Canada, provide an in-depth review of the endoscopic management of peptic ulcer bleeding. Drs Eric Tjwa, I. Lisanne Holster, and Ernst Kuipers from the Erasmus Medical Center University Hospital, Rotterdam, The Netherlands, review the endoscopic management of all other causes of acute nonvariceal upper GI bleeding, and in addition, Drs Louis Wong Kee Song and Michael Levy from the Mayo Clinic, Rochester, Minnesota discuss emerging endoscopic hemostasis treatments, such as topical sprays and over-the-scope clipping devices. Although endoscopic hemostasis is very highly effective, there are unfortunately cases

Gastroenterol Clin N Am 43 (2014) xv–xvi
http://dx.doi.org/10.1016/j.gtc.2014.09.001
0889-8553/14/$ – see front matter © 2014 Published by Elsevier Inc.

where bleeding is unable to be controlled or when significant rebleeding occurs that is not amenable to endoscopic therapy. Therefore, I have included two articles that provide insight into the question…what if endoscopic hemostasis fails? The first article, written by Drs Philip Wai Yan Chiu and James Yun Wong Lau, from Prince of Wales Hospital, The Chinese University of Hong Kong, focuses on tried and true surgical treatment options. The second article, by Dr Sujal Nanavati, University of California at San Francisco, Department of Radiology and Biomedical Imaging, addresses the alternative treatment strategy of angiographic embolization, which has now emerged as the often preferred salvage treatment strategy.

One of the most feared complications of cirrhosis and portal hypertension is variceal hemorrhage. In Section II of this issue, the focus is on variceal causes of acute upper GI bleeding. Usually due to esophageal variceal rupture, this complication occurs in an entirely different epidemiologic and clinical setting than nonvariceal upper GI bleeding. Thus, this topic requires an understanding of many critical issues, including diagnosis and management. We begin Section II with a review of the epidemiology, diagnosis, and early patient management strategies in bleeding esophagogastric varices by Drs Sumit Kumar, Sumeet Asrani, and Patrick Kamath from Mayo Clinic, Rochester, Minnesota. Drs Jawad Ilyas and Fasiha Kanwal from the Baylor College of Medicine, Houston, Texas go on to present the latest evidence on primary prophylaxis of variceal bleeding, both medical and endoscopic. However, for those patients who present with acute esophagogastric variceal bleeding, endoscopic management is the cornerstone of patient management. Drs Andrés Cárdenas, Anna Baiges, Virginia Hernandez-Gea, and Juan Carlos Garcia-Pagan from the GI/Endoscopy Unit and Barcelona Hepatic Hemodynamic Laboratory, Liver Unit, Barcelona, Spain, provide an evidence-based review of endoscopic hemostasis techniques in acute esophageal variceal bleeding, and Drs Frank Weilert and Kenneth Binmoeller from Waikato Hospital, Hamilton, New Zealand and the California Pacific Medical Center, San Francisco, respectively, discuss the recommended endoscopic management of bleeding gastric varices, including emerging techniques such as EUS-guided intravascular therapies. Next, Drs Sanjaya Satapathy and Arun Sanyal contribute a comprehensive review of nonendoscopic management strategies for esophagogastric variceal bleeding, and last but not least, Drs Kamran Qureshi and Abdullah Al-Osaimi, from Temple University, Philadelphia, Pennsylvania, discuss how to manage the patient with portal hypertensive gastropathy and gastric antral vascular ectasia (also known as watermelon stomach).

I am sincerely grateful to all of the authors who so willingly contributed to this issue. Of note, this is a true international effort since the distinguished guest authors of this issue come from five continents around the world and graciously provide their clinical expertise on this very important topic. We have attempted to put together a comprehensive issue on "Upper Gastrointestinal Bleeding" and I hope that you will find this issue as informative and helpful in your practice of gastroenterology as I have.

Ian M. Gralnek, MD, MSHS, FASGE
Hospital-Wide Ambulatory Care Services
GI Outcomes Unit
Department of Gastroenterology
Rambam Health Care Campus
Rappaport Faculty of Medicine
Technion-Israel Institute of Technology
Haifa, Israel

E-mail address:
i_gralnek@rambam.health.gov.il

Epidemiology and Diagnosis of Acute Nonvariceal Upper Gastrointestinal Bleeding

Gianluca Rotondano, MD

KEYWORDS

- Nonvariceal bleeding • Epidemiology • Diagnosis • Risk factors • Peptic ulcer
- Endoscopy • Timing

KEY POINTS

- There is a trend toward a decrease in the overall incidence and hospitalization for nonvariceal upper gastrointestinal bleeding (UGIB) worldwide. Peptic ulcer is still the most common cause of hemorrhage.
- The changing epidemiology is characterized by an aging population, with multiple comorbidities and increased use of aspirin, nonsteroidal antiinflammatory drugs (NSAIDs), or other antiplatelets/anticoagulants.
- Mortality for UGIB is still approximately 5% and is usually related to multiorgan failure, cardiopulmonary conditions, and end-stage malignancy.
- Endoscopy is the mainstay in the management of UGIB, allowing for proper diagnosis, risk stratification, and treatment of the bleeding lesion.
- Unless contraindicated, endoscopy should be performed within 24 hours of patient presentation to maximize benefits and improve economic outcomes.

EPIDEMIOLOGY OF ACUTE NONVARICEAL UPPER GASTROINTESTINAL BLEEDING

UGIB is predominantly nonvariceal in origin and remains one of the most common challenges faced by gastroenterologists and endoscopists in daily clinical practice. Despite major advances in the approach to the management of nonvariceal UGIB over the past 2 decades, including prevention of peptic ulcer bleeding, optimal use of endoscopic therapy, and adjuvant high-dose proton pump inhibitors (PPIs), it still carries considerable morbidity, mortality, and health economic burden.

The author has no conflict of interest to disclose.
Division of Gastroenterology & Digestive Endoscopy, Hospital Maresca, ASLNA3sud, Via Montedoro, Torre del Greco 80059, Italy
E-mail address: gianluca.rotondano@virgilio.it

Gastroenterol Clin N Am 43 (2014) 643–663
http://dx.doi.org/10.1016/j.gtc.2014.08.001
0889-8553/14/$ – see front matter © 2014 Elsevier Inc. All rights reserved.

gastro.theclinics.com

Incidence of Acute Upper Gastrointestinal Bleeding

With more than 300,000 hospital admissions annually in the United States,[1,2] UGIB is one of the most common gastrointestinal (GI) emergencies. A 2012 update on the burden of GI disease in the United States reports that GI hemorrhage still ranked 7th among the principal GI discharge diagnoses from hospital admissions in 2009, with a 22% increase compared with year 2000, and 10th among causes of death from GI and liver diseases.[3]

The incidence rates of UGIB demonstrate a large geographic variation, ranging from 48 to 160 cases per 100,000 population per year, with consistent reports of higher incidences among men and the elderly.[4–10] Possible explanations for the reported geographic variations in incidence are differences in definition of UGIB in various studies, population characteristics, prevalence of gastroerosive medications, in particular aspirin and NSAIDs, and *Helicobacter pylori* prevalence.

Some but not all time-trend studies have reported a significant decline in incidence of all-cause acute UGIB, especially peptic ulcer bleeding, in recent years. In the Netherlands, the incidence of UGIB decreased from 61.7/100,000 in 1993/1994 to 47.7/100,000 persons annually in 2000, corresponding to a 23% decrease in incidence after age adjustment.[6,7] This was confirmed in a population-based study carried out in Northern Italy in which the overall incidence of UGIB decreased from 112.5 to 89.8/100,000 per year, which corresponds to a 35.5% decrease after adjustment for age.[8] Trends for incidence of hospitalization due to GI complications in the United States from 2001 to 2009 confirm decreases in UGIB (78.4–60.6/100,000) and peptic ulcer bleeding (48.7–32.1/100,000).[11] The reasons for the observed decrease in hospitalizations due to nonvariceal UGIB are not well defined, but it is reasonable to assume that the use of eradication therapy in patients with ulcer disease and the progressive increase in the implementation of preventive strategies in patients taking aspirin and NSAIDs may have played a role.[12–14]

Outcome data from multicenter observational registries of UGIB, originating from Italy,[15] Canada,[16] and the United Kingdom,[17] reported a mean age of bleeders over 60 years and a prevalence of UGIB in men. In-hospital bleeding (ie, GI hemorrhage that occurs in patients already hospitalized for another medical-surgical condition) occurs in 10% to 25%.[7,18–20]

Causes of Acute Upper Gastrointestinal Bleeding

Peptic ulcer bleeding is still the most common cause of nonvariceal UGIB, responsible for approximately 31% to 67% of all cases, followed by erosive disease, esophagitis, malignancy, and Mallory-Weiss tears. In 2% to 8% of cases, uncommon causes, such as Dieulafoy lesion, hemobilia, angiodysplasia, vascular-enteric fistula, and gastric antral vascular ectasia are found (**Table 1**).[6–9,15–17,21–26]

In recent years, there has been an overall decrease in the incidence of UGIB related to bleeding peptic ulcers, at least in subjects under 70 years of age,[8] whereas its incidence is stable or even higher among patients of more advanced age.[27] A study from Australia on bleeding ulcers over a 10-year period (1997–2007) confirmed that the number of bleeding ulcers remained unchanged despite a decreased incidence of uncomplicated peptic ulcer.[28] Gastric ulcers increased significantly in both bleeding and nonbleeding patients whereas the proportion of duodenal ulcers fell significantly. The proportion of bleeding ulcers related to NSAIDs or aspirin increased significantly over 10 years, from 51% to 71%. Gastroduodenal ulcers are also the most frequent causes of nonvariceal bleeding in cirrhotic patients (48%–51%).[29,30]

Table 1	
Causes of upper gastrointestinal bleeding according to recent epidemiologic studies	
	%
Peptic ulcer	31–67
Erosive disease	7–31
Variceal bleeding	4–20
Esophagitis	3–12
Mallory-Weiss tears	4–8
Malignancy	2–8
Vascular lesions	2–8
None (no lesion identified)	3–19

Data from Refs.[8,15–17,24,33]

Nonvariceal UGIB is not just about peptic ulcers. According to different registries, nonvariceal nonulcer bleeding accounts for 34% to 64% of all presenting cases of nonvariceal UGIB.[15–17] Recent data from Italy[31] show that patients with Dieulafoy lesions have high rebleeding rates (19.1%); although they are rare causes of nonvariceal UGIB, they can cause torrential bleeding and can be difficult to locate. Patients with Dieulafoy lesions were more likely to present with hematemesis, shock, syncope, and a lower hemoglobin concentration and require blood transfusion compared with patients presenting with other endoscopic diagnoses. Of greater concern was the reported rebleeding rate for Mallory-Weiss tears (6.3%), traditionally considered benign, low-risk, and self-limiting lesions. It is possible that this may represent endoscopic undertreatment because of the perceived low-risk nature of Mallory-Weiss tears but also raises questions regarding uniform diagnostic criteria.

The source and outcomes of UGIB in oncologic patients are poorly investigated. The causes of UGIB in oncologic patients seem to be different from those in the general population. Retrospective data on 324 patients with cancer referred for endoscopy due to UGIB[32] showed that tumor was the most common cause of bleeding (23.8%), followed by varices (19.7%), peptic ulcer (16.3%), and gastroduodenal erosions (10.9%). If considering only patients with tumors outside the GI tract, however, the most common causes of UGIB are similar to those in the general population, that is, peptic ulcer, gastroduodenal erosions, and varices. On the other hand, even in patients with tumors outside the GI tract, metastases were the source of bleeding in a significant number of patients (11%).

Risk Factors for Acute Nonvariceal Upper Gastrointestinal Bleeding

Risk factors for peptic ulcer bleeding are *H pylori* infection, use of NSAIDs, use of low-dose aspirin, and other antiplatelet medications or oral anticoagulants.

Helicobacter pylori infection

H pylori infection is found in 43% to 56% of peptic ulcer bleeding patients.[15–17,23,33] The true *H pylori* prevalence in bleeding peptic ulcer is probably underestimated: in a recent meta-regression on 71 studies, including 8496 patients, the mean prevalence of *H pylori* infection in peptic ulcer bleeding was 72%.[34] The most significant variables associated with a high prevalence of *H pylori* infection were the use of a diagnostic test delayed until at least 4 weeks after the bleeding episode (odds ratio [OR] 2.08; 95% CI, 1.10–3.93) and a lower mean age of patients (OR 0.95 per additional year; 95% CI, 0.92–0.99). The low prevalence of *H pylori* infection reported in peptic ulcer bleeding may be due to the methodology of the studies and to patient characteristics. These data also support the recent recommendations of an international consensus on nonvariceal UGIB[35] regarding the performance of a delayed diagnostic test when *H pylori* tests carried out during the acute bleeding episode are negative.

The incidence of *H pylori*–negative idiopathic bleeding ulcers (ie, those not related to NSAIDs or other gastroerosive medications) is rising. These bleeding ulcers account for 16.1% of patients admitted for UGIB and 42.4% of patients who bled while in the hospital.[36] These ulcers are also prone to recurrent complications at 12 months: 13.4% (95% CI, 7.3%–19.5%) versus 2.5% (95% CI, 0.4%–4.6%) in patients with *H pylori*–positive ulcers who received eradication therapy.[36]

H pylori–negative bleeding ulcers are also associated with poorer outcomes regardless of use of NSAIDs. In a study from the University of Texas, patients without *H pylori* infection had significantly more comorbid medical conditions and higher Charlson index comorbidity scores than those with *H pylori*. Recurrent bleeding within 30 days was more frequent (11% vs 5%, $P = .009$) and hospital length of stay was significantly longer compared with *H pylori*–positive patients.[37] Such outcome data confirm previous findings of significantly higher incident rates of rebleeding and death in patients with *H pylori*-negative idiopathic ulcers than in controls with *H pylori*–positive bleeding ulcers. Moreover, gastroprotective agents, such as PPIs or H_2-receptor antagonists, did not reduce the risk of recurrent bleeding or mortality for patients with *H pylori*–negative idiopathic bleeding ulcers.[38]

Current guidelines recommend testing for *H pylori* infection among users of low-dose aspirin who are at high risk for developing ulcers, because the long-term incidence of rebleeding with aspirin use is reduced after *H pylori* is eradicated.[35] This was confirmed by a recent prospective study from Hong Kong,[39] in which the incidence of ulcer bleeding (per 100 patient-years) in the *H pylori*–eradicated cohort did not differ significantly from that of the average-risk cohort (no history of ulcers). Aspirin users without current or past *H pylori* infections who develop ulcer bleeding have a 5-fold incidence of recurrent bleeding.

Low-dose aspirin, antiplatelets, and nonsteroidal antiinflammatory drugs

Long-term use of aspirin is recommended for prevention of cardiovascular events among patients with prior cardiovascular disease or multiple risk factors.[40] Regular aspirin use is associated with an increased risk of major GI bleeding. A recent meta-analysis found an approximately 2-fold higher risk of GI bleeding among individuals regularly using aspirin compared with placebo, with no difference between 75 to 162.5 mg/d and greater than 162.5 to 325 mg/d.[41] Such a magnitude of risk is confirmed by a large prospective study of 87,680 women in which the relative risk (RR) of major UGIB requiring hospitalization or blood transfusion was 1.43 (95% CI, 1.29–1.59) over a 24-year follow-up period.[42] Furthermore, when used for primary prevention of cardiovascular disease, the absolute harms of aspirin seem to exceed its benefits: a meta-analysis of 27 studies showed that 60 to 84 major cardiovascular events per 100,000 person-years were averted, whereas 68 to 117 GI bleeds were incurred. There was a nonsignificant change in total cardiovascular disease, whereas risks were increased by 37% for GI bleeds.[43] Risk factors for UGIB among low-dose aspirin users include (1) a history of peptic ulcer disease or GI bleeding; (2) older age; (3) concomitant use of NSAIDs, including cyclooxygenase (COX)-2 inhibitors; (4) concomitant use of anticoagulants or other platelet aggregation inhibitors; (5) the presence of severe medical comorbidities; and (6) high aspirin dose. *H pylori* and aspirin seem to be independent risk factors for peptic ulcer bleeding, so that in patients with a history of peptic ulcer disease, H pylori infection should be assessed and treated if present.[44]

At-risk low-dose aspirin users are recommended to take gastroprotective agents. PPIs seem superior to eradication only to prevent recurrent ulcer bleeding in patients using low-dose aspirin.[35] Moreover, in patients with acute coronary syndrome or myocardial infarction receiving aspirin, clopidogrel, enoxaparin, or thrombolytics, PPIs are superior to H_2-receptor antagonists.[45]

Population-based epidemiologic data confirm that the use of low-dose aspirin, NSAIDs, warfarin, and the combination thereof are significantly more common among UGI bleeders than nonbleeders.[8,15–17,21,22,25] An increasing proportion of patients are nowadays hospitalized due to medication-related UGIB. Comparing data from Italy and the United Kingdom, the proportion of UGIB patients taking NSAIDs or antiplatelet agents and that of patients on anticoagulants was almost identical (46.4% vs 44.2% and 11.7% vs 13.2%, respectively).[8,17] The increased risk of UGIB associated with NSAIDs seems lower than previously reported: in a Spanish primary care research database study of more than 660,000 subjects,[46] increased risks were found with current use of NSAIDs (RR 1.72; 95% CI, 1.41–2.09), low-dose aspirin (RR 1.74; 95% CI, 1.37–2.21), other antiplatelet drugs (RR 1.73; 95% CI, 1.27–2.36), and oral anticoagulants (RR 2.00; 95% CI, 1.44–2.77). The use of oral corticosteroids, selective serotonin reuptake inhibitors, or acetaminophen was not associated with an increased risk.

In patients at risk for GI bleeding and using NSAIDs, a protective drug is recommended.[35] Acid-suppressing drugs reduce the risk among users of NSAIDs (OR 0.58; 0.39–0.85), particularly in users with antecedent peptic ulcer (OR 0.16; 0.05–0.58).[47] Unfortunately, despite several society and national guidelines that have been formulated, these are poorly followed in clinical practice and gastroprotection is largely underused. Data from Europe show that although approximately one-half of all patients with peptic ulcer bleeding were using NSAIDs or aspirin, an effective gastroprotective agent was only used in 10% to 15% of at-risk patients.[7,23,47,48] A multinational study from the United Kingdom, Italy, and the Netherlands confirmed that the risk of UGIB is significantly higher in nonselective NSAID users with gastroprotective nonadherence. Among 618,684 nonselective NSAID users, nonadherers to gastroprotection had a 2-fold risk of UGIB (OR 1.89; 95% CI, 1.09–3.28).[49] Selective cyclooxygenase (COX)-2 inhibitors are associated with a lower risk of clinically significant UGIB than nonselective NSAIDs[7,48]; however, concerns over the possible cardiovascular adverse effects of some of these agents should be taken into account. Moreover, switching to selective COX-2 inhibitors in patients with previous bleeding is not completely risk-free, and concomitant PPI therapy may also be needed. The combination of COX-2 inhibitors with PPIs promotes the greatest risk reduction for NSAID-related UGIB.[48]

A retrospective study among general practitioners in France[50] documented that within 2 years after prescribing a PPI, physicians did not renew this prescription for approximately 33% of those patients at risk for GI events (>65 years, past history of GI ulcer, or receiving antiplatelet agents) receiving continuous NSAIDs. Predictors for no longer receiving a prescription for a PPI included switching to a COX-2 selective inhibitor or to a nonselective NSAID and female gender. The risk for upper GI injury was higher among patients with discontinued PPI prescriptions (OR 1.45; 95% CI, 1.06–2.09).

UGIB is a rare but serious potential side effect of bisphosphonate therapy. In a population-based nested cohort study in Canada within an exposure cohort of 26,223 subjects,[51] 117 individuals suffered a serious UGIB within 120 days of starting a bisphosphonate (0.4%). Age greater than 80 (adjusted OR 2.03; 95% CI, 1.40–2.94) and a past history of serious UGIB (adjusted OR 2.28; 95% CI, 1.29–4.03) were the strongest predictors. Men were 70% more likely to suffer an UGIB compared with women (adjusted OR 1.69; 95% CI, 1.05–2.72).

Patients with UGIB have increasing non-GI comorbidities. Results of a matched case-control study on 16,355 patients with nonvariceal UGIB and 81,636 controls showed that non-GI comorbidity had a strong association with UGIB; the adjusted OR for a single comorbidity was 1.43 (95% CI, 1.35–1.52) and for multiple or severe comorbidity was 2.26 (95% CI, 2.14–2.38). The additional population attributable fraction for comorbidity (19.8%; 95% CI, 18.4–21.2) was considerably larger than that for any other measured risk factor, including aspirin or NSAIDs use (3.0% and 3.1%, respectively).[52] Non-GI comorbidity is an independent risk factor for UGIB and contributes to a greater proportion of patients with bleeding in the population than other recognized risk factors. These findings could explain why the incidence of nonvariceal bleeding remains high in older populations.

Mortality from Acute Upper Gastrointestinal Bleeding

Despite advances in endoscopic hemostasis and adjuvant pharmacologic treatment, the overall mortality from UGIB remains 5% to 14%, although most studies from the United States, Europe, and Asia place that figure closer to 5%.[15–17,22,25] A systematic review of 18 studies (10 using administrative databases and 8 using bleeding registries) showed mortality rates from acute UGIB ranging from 1.1% in Japan to 11% in Denmark.[53] The 28-day mortality after nonvariceal UGIB in England decreased from 14.7% in 1999 to 13.1% in 2007.[54] A recent analysis of the trends for incidence of hospitalization and death due to UGIB in the United States from 2001 to 2009 confirmed that age/gender-adjusted case fatality owing to bleeding is low (2.5%) and increases with age but remains less than 5% even in elderly patients.[11] These discrepancies in reported mortality rates of nonvariceal UGIB are attributable to differences in study methodologies and populations studied (heterogeneous definitions of case ascertainment, differing patient populations with regard to severity of presentation and associated comorbidities, varying durations of follow-up, and different health care system-related practices). More uniform standards in reporting would enable a better understanding of causes of death and the apparent discrepant outcome in endoscopic end points versus clinical end points. Nonvariceal UGIB is now predominantly a disease of the elderly, with more than 60% of patients over the age of 60 years and approximately 20% over the age of 80 years.[8,15] Because elderly patients have more comorbid illness, are more likely users of aspirin and NSAIDs, and are less tolerant of hemodynamic insult, the management of this high-risk population is a major challenge.[55] Current evidence indicates that most peptic ulcer bleeding–linked deaths are not a direct sequela of the bleeding ulcer itself. Instead, mortality derives from multiorgan failure, cardiopulmonary conditions, or end-stage malignancy, suggesting that improving further current treatments for the bleeding ulcer may have a limited impact on mortality unless supportive therapies are developed for the global management of these patients.[18] In a prospective cohort study enrolling more than 10,000 cases of peptic ulcer bleeding at the Prince of Wales Hospital in Hong Kong,[22] one of the most reputed bleeding centers worldwide, overall mortality was 6.2%. The study reported that approximately 80% of deceased patients died of non–bleeding-related causes.

Risk factors for mortality after nonvariceal UGIB[6,15–17,22,24,25,55–57] are

- Increasing age
- Hemodynamic instability on admission
- Presence of severe and life-threatening comorbid medical conditions

Recent data from Italy also identified an American Society of Anesthesiologists (ASA) score of 3 or 4 versus 1 or 2 as the variable with the greatest OR for predicting mortality (OR 3.92; 95% CI, 2.37–6.50).[31] One or more comorbidities are present in almost two-thirds of UGIB patients.[15–17,21] Underlying comorbidity is consistently associated with an increased short-term mortality in patients with peptic ulcer bleeding. A systematic review and meta-analysis of 16 studies[58] showed that the risk of 30-day or in-hospital mortality was significantly greater in patients with comorbidity than in those without (RR 4.44; 95% CI, 2.45–8.04). Patients with 3 or more comorbidities had a greater risk of dying than those with 1 or 2 (RR 3.46; 95% CI, 1.34–8.89). Among individual comorbidities that significantly increased the risk of death, RRs were higher for hepatic, renal, and malignant disease (RR range, 4.04–6.33) than for cardiovascular and respiratory disease and diabetes (2.39, 2.45, and 1.63, respectively). Coagulation disorders are also independently associated with more than a 5-fold increase in the odds of in-hospital mortality.[59]

Cirrhotic patients suffering a nonvariceal bleed have significantly greater in-hospital mortality than noncirrhotic patients.[29,30,60] The presence of cirrhosis independently increased mortality (adjusted OR 3.3; 95% CI, 2.2–4.9). Decompensated cirrhosis had higher mortality than compensated cirrhosis.[60] Cryptogenic etiology of cirrhosis, renal dysfunction, actively bleeding ulcers on hospital admission, concurrent presence of duodenal ulcer and erosive disease, and bleeding from vascular lesions are all independent predictors of mortality.[29,30]

Impaired renal function is an independent risk factor for UGIB. Crude rates of acute nonvariceal UGIB among patients undergoing dialysis have not decreased in the past 10 years.[61] Although 30-day mortality related to UGIB declined, the burden on the end-stage renal disease population remains substantial. Overall 30-day mortality is 4.8% to 13.7%, with a 2-fold risk of death in peptic ulcer bleeding patients with end-stage renal disease compared with those without.[62,63] Such a high mortality in patients undergoing dialysis was significantly correlated with older age, female gender, infection during hospitalization, single episodic UGIB, abnormal white blood cell count, and albumin level less than or equal to 3 g/dL.[62]

Mortality is also increased in patients who are already admitted in hospital for another medical problem. In-hospital bleeding accounts for 10% to 25% of the overall nonvariceal bleeding population[7,19,20,33] and is associated with poorer outcome, with mortality rates as high as 26%.[8,15–17,19,21] Nonetheless, the reasons for increased mortality in this subgroup of patients have not been consistently identified. Guidelines on optimal management of inpatients who develop nonvariceal UGIB[35,64–66] have been derived essentially from studies on outpatient bleeding, whereas few data are available that focus on in-hospital bleeding and its management. Recent data from Italy shed some light on the issue, showing that the mortality rate for in-hospital bleeding was significantly higher than that of outpatient bleeding (8.9% vs 3.8%; OR 2.44; 95% CI, 1.57–3.79). Hemodynamic instability on presentation and the presence of severe comorbidity were the strongest predictors of mortality for in-hospital bleeders.[20]

The risk of mortality increases with rebleeding, which is thus another major outcome parameter. Rebleeding rates, using a combination of endoscopic hemostasis and adjuvant acid-suppressing therapy, have been shown to be reduced to less than 10%[21,22,25] and it would be difficult, if not impossible, to reduce this further. Because a majority of nonvariceal UGIB patients today are of advanced age, users of NSAIDs and aspirin, and with multiple comorbid illnesses, the "endeavor to further reduce this rebleeding rate is an uphill battle."[22]

Little is known about mortality associated with nonulcer, nonvariceal UGIB. This may stem from a perception among clinicians that, other than those patients with a GI malignancy as the causative bleeding lesion, outcomes of patients with nonulcer bleeding are favorable. Therefore, it is possible that the usual algorithms of postendoscopy care, pharmacotherapy, and monitoring that are applied to patients in whom endoscopic hemostasis has been achieved after peptic ulcer bleeding may not be applied with the same rigor to those with nonulcer bleeding. A large prospective, multicenter study of 3207 patients with documented nonulcer UGIB have a risk of death similar to bleeding peptic ulcers.[20] Mortality was 9.8% for neoplasia, 4.8% for Mallory-Weiss tears, 4.8% for vascular lesions, 4.4% for gastroduodenal erosions, 4.4% for duodenal ulcer, and 3.1% for gastric ulcer. Frequency of death was not different among benign endoscopic diagnoses. The strongest predictor of mortality was the overall ASA score. After adjusting for ASA score, the endoscopic diagnosis had no impact on mortality, suggesting that nonulcer causes of bleeding carry a risk of mortality similar to that of peptic ulcers. Therefore, even a bleed from what is perceived to be a minor lesion in a high-risk patient can be a sufficient precipitant to initiate a downward cascade of clinical events, resulting in multiorgan failure and death. The message could not be clearer: treat the patient and not just the source of GI bleeding.

DIAGNOSIS OF ACUTE NONVARICEAL UPPER GASTROINTESTINAL BLEEDING

Upper GI endoscopy is an essential part of UGIB management and is the mainstay of diagnosis and treatment of most causes of UGIB.[26]

Endoscopy seems to reduce mortality among patients hospitalized for UGIB and specialty care in a gastroenterology ward offers additional protective effects. In a prospective study on 13,427 hospitalizations for UGIB in Italy, the 30-day mortality was 6.9%. Significantly lower rates were observed among hospitalizations that included endoscopy (OR 0.30; 95% CI, 0.26–0.34), specialist care (OR 0.55; 95% CI, 0.37–0.82), or both (OR 0.12; 95% CI, 0.07–0.22). The protective effects of endoscopy and specialist care remained strong after adjustment for potential confounders.[67]

Endoscopy provides crucial prognostic data as to the risk for recurrent bleeding through the assessment of the stigmata of recent hemorrhage (ie, endoscopic appearance of the ulcer crater). These are categorized according to the Forrest classification, developed 4 decades ago and first published by Forrest and colleagues in *The Lancet* in 1974.[68] The purpose of the classification was initially to uniformly describe lesions that are or have been bleeding. The Forrest classification, however, has since been mostly used to stratify patients with ulcer bleeding into high- and low-risk categories for rebleeding and mortality (**Table 2**).[69] Several endoscopic findings portend a higher risk for recurrent bleeding and their recognition is essential for proper therapeutic planning. Endoscopic treatment is indicated for patients found to have active spurting (Forrest Ia) or oozing bleeding (Forrest Ib) (**Fig. 1**) and for those with a nonbleeding visible vessel (Forrest IIa, NBVV) (**Fig. 2**) in an ulcer. Overlying adherent clots (Forrest IIb) (**Fig. 3**) should be vigorously irrigated to evaluate and potentially treat any underlying lesion. The management of peptic ulcers with adherent clots that are resistant to removal by vigorous irrigation remains, however, controversial.[35] Ulcers with low-risk stigmata (ie, those with flat pigmented spots [Forrest IIc] of hematin or fibrin-covered clean base [Forrest III] [**Fig. 4**]) do not warrant any endoscopic intervention.[26,35,64–66]

A recent prospective reassessment of the predictive value of Forrest classification documented that it still has predictive value for rebleeding of peptic ulcers, especially

Table 2
The Forrest classification of peptic ulcer hemorrhage

Active hemorrhage	
Forrest Ia	Active spurting hemorrhage
Forrest Ib	Oozing hemorrhage
Signs of recent hemorrhage	
Forrest IIa	NBVV
Forrest IIb	Adherent clot
Forrest IIc	Flat pigmented spot on ulcer base
Lesions without active bleeding	
Forrest III	Clean-base ulcer

Data from Forrest JA, Finlayson ND, Shearman DJ. Endoscopy in gastrointestinal bleeding. Lancet 1974;2:394–7.

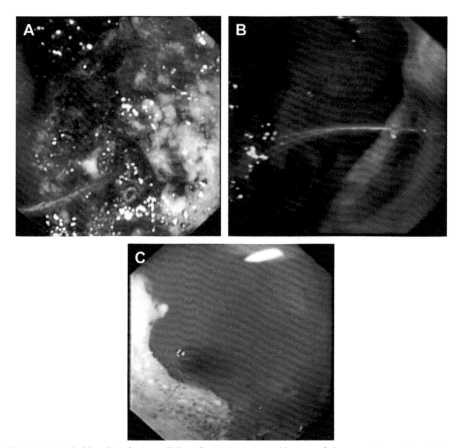

Fig. 1. Actively bleeding lesions: (*A*) malignant ulcerated lesion of the gastric angulus with a spurting arterial vessel; (*B*) an NSAID-related gastric ulcer in the upper portion of the gastric body with a brisk flow of arterial blood; and (*C*) oozing bleeding from an exposed vessel in a duodenal ulcer.

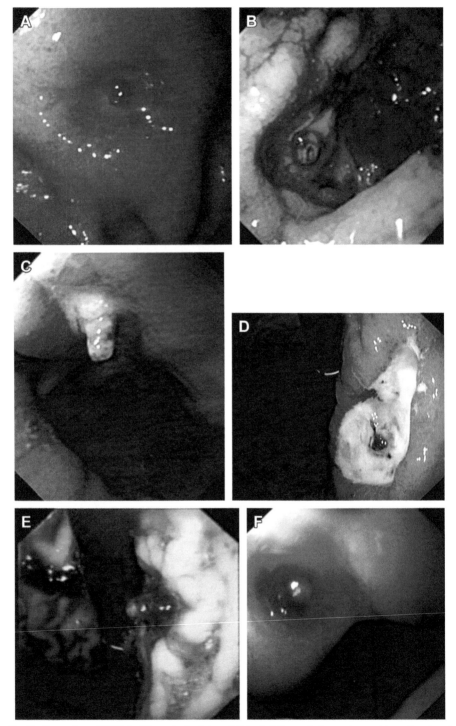

Fig. 2. Examples of NBVVs: (A) central pink-reddish slightly protuberant vessel in a duodenal ulcer; (B) ulcer of the pyloric channel with a white translucent eccentric vessel; (C) ulcer of the lesser curvature of the stomach with a protuberant white vessel; (D) retroflexed view of a gastric ulcer in the corpus with a brownish consolidated flattened vessel (sentinel clot); (E) ulcer of the gastric body showing a large protuberant aneurysmic dark red vessel seen in retroflexion; and (F) ulcer of the duodenal bulb with a red protuberant vessel.

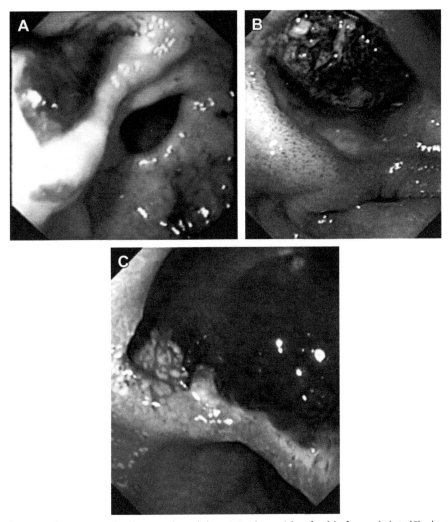

Fig. 3. Various types of adherent clots: (*A*) gastric ulcer with a freshly formed clot; (*B*) ulcer of the anterosuperior duodenal wall with an organized clot covering the ulcer base; and (*C*) a black hardened clot overlying the base of a duodenal bulb ulcer.

for gastric ulcers; however, it does not predict mortality.[70] Another study finding was that a proposed simplified classification into high risk (Forrest Ia), increased risk (Forrest Ib–IIc), and low risk (Forrest III) had similar test characteristics to the original Forrest classification.

The finding of an NBVV has been touted as a reliable predictor of the risk of recurrent bleeding and poor outcome.[69,71–73] Not all exposed vessels carry the same risk of recurrent bleeding, however, with pale, protuberant vessels shown much more risky than dark, flattened ones.[74] The distinction between NBVV and clots can be difficult[75,76]; hence the presence of an NBVV may not be in itself a sufficiently reliable indicator to select patients for invasive therapy. Enhanced endoscopic imaging of bleeding ulcers to identify and characterize an involved buried vessel may allow for more cost-effective management. Although the endoscopic Doppler ultrasound

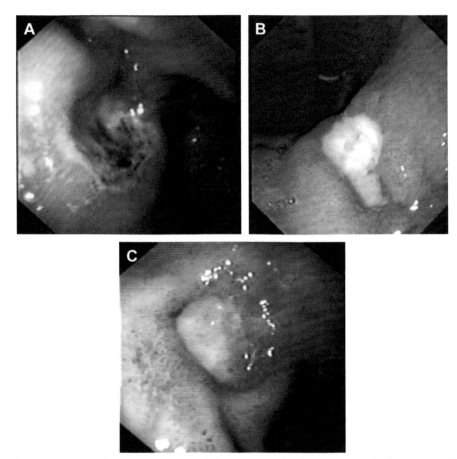

Fig. 4. Low-risk endoscopic stigmata: (*A*) flat gray sloughs of hematin on the base of an ulcer in the gastric antrum; (*B*) endoscopic view in retroflexion of a clean-base ulcer on the angulus of the stomach; and (*C*) clean-base duodenal bulb ulceration.

probes[77] have been proposed to evaluate the size and patency of underlying vessels, these systems have not gained widespread popularity. A pilot study from Italy investigated the role of magnification endoscopy in improving the characterization of exposed vessels in ulcer hemorrhage.[78] Zoom endoscopy after methylene blue staining provided clear images of the vessel and allowed visualization of the artery, the site of rupture, and the presence of a clot plugging the hole. A diagnostic gain (ie, an upgrading from low-to high-risk category of the vessel) was achieved in 33% of cases. No lesion was downstaged, possibly because frankly protruding reddish or pale vessels are already very clear under standard endoscopic visualization. The vessels that appear only slightly protuberant or that resemble clots or pigment spots were the ones most likely to be upgraded by magnification endoscopy.

Upper GI endoscopy in a bleeding patient should be carried out in an adequately equipped setting—the endoscopy suite or operating theater—by qualified endoscopists. A therapeutic endoscope with 3.7-mm operative working channel should be used. Scopes with 6-mm jumbo channels or double-channel scopes may occasionally be required. All devices for endoscopic hemostasis (injection needles and solutions, monopolar or bipolar thermal probes, and mechanical devices, such as hemoclips) should be available and ready to be used by skilled personnel. The use of modern high-frequency generators with built-in argon plasma coagulation modules is advisable. Patients should ideally be hemodynamically stable at the time of upper endoscopy. The assistance of an anesthesiologist is required in patients with severe hematemesis and endotracheal intubation should be considered in such selected cases to prevent aspiration.

The quality of endoscopy can be adversely affected by poor visibility in patients requiring urgent endoscopy with UGIB due to obscuring blood in the gastric lumen. In 3% to 19% of cases, no apparent cause of UGIB can be identified.[15,17,21,23,33] This may be related either to the aforementioned presence of food or blood debris hampering proper endoscopic visualization (in particular for awkwardly positioned lesions) or to the presence of faint lesions that are difficult to identify if not actively bleeding, specifically vascular lesions (**Fig. 5**). Apart from the routine use of

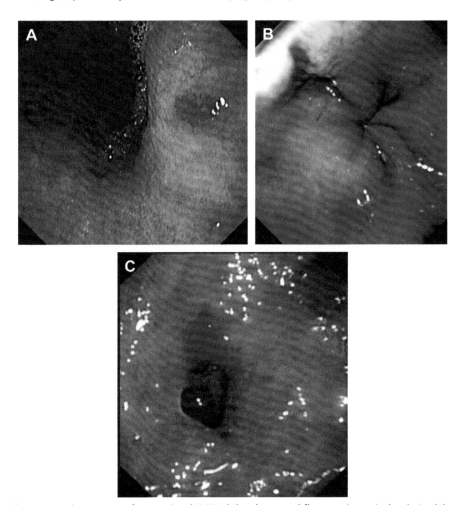

Fig. 5. Nonulcer causes of nonvariceal UGIB: (*A*) a cherry-red flat gastric angiodysplasia; (*B*) a Mallory-Weiss tear covered with hematin; and (*C*) a Dieulafoy lesion of the gastric fundus with an overlying clot.

water-jet irrigation and adequate suction applied to the endoscope, a patient may need to be rolled over in different positions to improve visibility. In cases of large fundic blood clots, a large-bore nasogastric or orogastric tube should be considered for inserting to empty the stomach and repeat the examination shortly thereafter. The systematic use of a nasogastric tube before endoscopy is not recommended,[35] but in selected patients it may offer important prognostic information. The presence of blood in the nasogastric aspirate is a significant predictor of high-risk stigmata at index upper endoscopy.[79]

Pre-endoscopic administration of intravenous erythromycin or metoclopramide (20–120 minutes before endoscopy) has been shown to reduce the need for repeat endoscopy to determine the site and cause of bleeding in patients with UGIB (OR 0.55; 95% CI, 0.32–0.94).[80] This is an important adjunct to treatment with regard to the ability to make a diagnosis, apply definitive treatment, and avoid unnecessary exposure of patients to repeat procedures; additional data show that the use of prokinetic agents may also decrease the duration of hospitalization,[81] so although not routinely recommended, they should be used in patients with a high probability of having fresh blood or a clot in the stomach when undergoing upper endoscopy to improve diagnostic yield.

Timing of Endoscopy: When Should Endoscopy Be Performed?

Urgent EGD has been proposed as the standard of care in patients with acute UGIB, although the optimal timing for early endoscopy is still uncertain. A 24-hour time frame for endoscopic examination is internationally recommended as the optimal window of opportunity,[35,64,66] especially for patients with a history of malignancy or cirrhosis, presentation with hematemesis, and signs of hypovolemia, including hypotension, tachycardia, hemodynamic shock, and hemoglobin less than 8 g/dL.[26]

Although no study has been able to show a direct reduction in mortality through performance of early endoscopy, available data from observational studies favor a reduction in length of hospital stay, recurrent bleeding, and need for surgery,[82–85] with decreased mortality in a subgroup analysis of patients at particularly high risk of a negative outcome.[57,85,86] Early endoscopy aids in risk stratification; however, it may also expose additional cases of active bleeding and hence increase the use of therapeutic intervention. No evidence exists that earlier endoscopy, performed less than 12 hours of patient presentation, can reduce the risk of rebleeding or improve survival compared with later (>24 hours) endoscopy.[87,88] In the UK audit, only 50% of all patients underwent endoscopy within 24 hours of presentation (a figure that had not improved from the previous audit performed 14 years earlier), probably related to the lack of 24-hour provision of emergency endoscopy in 48% of hospitals at the time of the audit in 2007.[17] These figures are better in Canada (76%)[16] and in other European countries (78%–81%),[15,21,24] despite a wide between-country variability in the area and speciality of the nonvariceal UGIB management team. The mean time from admission to endoscopy was less than 1 day only in Italy and Spain.[89] Therefore, there seems to be room for considerable improvement in this aspect of care delivery and this could be used as a key parameter to monitor standards and organization of care delivery in future studies of UGIB.

In a variation on this theme, several studies indicate that patients with nonvariceal UGIB admitted on weekends have higher in-hospital mortality (adjusted OR ranging from 1.08 to 2.68) and significantly lower rates of early endoscopy compared with patients admitted on weekdays.[10,90–92] The higher mortality for weekend and public holiday admissions could not be explained by measures of case mix and may indicate a possible impact of reduced staffing levels and delays to endoscopy on weekends in some hospitals. Also, when the quality of care did not seem to differ between week-day/weekend admissions, UGIB patients admitted during the weekend were at higher risk of an adverse outcome,[93] possibly because this subgroup is more likely to present with hemodynamic shock and hematemesis and receive red blood cell transfusion.[94] Nonetheless, in the UK audit there was no evidence of increased mortality for week-end versus weekday presentation despite patients being more critically ill and having greater delays to endoscopy on the weekends. The absence of a weekend effect on mortality from peptic ulcer bleeding was confirmed in a large Asian cohort of 8222 patients.[95] An overall 19.1% of patients were admitted on holidays and there was no difference in mortality between holiday versus weekday admissions (4.1% vs 4.0%). The waiting time for endoscopy was correlated with the risk of 30-day mortality. When therapeutic endoscopy can be offered within 1 day of hospital admission, holiday admission does not adversely affect bleeding mortality.[95]

In theory, the availability both of on-call physicians proficient in endoscopic hemostasis and on-call support staff with technical expertise in usage of endoscopic devices enables performance of endoscopy on a 24/7 basis. This is especially important to achieve in those countries that have demonstrated evidence of a weekend effect for UGIB mortality, including the United States[90–92] and Wales.[10] In contrast, no evidence of a weekend effect for mortality was found in Hong Kong[95] or in the United Kingdom.[94] In the latter case, there was even no difference in the risk of death for weekend compared with weekday presentation between patients presenting to hospitals with an out-of-hours endoscopy rota compared with those presenting to hospitals without such a facility, questioning the need for provision of 24/7 access to emergency endoscopy.

In appropriate settings, endoscopy can be used to assess the need for inpatient admission. Hemodynamically stable patients who are evaluated for UGIB with upper endoscopy and subsequently found to have low-risk stigmata for recurrent bleeding can be safely discharged and followed as outpatients, reducing the need for hospitalization and consequently hospital costs.[96,97]

In conclusion, upper GI endoscopy is the cornerstone of diagnosis and management of patients with UGIB. Early endoscopy (within 24 hours of patient presentation) ensures a correct identification of the bleeding source and allows risk stratification, valuable in allocating the patient to the adequate level of care. High-risk patients should be treated endoscopically and followed in monitored or high-dependency units. Low-risk patients can be safely discharged home or even be treated as outpatients.

REFERENCES

1. Yavorski RT, Wong RK, Maydonovitch C, et al. Analysis of 3,294 cases of upper gastrointestinal bleeding in military medical facilities. Am J Gastroenterol 1995; 90:568–73.
2. Longstreth GF. Epidemiology of hospitalization for acute upper gastrointestinal hemorrhage: a population-based study. Am J Gastroenterol 1995;90:206–10.
3. Peery AF, Dellon ES, Lund J, et al. Burden of gastrointestinal disease in the United States: 2012 update. Gastroenterology 2012;143:1179–87.
4. Targownik LE, Nabalamba A. Trends in management and outcomes of acute nonvariceal upper gastrointestinal bleeding: 1993-2003. Clin Gastroenterol Hepatol 2006;4:1459–66.
5. Theocharis GJ, Thomopoulos KC, Sakellaropoulos G, et al. Changing trends in the epidemiology and clinical outcome of acute upper gastrointestinal bleeding in a defined geographical area in Greece. J Clin Gastroenterol 2008;42:128–33.

6. van Leerdam ME, Vreeburg EM, Rauws EA, et al. Acute upper GI bleeding: did anything change? Time trend analysis of incidence and outcome of acute upper GI bleeding between 1993/1994 and 2000. Am J Gastroenterol 2003;98:1494–9.

7. van Leerdam ME. Epidemiology of acute upper gastrointestinal bleeding. Best Pract Res Clin Gastroenterol 2008;22:209–24.

8. Loperfido S, Baldo V, Piovesana E, et al. Changing trends in acute upper-GI bleeding: a population-based study. Gastrointest Endosc 2009;70:212–24.

9. Hreinsson JP, Kalaitzakis E, Gudmundsson S, et al. Upper gastrointestinal bleeding: incidence, etiology and outcomes in a population-based setting. Scand J Gastroenterol 2013;48:439–47.

10. Button LA, Roberts SE, Evans PA, et al. Hospitalized incidence and case fatality for upper gastrointestinal bleeding from 1999 to 2007: a record linkage study. Aliment Pharmacol Ther 2011;33:64–76.

11. Laine L, Yang H, Chang SC, et al. Trends for incidence of hospitalization and death due to GI complications in the United States from 2001 to 2009. Am J Gastroenterol 2012;107:1190–5.

12. Lanas A, García-Rodríguez LA, Polo-Tomás M, et al. Time trends and impact of upper and lower gastrointestinal bleeding and perforation in clinical practice. Am J Gastroenterol 2009;104:1633–41.

13. Sonnenberg A. Time trends of ulcer mortality in Europe. Gastroenterology 2007; 132:2320–7.

14. Chan FK, Abraham NS, Scheiman JM, et al. Management of patients on nonsteroidal anti-inflammatory drugs: a clinical practice recommendation from the First International Working Party on Gastrointestinal and Cardiovascular Effects of Nonsteroidal Anti-inflammatory Drugs and Anti-platelet Agents. Am J Gastroenterol 2008;103:2908–18.

15. Marmo R, Koch M, Cipolletta L, et al, PNED Investigators. Predictive factors of mortality from nonvariceal upper gastrointestinal hemorrhage: a multicenter study. Am J Gastroenterol 2008;103:1639–47.

16. Barkun A, Sabbah S, Enns R, et al. The Canadian Registry on Nonvariceal Upper Gastrointestinal Bleeding and Endoscopy (RUGBE): endoscopic hemostasis and proton pump inhibition are associated with improved outcomes in a real-life setting. Am J Gastroenterol 2004;99:1238–46.

17. Hearnshaw SA, Logan RF, Lowe D, et al. Acute upper gastrointestinal bleeding in the UK: patient characteristics, diagnoses and outcomes in the 2007 UK audit. Gut 2011;60:1327–35.

18. Sostres C, Lanas A. Epidemiology and demographics of upper gastrointestinal bleeding: prevalence, incidence, and mortality. Gastrointest Endosc Clin N Am 2011;21:567–81.

19. Müller T, Barkun AN, Martel M. Non-variceal upper GI bleeding in patients already hospitalized for another condition. Am J Gastroenterol 2009;104:330–9.

20. Marmo R, Koch M, Cipolletta L, et al. Predicting mortality in patients with in-hospital nonvariceal upper GI bleeding: a prospective, multicenter database study. Gastrointest Endosc 2014;79(5):741–9.e1.

21. Marmo R, Koch M, Cipolletta L, et al, Italian Registry on Upper Gastrointestinal Bleeding (PNED2). Predicting mortality in non-variceal upper gastrointestinal bleeders: validation of the Italian PNED score and prospective comparison with the Rockall Score. Am J Gastroenterol 2010;105:1284–91.

22. Sung JJ, Tsoi KK, Ma TK, et al. Causes of mortality in patients with peptic ulcer bleeding: a prospective cohort study of 10,428 cases. Am J Gastroenterol 2010; 105:84–9.

23. Enestvedt BK, Gralnek IM, Mattek N, et al. An evaluation of endoscopic indications and findings related to nonvariceal upper-GI hemorrhage in a large multicenter consortium. Gastrointest Endosc 2008;67:422–9.
24. Nahon S, Hagège H, Latrive JP, et al, Groupe des Hémorragies Digestives Hautes de l'ANGH. Epidemiological and prognostic factors involved in upper gastrointestinal bleeding: results of a French prospective multicenter study. Endoscopy 2012;44:998–1008.
25. Del Piano M, Bianco MA, Cipolletta L, et al, Prometeo Study Group of the Italian Society of Digestive Endoscopy (SIED). The "Prometeo" study: online collection of clinical data and outcome of Italian patients with acute nonvariceal upper gastrointestinal bleeding. J Clin Gastroenterol 2013;47:33–7.
26. Hwang JH, Fisher DA, Ben-Menachem T, et al, Standards of Practice Committee of the American Society for Gastrointestinal Endoscopy. The role of endoscopy in the management of acute non-variceal upper GI bleeding. Gastrointest Endosc 2012;75:1132–8.
27. Yachimski PS, Friedman LS. Gastrointestinal bleeding in the elderly. Nat Clin Pract Gastroenterol Hepatol 2008;5:80–93.
28. Gururatsakul M, Ching KJ, Talley NJ, et al. Incidence and risk factors of uncomplicated peptic ulcer and bleeding peptic ulcer over a 10-year period. Gastrointest Endosc 2009;69:AB607.
29. González-González JA, García-Compean D, Vázquez-Elizondo G, et al. Nonvariceal upper gastrointestinal bleeding in patients with liver cirrhosis. Clinical features, outcomes and predictors of in-hospital mortality. A prospective study. Ann Hepatol 2011;10:287–95.
30. Marmo R, del Piano M, Cipolletta L, et al. Mortality from non variceal upper gastrointestinal bleeding in patients with liver cirrhosis: an individual patient data meta-analysis. Gastrointest Endosc 2013;77:AB180.
31. Marmo R, Del Piano M, Rotondano G, et al. Mortality from nonulcer bleeding is similar to that of ulcer bleeding in high-risk patients with nonvariceal hemorrhage: a prospective database study in Italy. Gastrointest Endosc 2012;75: 263–72.
32. Maluf-Filho F, da Costa Martins B, Simas de Lima M, et al. Etiology, endoscopic management and mortality of upper gastrointestinal bleeding in patients with cancer. United European Gastroenterol J 2013;1:60–7.
33. Holster IL, Kuipers EJ. Management of acute nonvariceal upper gastrointestinal bleeding: current policies and future perspectives. World J Gastroenterol 2012; 18:1202–7.
34. Sánchez-Delgado J, Gené E, Suárez D, et al. Has H. pylori prevalence in bleeding peptic ulcer been underestimated? A meta-regression. Am J Gastroenterol 2011;106:398–405.
35. Barkun AN, Bardou M, Kuipers EJ, et al. International consensus recommendations on the management of patients with nonvariceal upper gastrointestinal bleeding. Ann Intern Med 2010;152:101–13.
36. Hung LC, Ching JY, Sung JJ, et al. Long-term outcome of Helicobacter pylori-negative idiopathic bleeding ulcers: a prospective cohort study. Gastroenterology 2005;128:1845–50.
37. Chason RD, Reisch JS, Rockey DC. More favorable outcomes with peptic ulcer bleeding due to Helicobacter pylori. Am J Med 2013;126:811–8.
38. Wong GL, Au KW, Lo AO, et al. Gastroprotective therapy does not improve outcomes of patients with Helicobacter pylori-negative idiopathic bleeding ulcers. Clin Gastroenterol Hepatol 2012;10:1124–9.

39. Chan FK, Ching JY, Suen BY, et al. Effects of Helicobacter pylori infection on long-term risk of peptic ulcer bleeding in low-dose aspirin users. Gastroenterology 2013;144:528–35.
40. US Preventive Services Task Force. Aspirin for the prevention of cardiovascular disease: U.S. Preventive Services Task Force recommendation statement. Ann Intern Med 2009;150:396–404.
41. McQuaid KR, Laine L. Systematic review and meta-analysis of adverse events of low-dose aspirin and clopidogrel in randomized controlled trials. Am J Med 2006;119:624–38.
42. Huang ES, Strate LL, Ho WW, et al. Long-term use of aspirin and the risk of gastrointestinal bleeding. Am J Med 2011;124:426–33.
43. Sutcliffe P, Connock M, Gurung T, et al. Aspirin in primary prevention of cardiovascular disease and cancer: a systematic review of the balance of evidence from reviews of randomized trials. PLoS One 2013;8:e81970.
44. Valkhoff VE, Sturkenboom MC, Kuipers EJ. Risk factors for gastrointestinal bleeding associated with low-dose aspirin. Best Pract Res Clin Gastroenterol 2012;26:125–40.
45. Ng FH, Tunggal P, Chu WM, et al. Esomeprazole compared with famotidine in the prevention of upper gastrointestinal bleeding in patients with acute coronary syndrome or myocardial infarction. Am J Gastroenterol 2012;107:389–96.
46. de Abajo FJ, Gil MJ, Bryant V, et al. Upper gastrointestinal bleeding associated with NSAIDs, other drugs and interactions: a nested case-control study in a new general practice database. Eur J Clin Pharmacol 2013;69:691–701.
47. Ramsoekh D, van Leerdam ME, Rauws EA, et al. Outcome of peptic ulcer bleeding, nonsteroidal anti-inflammatory drug use, and Helicobacter pylori infection. Clin Gastroenterol Hepatol 2005;3:859–64.
48. Targownik LE, Metge CJ, Leung S, et al. The relative efficacies of gastroprotective strategies in chronic users of nonsteroidal anti-inflammatory drugs. Gastroenterology 2008;134:937–44.
49. van Soest EM, Valkhoff VE, Mazzaglia G, et al. Suboptimal gastroprotective coverage of NSAID use and the risk of upper gastrointestinal bleeding and ulcers: an observational study using three European databases. Gut 2011;60:1650–9.
50. Le Ray I, Barkun AN, Vauzelle-Kervroëdan F, et al. Failure to renew prescriptions for gastroprotective agents to patients on continuous nonsteroidal anti-inflammatory drugs increases rate of upper gastrointestinal injury. Clin Gastroenterol Hepatol 2013;11:499–504.
51. Knopp-Sihota JA, Cummings GG, Homik J, et al. The association between serious upper gastrointestinal bleeding and incident bisphosphonate use: a population-based nested cohort study. BMC Geriatr 2013;13:36.
52. Crooks CJ, West J, Card TR. Comorbidities affect risk of non variceal upper gastrointestinal bleeding. Gastroenterology 2013;144:1384–93.
53. Jairath V, Martel M, Logan RF, et al. Why do mortality rates for nonvariceal upper gastrointestinal bleeding differ around the world? A systematic review of cohort studies. Can J Gastroenterol 2012;26:537–43.
54. Crooks C, Card T, West J. Reductions in 28-day mortality following hospital admission for upper gastrointestinal hemorrhage. Gastroenterology 2011;141:62–70.
55. Lau JY, Barkun A, Fan DM, et al. Challenges in the management of acute peptic ulcer bleeding. Lancet 2013;381:2033–43.
56. Rosenstock SJ, Møller MH, Larsson H, et al. Improving quality of care in peptic ulcer bleeding: nationwide cohort study of 13,498 consecutive patients in the

Danish Clinical Register of Emergency Surgery. Am J Gastroenterol 2013;108: 1449–57.

57. Wysocki JD, Srivastav S, Winstead NS. A nationwide analysis of risk factors for mortality and time to endoscopy in upper gastrointestinal haemorrhage. Aliment Pharmacol Ther 2012;36:30–6.

58. Leontiadis GI, Molloy-Bland M, Moayyedi P, et al. Effect of comorbidity on mortality in patients with peptic ulcer bleeding: systematic review and meta-analysis. Am J Gastroenterol 2013;108:331–45.

59. Jairath V, Kahan BC, Stanworth SJ, et al. Prevalence, management, and outcomes of patients with coagulopathy after acute nonvariceal uppergastrointestinal bleeding in the United Kingdom. Transfusion 2013;53:1069–76.

60. Venkatesh PG, Parasa S, Njei B, et al. Increased mortality with peptic ulcer bleeding in patients with both compensated and decompensated cirrhosis. Gastrointest Endosc 2014;79(4):605–14.

61. Yang JY, Lee TC, Montez-Rath ME, et al. Trends in acute nonvariceal upper gastrointestinal bleeding in dialysis patients. J Am Soc Nephrol 2012;23: 495–506.

62. Weng SC, Shu KH, Tarng DC, et al. In-hospital mortality risk estimation in patients with acute nonvariceal upper gastrointestinal bleeding undergoing hemodialysis: a retrospective cohort study. Ren Fail 2013;35:243–8.

63. Parasa S, Navaneethan U, Sridhar AR, et al. End-stage renal disease is associated with worse outcomes in hospitalized patients with peptic ulcer bleeding. Gastrointest Endosc 2013;77:609–16.

64. Gralnek IM, Barkun AN, Bardou M. Management of acute bleeding from a peptic ulcer. N Engl J Med 2008;359:928–37.

65. Sung JJ, Chan FK, Chen M, et al. Asia-Pacific Working Group consensus on non-variceal upper gastrointestinal bleeding. Gut 2011;60:1170–7.

66. Laine L, Jensen DM. Management of patients with ulcer bleeding. Am J Gastroenterol 2012;107:345–60.

67. Kohn A, Ancona C, Belleudi V, et al. The impact of endoscopy and specialist care on 30-day mortality among patients with acute non-variceal upper gastrointestinal hemorrhage: an Italian population-based study. Dig Liver Dis 2010;42: 629–34.

68. Forrest JA, Finlayson ND, Shearman DJ. Endoscopy in gastrointestinal bleeding. Lancet 1974;2:394–7.

69. Laine L, Peterson WL. Bleeding peptic ulcer. N Engl J Med 1994;331:717–27.

70. de Groot NL, van Oijen MG, Kessels K, et al. Reassessment of the predictive value of the Forrest classification for peptic ulcer rebleeding and mortality: can classification be simplified? Endoscopy 2014;46:46–52.

71. Griffiths WJ, Neumann DA, Welsh JD. The visible vessel as an indicator of uncontrolled or recurrent gastrointestinal hemorrhage. N Engl J Med 1979;300: 1411–3.

72. Wara P. Endoscopic prediction of major rebleeding - a prospective study of stigmata of hemorrhage in bleeding ulcer. Gastroenterology 1985;88(5 Pt 1):1209–14.

73. Freeman ML. Stigmata of hemorrhage in bleeding ulcers. Gastrointest Endosc Clin N Am 1997;7:559–74.

74. Freeman ML, Cass OW, Peine CJ, et al. The non-bleeding visible vessel versus the sentinel clot: natural history and risk of rebleeding. Gastrointest Endosc 1993;39:359–66.

75. Laine L, Freeman M, Cohen H. Lack of uniformity in evaluation of endoscopic prognostic features of bleeding ulcers. Gastrointest Endosc 1994;40:411–7.

76. Lau JY, Sung JJ, Chan AC, et al. Stigmata of hemorrhage in bleeding peptic ulcers: an interobserver agreement study among international experts. Gastrointest Endosc 1997;46:33–6.

77. Wong RC. Endoscopic Doppler US probe for acute peptic ulcer hemorrhage. Gastrointest Endosc 2004;60:804–12.

78. Cipolletta L, Bianco MA, Salerno R, et al. Improved characterization of visible vessels in bleeding ulcers by using magnification endoscopy: results of a pilot study. Gastrointest Endosc 2010;72:413–8.

79. Wyse JM, Barkun AN, Bardou M, et al. Can the presence of endoscopic high-risk stigmata be confidently predicted before gastroscopy? Gastrointest Endosc 2009;69:AB181.

80. Barkun AN, Bardou M, Martel M, et al. Prokinetics in acute upper GI bleeding: a meta-analysis. Gastrointest Endosc 2010;72:1138–45.

81. Altraif I, Handoo FA, Aljumah A, et al. Effect of erythromycin before endoscopy in patients presenting with variceal bleeding: a prospective, randomized, double-blind, placebo-controlled trial. Gastrointest Endosc 2011;73:245–50.

82. Cooper GS, Chak A, Way LE, et al. Early endoscopy in upper gastrointestinal hemorrhage: associations with recurrent bleeding, surgery, and length of hospital stay. Gastrointest Endosc 1999;49:145–52.

83. Chak A, Cooper GS, Lloyd LE, et al. Effectiveness of endoscopy in patients admitted to the intensive care unit with upper GI hemorrhage. Gastrointest Endosc 2001;53:6–13.

84. Cooper GS, Kou TD, Wong RC. Use and impact of early endoscopy in elderly patients with peptic ulcer hemorrhage: a population-based analysis. Gastrointest Endosc 2009;70:229–35.

85. Lim LG, Ho KY, Chan YH, et al. Urgent endoscopy is associated with lower mortality in high-risk but not low-risk nonvariceal upper gastrointestinal bleeding. Endoscopy 2011;43:300–6.

86. Karsan SS, Kanwal F, Huang ES, et al. Early endoscopy predicts lower mortality in acute gastrointestinal haemorrhage. Gastroenterology 2009;136(5 Suppl 1): A606.

87. Tsoi KK, Ma TK, Sung JJ. Endoscopy for upper gastrointestinal bleeding: how urgent is it? Nat Rev Gastroenterol Hepatol 2009;6:463–9.

88. Jairath V, Kahan BC, Logan RF, et al. Outcomes following acute nonvariceal upper gastrointestinal bleeding in relation to time to endoscopy: results from a nationwide study. Endoscopy 2012;44:723–30.

89. Lanas A, Aabakken L, Fonseca J, et al. Variability in the management of nonvariceal upper gastrointestinal bleeding in Europe: an observational study. Adv Ther 2012;29:1026–36.

90. Ananthakrishnan AN, McGinley EL, Saeian K. Outcomes of weekend admissions for upper gastrointestinal hemorrhage: a nationwide analysis. Clin Gastroenterol Hepatol 2009;7:296–302.

91. Shaheen AA, Kaplan GG, Myers RP. Weekend versus weekday admission and mortality from gastrointestinal hemorrhage caused by peptic ulcer disease. Clin Gastroenterol Hepatol 2009;7:303–10.

92. Dorn SD, Shah ND, Berg BP, et al. Effect of weekend hospital admission on gastrointestinal hemorrhage outcomes. Dig Dis Sci 2010;55:1658–66.

93. de Groot NL, Bosman JH, Siersema PD, et al, RASTA Study Group. Admission time is associated with outcome of upper gastrointestinal bleeding: results of a multicentre prospective cohort study. Aliment Pharmacol Ther 2012;36:477–84.

94. Jairath V, Kahan BC, Logan RF, et al. Mortality from acute upper gastrointestinal bleeding in the United Kingdom: does it display a "weekend effect"? Am J Gastroenterol 2011;106:1621–8.
95. Tsoi KK, Chiu PW, Chan FK, et al. The risk of peptic ulcer bleeding mortality in relation to hospital admission on holidays: a cohort study on 8,222 cases of peptic ulcer bleeding. Am J Gastroenterol 2012;107:405–10.
96. Lee JG, Turnipseed S, Romano PS, et al. Endoscopy-based triage significantly reduces hospitalization rates and costs of treating upper GI bleeding: a randomized controlled trial. Gastrointest Endosc 1999;50:755–61.
97. Cipolletta L, Bianco MA, Rotondano G, et al. Outpatient management for low-risk nonvariceal upper GI bleeding: a randomized controlled trial. Gastrointest Endosc 2002;55:1–5.

Upper Gastrointestinal Bleeding

Patient Presentation, Risk Stratification, and Early Management

Andrew C. Meltzer, MD, MS*, Joshua C. Klein, BS

KEYWORDS

- Gastrointestinal hemorrhage • Hemorrhage • Risk stratification • Early management
- Variceal • Nonvariceal

KEY POINTS

- Early resuscitation including support for airway, breathing, and circulation is critical in the initial evaluation of a patient with a suspected upper gastrointestinal (GI) hemorrhage.
- Early risk stratification for mortality and rebleeding should be performed using validated decision tools such as the Glasgow-Blatchford Score or the Clinical Rockall Score.
- Early administration of proton pump inhibitors decreases the need for endoscopic intervention.
- Vasoactive medications such as somatostatin, vasopressin, and their analogues should be given in cases of acute variceal upper GI hemorrhage and considered in cases of acute nonvariceal upper GI hemorrhage.
- Improved survival has been shown to be associated with a restrictive strategy of blood transfusion.

BACKGROUND

Acute upper gastrointestinal (GI) hemorrhage is a common presentation in hospital-based emergency departments (EDs) in the United States and around the world. According to data from the Healthcare Cost and Utilization Project, there were 863,000 US hospital admissions for GI hemorrhage in 2008, which included both upper and lower GI bleeding.[1] The mean length of stay for patients discharged from the hospital with a diagnosis of GI hemorrhage is 4.5 days and the mean hospital

Disclosures: Investigator-Initiated Research; Exalenz Inc, Consultant, Medical Device Company.
Department of Emergency Medicine, George Washington University, 2120 L Street Northwest, Suite 450, Washington, DC 20037, USA
* Corresponding author.
E-mail address: ameltzer@mfa.gwu.edu

charges are $26,210 per admission. Acute upper GI hemorrhage is a particularly severe manifestation of GI hemorrhage and is associated with mortalities ranging from 15% to 20%.[2] Acute upper GI hemorrhage is blood loss that has a source proximal to the ligament of Treitz, and is divided into variceal and nonvariceal sources. On initial evaluation of a patient with a suspected acute upper GI hemorrhage, the physician must perform a rapid clinical assessment in order to estimate the source of bleeding and the severity. However, early management is a challenge because the patient presentation is variable, the risk stratification is imperfect, and the tools to stop the bleeding before an esophagogastroduodenoscopy (EGD) are limited.

PRESENTATION

The most common presentation for an upper GI hemorrhage is hematemesis, coffee-ground emesis, or melena. For a lower GI hemorrhage, the most common presentation is bright red blood per rectum. However, the distinction between an upper and lower source of hemorrhage is not always obvious. Bright red blood per rectum may be the presenting symptom in an especially brisk upper GI hemorrhage.[3] In addition, several conditions and medications may mimic a GI hemorrhage. Nosebleeds, dental bleeding, tonsilar bleeding, and red drinks or food can be mistaken for hematemesis; bismuth-containing medications such as Pepto-Bismol can mimic melena; and vaginal bleeding and gross hematuria can mimic bright red blood per rectum. Although the occult blood test can be used to confirm the presence of blood in the stool, false-positive occult blood tests can occur with red meat, turnips, horseradish, and vitamin C (**Table 1**).[4] Oral iron supplements do not cause a false-positive occult blood result.[5] In addition, patients may have bleeding lesions and only present with systemic signs of blood loss such as weakness, light-headedness, chest pain, or syncope.

The most common type of acute upper GI hemorrhage is the nonvariceal hemorrhage, which includes peptic ulcer disease, Mallory-Weiss tears, and Dieulafoy lesions. Variceal hemorrhage usually occurs in patients with portal hypertension and is always considered high risk for rebleeding and mortality. Nonvariceal upper GI hemorrhage can present with a range of severity from self-limiting to life threatening. As part of the natural course of the disease, 80% of the nonvariceal hemorrhages resolve spontaneously but 10% lead to death.[6] Upper endoscopy, also called EGD, is the diagnostic and therapeutic test of choice for patients who present with an upper GI hemorrhage; however, the EGD is not always feasible at initial presentation.

INITIAL MANAGEMENT

As with all critically ill patients, early assessment begins with the A, B, Cs: airway, breathing and circulation. In the setting of GI hemorrhage, airway control is especially important because aspiration of vomited blood is associated with significant morbidity and mortality.[7] The placement of an advanced airway may be indicated in cases of profuse vomiting or altered mental status. Rapid sequence intubation, a method of

Table 1 Mimics of GI bleeding	
Mimics for hematemesis	Nosebleeds, tonsilar bleeding, red drinks and food
Mimics for melena	Bismuth medications such as Pepto-Bismol
Mimics for bright red blood	Red food, vaginal bleeding, gross hematuria
False-positive occult blood test	Red meat, turnips, horseradish, vitamin C

intubation that quickly induces unconsciousness and paralysis, is the ideal method to perform endotracheal intubation because it is associated with a reduced risk of aspiration. Breathing is evaluated by clinical criteria such as chest rise, absence of cyanosis, and normal oxygen saturation levels by pulse oximetry. Circulatory or hemodynamic status is assessed with blood pressure, heart rate, and signs of end organ hypoperfusion such as altered mental status, increased capillary refill, decreased urine output, and increased lactate (**Table 2**). Elderly patients and patients on hypertensive medications may not become tachycardic in response to volume loss. Abnormal changes in vital signs measured while patients are lying, sitting, and standing (orthostatics) support the presence of volume loss and augments the information gathered from standard vital signs. Potential volume loss should be addressed with 2 large-bore (16 gauge or 18 gauge) intravenous angiocatheters to enable fluid resuscitation and targeted blood transfusion. The initial fluid replacement should be crystalloid and a complete blood count, metabolic panel, coagulation panel, and type and screen should be ordered with initial intravenous access.

Once hemodynamic stability has been established, a thorough history and secondary survey should be conducted with specific questions regarding prior episodes of bleeding, including the amount of blood and color of the blood. However, a patient's assessment of blood loss is frequently inaccurate.[8] Comorbidities such as congestive heart failure, renal disease, liver disease, or vascular disease increase overall mortality risk and help determine the source of bleeding. Recent vascular surgery increases the risk for an aortoenteric fistula, a particularly severe cause of upper GI hemorrhage.[9] In addition, medications such as steroids, nonsteroidal antiinflammatory drugs, and anticoagulants also increase the risk of bleeding. Patients should be examined for signs of liver failure that might indicate that the bleed has a variceal source. Stigmata of liver disease include vascular collaterals (caput medusa), ascites, asterixis, gynecomastia, hepatomegaly, jaundice, scleral icterus, vascular spiders (spider telangiectasias, spider angiomata), and splenomegaly.

RISK STRATIFICATION

An early challenge in the initial evaluation is to distinguish the severe from the benign causes of upper GI hemorrhage. Lacking the ability to directly visualize the bleeding source with an EGD, surrogate diagnostic techniques such as clinical decision rules

Table 2
Blood loss based on patient presentation

	Class 1	Class 2	Class 3	Class 4
Blood loss (mL)	<750	750–1500	1500–2000	>2000
Heart rate (BPM)	<100	100–120	120–140	>140
BP	Normal	Normal	Decreased	Decreased
Pulse pressure	Normal/Increased	Decreased	Decreased	Decreased
Respiratory rate (breaths/min)	14–20	20–30	30–40	>40
Urine output (mL/h)	>30	20–30	5–15	Negligible
Mental status	Slightly anxious	Mildly Anxious	Anxious, confused	Lethargic

Abbreviation: BP, blood pressure.
From Spahn DR, Cerny V, Coats TJ, et al. Management of bleeding following major trauma: a European guideline. Crit Care 2007;11(1):R17.

and nasogastric aspiration (NGA) are often used at initial presentation. Clinical decision rules such as the Clinical Rockall Score (CRS) and the Glasgow-Blatchford Score (GBS) that incorporate vital signs, laboratory values, and comorbidities to risk stratify patients have been derived and validated to identify low-risk patients before endoscopy (**Tables 3** and **4**).[10–15] Both have been validated to help predict high risk and low risk for rebleeding and mortality. The GBS has been shown to be useful in discharging some patients with a very low risk who can be followed as outpatients. In a prospective study of 676 patients, 16% had a GBS of zero and none of these patients were required to have an endoscopic interventions or died at outpatient follow-up.[16] In addition to identifying some patients who may be managed as outpatients, the GBS can predict the risk of rebleeding, the need for transfusion, and the need for surgery.[17] GBS seems to be superior to the CRS at predicting rebleeding but both GBS and CRS have been shown to be effective at predicting the risk of death.[17] Limitations to the GBS are the low adoption by US physicians and the low specificity of the test.[18,19] An additional limitation is that an endoscopic view (using traditional EGD) still seems to be desired by physicians and patients regardless of the risk score.[20]

NGA is a diagnostic tool that has been used to risk stratify patients for many years. Despite the claim that insertion of the tube is the single most disliked procedure by

Table 3
GBS

Risk Marker	Score Value
BUN (mmol/L)	
6.5–8.0	2
8.0–10.0	3
10.0–25.0	4
≥25.0	6
Hemoglobin (g/L) for Men	
120–130	1
100–120	3
<100	6
Hemoglobin (g/L) for Women	
100–120	1
≤100	6
SBP (mm Hg)	
100–109	1
90–99	2
<90	3
Other Markers	
Pulse ≥100 BPM	1
Melena	1
Syncope	2
Hepatic disease	2
Cardiac failure	2

Abbreviations: BPM, beats per minute; BUN, blood urea nitrogen; SBP, systolic blood pressure.
From Blatchford, O, Murray, WR, and Blatchford, M. A risk score to predict need for treatment for upper gastrointestinal haemorrhage. Lancet. 2000;356:1319.

Table 4 Rockall Score				
	Score			
Variable	0	1	2	3
Age (y)	<60	60–79	≥80	—
Shock	No shock	SBP ≥100 Pulse ≥100 BPM	Hypotension	—
Comorbidity	No major	—	Cardiac failure, ischemic heart disease, major comorbidities	Renal failure, liver failure, disseminated malignancy
Diagnosis	Mallory-Weiss tear, no lesion identified, and no stigmata	All other diagnoses	Malignancy upper GI tract	—
Major stigmata of recent hemorrhage	None or dark Spot only	—	Blood in GI tract, adherent clot, visible or bleeding vessel	—

From Rockall T, Logan R, Devlin H, et al. Risk assessment after acute upper gastrointestinal haemorrhage. Gut 1996;38(3):318; with permission.

patients in EDs, NGA is often used to predict the presence of a high-risk lesion that requires endoscopic hemostasis.[21] The sensitivity of a bloody aspirate is estimated at 45% and specificity 72% for a high-risk lesion.[22,23] False-positives can occur from epistaxis caused by the tube insertion and false-negatives occur when the lesion is in the duodenum or a nonbleeding visible vessel.[24] In general, a positive NGA is a good indicator of an upper GI hemorrhage, whereas a negative NGA is insufficient to rule out an acute bleed. NGA has not been shown to have an effect on clinical outcomes such as mortality, surgery, and length of hospital stay, or transfusion requirements. The only clinical outcome that is affected by the NGA is a decreased time to endoscopy, which may reflect a belief that a positive aspiration indicates the need for expedited care.[25] There is no evidence that placement of a nasogastric tube leads to bleeding by esophageal varices.[26]

A novel approach to risk stratify an upper GI hemorrhage in the ED is to use video capsule endoscopy to directly visualize the bleeding. In 3 small ED-based studies, video capsule endoscopy showed good patient tolerance and good sensitivity for detecting acute upper GI hemorrhage.[27,28] Potential advantages of video capsule endoscopy include improved patient tolerance compared with NGA, point-of-care results obtained without a specialist at the bedside, and decreased hospitalization rates. Potential barriers to adoption include the cost of the equipment, the need to train ED physicians to interpret the videos, the need to create a secure means to transmit images to on-call GI specialists, and the increased ED length of stay that may be required to use video capsule endoscopy in an ED. Further studies are needed to confirm the sensitivity of the test in multiple settings for detecting high-risk bleeding lesions and as a means to guide clinical decisions compared with standard of care.

PHARMACOLOGIC THERAPY

Although definitive management of a bleeding lesion requires endoscopic or surgical intervention, preendoscopic pharmacologic therapy may assist in achieving hemostasis. Six randomized controlled trials have been conducted to determine the effect of using preendoscopic proton pump inhibitors (PPIs) versus controls for patients with upper GI hemorrhage.[29–34] Reducing acid secretion may stabilize an upper GI bleeding lesion and possibly improve clinical outcomes. PPIs reduce the stigmata of high-risk lesions 9-fold and reduce the need for endoscopic intervention 3-fold, but do not reduce mortality, need for blood transfusion, need for surgery, or rebleeding rates (**Table 5**).[35] The use of PPIs should not replace emergent endoscopy but may improve outcomes when started early.[36] Future large-scale randomized control trials are still needed to determine whether acid suppression by intravenous PPIs promotes a benefit in mortality.

VASOACTIVE MEDICATIONS

The use of vasoactive medications such as somatostatin, vasopressin, and their analogues before EGD is well established for variceal sources of bleeding but is controversial for nonvariceal or undifferentiated sources of bleeding.[37] In general, vasoactive medications cause splanchnic vasoconstriction, reducing blood flow to the viscera and decreasing portal pressure. Somatostatin and vasopressin are most commonly used as adjunct therapy to endoscopic treatment in variceal upper GI hemorrhage, and they have been associated with a reduction in blood transfusion requirements and a lower risk of all-cause mortality in separate meta-analyses.[38–40] As first-line therapy, somatostatin analogues are as effective as emergency sclerotherapy.[41] In nonvariceal hemorrhage, no definitive studies have shown a benefit in terms of need for endoscopic therapy or mortality. Similar to PPIs, somatostatin and vasopressin are not substitutes for emergency EGD but can be considered before EGD in patients with either variceal or nonvariceal hemorrhage.[42]

ANTIBIOTICS IN VARICEAL HEMORRHAGE

In patients with a variceal upper GI bleeding caused by liver cirrhosis, prophylactic antibiotics have been shown to decrease the incidence of bacterial infections and all-cause mortality.[43] In a meta-analysis of 12 randomized control trials of 588 patients, the use of antibiotic prophylaxis showed a significant decrease in overall mortality (relative risk, 0.79; 95% confidence interval, 0.63–0.98).[43] This benefit is most pronounced in patients with severe liver disease.[44] Both oral quinolones and intravenous third-generation cephalosporins have been shown to be effective.[23,45–48]

Table 5 PPI before endoscopy			
Outcome Measure	PPI	Control	Odds Ratio (95% Confidence Interval)
Stigmata of recent hemorrhage	37.2%	46.5%	0.67 (0.54 to 0.84)
Need for Endoscopic therapy	8.6%	11.7%	0.68 (0.50 to 0.93)
Mortality Rates	6.1%	5.5%	1.12 (0.72 to 1.73)
Rebleeding	13.9%	16.6%	0.81 (0.61 to 1.09)
Surgery	9.9%	10.2%	0.96 CI (0.68 to 1.35)

From Sreedharan A, Martin J, Leontiadis GI, et al. Proton pump inhibitor treatment initiated prior to endoscopic diagnosis in upper gastrointestinal bleeding. Cochrane Database Syst Rev 2010;7(7):CD005415.

BLOOD TRANSFUSION

For patients with acute upper GI hemorrhage who are in shock or have active coronary artery disease, blood transfusions can be lifesaving. However, there is recent evidence that less aggressive transfusion strategies provide a mortality benefit for many patients with acute bleeding. The physiologic explanation is that aggressive blood transfusion leads to an increase in portal hypertension and a subsequent increase in bleeding.[49] A randomized controlled study of 921 patients compared the efficacy and safety of using a restrictive approach versus a liberal approach.[50] The restrictive approach, in which transfusion occurred if hemoglobin was within a range of 7.0 to 9.0 g/dL, required fewer total transfusions (51% vs 14%; $P<.05$), showed less rebleeding (16% vs 10%; $P<.05$), and had lower mortality (5% vs 9%; $P<.05$) than the liberal transfusion group, in which transfusion was initiated if hemoglobin within a range of 9.0 to 11.0 g/dL.[50]

Patients who present to the ED with upper GI hemorrhage while anticoagulated are in urgent need of reversal in order to stop the bleeding. However, oral vitamin K reversal takes approximately 24 hours; parenteral vitamin K reversal takes 4 to 6 hours.[51] Fresh frozen plasma (FFP) reverses the effects of Coumadin almost immediately but is limited because FFP must be thawed before administration and also carries the risk of transmission of disease and of allergic reactions, and of volume overload in patients with congestive heart failure. Prothrombin complex concentrate (PCC) is a possible alternative to FFP. PCC contains the vitamin K–dependent coagulation factors II, VII, IX, and X, which are deficient in patients on warfarin therapy. PCC may be the preferred choice for patients with active bleeding who have an International Normalized Ratio greater than 2.0 and are candidates for urgent surgery.[52,53] The most serious adverse outcome associated with PCC is a thromboembolic event.[54] Newer oral anticoagulants have recently gained popularity because of their more stable pharmacokinetics compared with warfarin. Both dabigatran, a direct thrombin inhibitor, and rivaroxaban, a direct factor Xa inhibitor, may be used to treat thromboembolic disease and can be dosed without regular blood monitoring. However, in the case of upper GI hemorrhage, there is no established reversal agent for these newer medications. PCC has shown some promising results in reversing dabigatran and rivaroxaban in a single study.[55]

BLAKEMORE TUBE

The Blakemore tube is a nonsurgical approach that is used rarely in the modern ED or intensive care unit (ICU) to temporarily treat active variceal hemorrhage. The enduring image of the Blakemore tube is the football helmet with the proximal end of the tube attached to the face mask to secure positioning. The tube works by being inflated inside the esophagus to tamponade the esophageal varices. The Blakemore tube is considered an eleventh-hour effort to temporarily control bleeding in a critically ill patient. A few limited studies have shown moderate effectiveness for the Blakemore tube to control bleeding before more definitive care such as transjugular intrahepatic portosystemic shunt or sclerotherapy.[56,57]

SUMMARY

The established quality indicators for early management of upper GI hemorrhage are based on rapid diagnosis, risk stratification, and early management (**Table 6**). Effective preendoscopic treatment may improve survivability of critically ill patients and improve resource allocation for all patients. Accurate risk stratification helps determine the need for hospital admission, hemodynamic monitoring, blood transfusion, and

Table 6
Preendoscopic quality indicators for upper GI hemorrhage

Diagnosis	Evidence
Perform following tests at initial evaluation: complete blood, electrolyte levels, blood type, and crossmatch	IC
Document risk stratification for rebleeding and mortality using either Glasgow-Blatchford or CRS for NVUGIH	IB
Document orthostatic vital signs in patients with normal resting vital signs for NVUGIH	IC
If the patient receives nasogastric aspiration, document findings as fresh red blood, coffee-ground blood, bilious or nonbilious aspirate	IB
Place large-bore intravenous lines at initial evaluation	IC
If patient shows signs of hypovolemia, administer crystalloids for fluid resuscitation at initial evaluation	IC
If patient has hypoxemia, administer supplemental oxygen	IC
If hypovolemia is not responsive to initial crystalloid fluid resuscitation, patient should be admitted to the ICU	IC
If patient has active hematemesis with mental status changes, patient should be admitted to the intensive care unit	IC
Acute GI hemorrhage in a patient with cirrhosis requires prompt attention with intravascular volume support and blood transfusions, being careful to maintain a hemoglobin of ~8 g/dL	IB
Short-term (maximum 7 d) antibiotic prophylaxis should be instituted in any patient with cirrhosis and GI hemorrhage. Oral norfloxacin (400 mg BID) or intravenous ciprofloxacin is the recommended antibiotic. In patients with advanced cirrhosis intravenous ceftriaxone (1 g/d) may be preferable	IA, I A, IB
Pharmacologic therapy (somatostatin or its analogues octreotide and vapreotide; terlipressin) should be initiated as soon as variceal hemorrhage is suspected and continued for 3–5 d after diagnosis is confirmed	IA
Balloon tamponade should be used as a temporizing measure (maximum 24 h) in patients with uncontrollable bleeding for whom a more definitive therapy (eg, TIPS or endoscopic therapy) is planned	IB

Abbreviations: BID, twice a day; NVUGIH, nonvariceal upper GI hemorrhage; TIPS, transjugular intrahepatic portosystemic shunt.

Adapted from Garcia-Tsao G, Sanyal AJ, Grace ND, et al. Prevention and management of gastroesophageal varices and variceal hemorrhage in cirrhosis. Am J Gastroenterol 2007;102(9):2086–102; and Kanwal F, Barkun A, Gralnek IM, et al. Measuring quality of care in patients with nonvariceal upper gastrointestinal hemorrhage: development of an explicit quality indicator set. Am J Gastroenterol 2010;105(8):1710–18.

endoscopic hemostasis before EGD via indirect measures such as laboratory studies, physiologic data, and comorbidities. Early management before the definitive EGD is essential to improving outcomes for patients with upper GI bleeding.

REFERENCES

1. AHRQ. Weighted national estimates from HCUP nationwide emergency department sample (NEDS). 2008. Available at: http://hcupnet.ahrq.gov/HCUPnet.jsp.
2. Crooks C, Card T, West J. Reductions in 28-day mortality following hospital admission for upper gastrointestinal hemorrhage. Gastroenterology 2011;141: 62–70.

3. British Society of Gastroenterology Endoscopy Committee. Non-variceal upper gastrointestinal haemorrhage: guidelines. Gut 2002;51(Suppl 4):iv1–6.

4. Jaffe RM, Kasten B, Young DS, et al. False negative stool occult blood test caused by ingestion of ascorbic acid (vitamin C). Ann Intern Med 1975;83(6): 824–6.

5. Kulbaski MJ, Goold SD, Tecce MA, et al. Oral iron and the hemoccult test: a controversy on the teaching wards. N Engl J Med 1989;320(22):1500.

6. Sugawa C, Steffes CP, Nakamura R, et al. Upper GI bleeding in an urban hospital: etiology, recurrence, and prognosis. Ann Surg 1990;212(4):521–6.

7. Rubin M, Hussain SA, Shalomov A, et al. Live view video capsule endoscopy enables risk stratification of patients with acute upper GI bleeding in the emergency room: a pilot study. Dig Dis Sci 2011;56:786–91.

8. Oliwa N, Mort TC. Is a rapid sequence intubation always indicated for emergency airway management of the upper GI bleeding patient?: 162-M. Crit Care Med 2005;33(12):A97.

9. Strote J. ED patient estimation of blood loss. Am J Emerg Med 2009;27(6): 709–11.

10. Rockall T, Logan R, Devlin H, et al. Risk assessment after acute upper gastrointestinal haemorrhage. Gut 1996;38(3):316–21.

11. Vreeburg E, Terwee C, Snel P, et al. Validation of the Rockall risk scoring system in upper gastrointestinal bleeding. Gut 1999;44(3):331–5.

12. Tham T, James C, Kelly M. Predicting outcome of acute non-variceal upper gastrointestinal haemorrhage without endoscopy using the clinical Rockall score. Postgrad Med J 2006;82(973):757–9.

13. Gralnek IM, Dulai GS. Incremental value of upper endoscopy for triage of patients with acute non-variceal upper-GI hemorrhage. Gastrointest Endosc 2004;60(1):9–14.

14. Blatchford O, Murray WR, Blatchford M. A risk score to predict need for treatment for upper-gastrointestinal haemorrhage. Lancet 2000;356(9238):1318–21.

15. Schiefer M, Aquarius M, Leffers P, et al. Predictive validity of the Glasgow Blatchford bleeding score in an unselected emergency department population in continental Europe. Eur J Gastroenterol Hepatol 2012;24(4):382–7.

16. Gralnek IM. Outpatient management of "low-risk" nonvariceal upper GI hemorrhage. Are we ready to put evidence into practice? Gastrointest Endosc 2002; 55(1):131–4.

17. Stanley AJ, Ashley D, Dalton HR, et al. Outpatient management of patients with low-risk upper-gastrointestinal haemorrhage: multicentre validation and prospective evaluation. Lancet 2009;373(9657):42–7.

18. Bryant RV, Kuo P, Williamson K, et al. Performance of the Glasgow-Blatchford score in predicting clinical outcomes and intervention in hospitalized patients with upper GI bleeding. Gastrointest Endosc 2013;78(4):576–83.

19. Meltzer AC, Pinchbeck C, Burnett S, et al. Emergency physicians accurately interpret video capsule endoscopy findings in suspected upper gastrointestinal hemorrhage: a video survey. Acad Emerg Med 2013;20(7):711–5.

20. Meltzer AC, Burnett S, Pinchbeck C, et al. Pre-endoscopic Rockall and Blatchford scores to identify which emergency department patients with suspected gastrointestinal bleed do not need endoscopic hemostasis. J Emerg Med 2013;44(6):1083–7.

21. Pang SH, Ching JY, Lau JY, et al. Comparing the Blatchford and pre-endoscopic Rockall score in predicting the need for endoscopic therapy in patients with upper GI hemorrhage. Gastrointest Endosc 2010;71(7):1134–40.

22. Witting MD, Magder L, Heins AE, et al. Usefulness and validity of diagnostic nasogastric aspiration in patients without hematemesis. Ann Emerg Med 2004;43(4):525–32.
23. Cuellar RE, Gavaler JS, Alexander JA, et al. Gastrointestinal tract hemorrhage. The value of a nasogastric aspirate. Arch Intern Med 1990;150(7):1381–4.
24. Singer AJ, Richman PB, Kowalska A, et al. Comparison of patient and practitioner assessments of pain from commonly performed emergency department procedures. Ann Emerg Med 1999;33:652–8.
25. Aljebreen AM, Fallone CA, Barkun AN. Nasogastric aspirate predicts high-risk endoscopic lesions in patients with acute upper-GI bleeding. Gastrointest Endosc 2004;59(2):172–8.
26. Huang ES, Karsan S, Kanwal F, et al. Impact of nasogastric lavage on outcomes in acute GI bleeding. Gastrointest Endosc 2011;74(5):971–80.
27. Gralnek IM, Ching JY, Maza I, et al. Capsule endoscopy in acute upper gastrointestinal hemorrhage: a prospective cohort study. Endoscopy 2013;45(1): 12–9.
28. Meltzer AC, Ali MA, Kresiberg RB, et al. Video capsule endoscopy in the emergency department: a prospective study of acute upper gastrointestinal hemorrhage. Ann Emerg Med 2013. http://dx.doi.org/10.1016/j.annemergmed.2012. 11.008.
29. Yachimski PS, Friedman LS. Gastrointestinal bleeding in the elderly. Nat Clin Pract Gastroenterol Hepatol 2008;5(2):80–93.
30. Daneshmend T, Hawkey C, Langman M, et al. Omeprazole versus placebo for acute upper gastrointestinal bleeding: randomised double blind controlled trial. BMJ 1992;304(6820):143.
31. Hawkey G, Cole A, McIntyre A, et al. Drug treatments in upper gastrointestinal bleeding: value of endoscopic findings as surrogate end points. Gut 2001;49(3): 372–9.
32. Hulagu S, Demirturk L, Gul S, et al. The effect of omeprazole or ranitidine intravenous on upper gastrointestinal bleeding. Endoscopy 1994;26:404.
33. Lau JY, Leung WK, Wu JC, et al. Omeprazole before endoscopy in patients with gastrointestinal bleeding. N Engl J Med 2007;356(16):1631–40.
34. Naumovski-Mihalic S, Katicic M, Colic-Cvlje V, et al. Intravenous proton pump inhibitor in ulcer bleeding in patients admitted to an intensive care unit. Gastroenterology 2005;128(Suppl 4):W1578.
35. Wallner G, Ciechanski A, Wesolowski M, et al. Treatment of acute upper gastrointestinal bleeding with intravenous omeprazole or ranitidine. European Journal of Clinical Research 1996;8:235–43.
36. Sreedharan A, Martin J, Leontiadis GI, et al. Proton pump inhibitor treatment initiated prior to endoscopic diagnosis in upper gastrointestinal bleeding. Cochrane Database Syst Rev 2010;(7):CD005415.
37. Wong SH, Sung J. Management of GI emergencies: peptic ulcer acute bleeding. Best Pract Res Clin Gastroenterol 2013;27(5):639–47.
38. Arabi Y, Al Knawy B, Barkun A, et al. Pro/con debate: octreotide has an important role in the treatment of gastrointestinal bleeding of unknown origin? Crit Care 2006;10(4):218.
39. Okan A, Simsek I, Akpinar H, et al. Somatostatin and ranitidine in the treatment of non-variceal upper gastrointestinal bleeding: a prospective, randomized, double-blind, controlled study. Hepatogastroenterology 2000;47:1325–7.
40. Gotzsche P, Hróbjartsson A. Somatostatin analogues for acute bleeding oesophageal varices. Cochrane Database Syst Rev 2008;(3):CD000193.

41. Wells M, Chande N, Adams P, et al. Meta-analysis: vasoactive medications for the management of acute variceal bleeds. Aliment Pharmacol Ther 2012; 35(11):1267–78.
42. D'Amico G, Pagliaro L, Pietrosi G, et al. Emergency sclerotherapy versus vasoactive drugs for bleeding oesophageal varices in cirrhotic patients. Cochrane Database Syst Rev 2010;(3):CD002233.
43. Barkun A, Bardou M, Marshall JK, Nonvariceal Upper GI Bleeding Consensus Conference Group. Consensus recommendations for managing patients with nonvariceal upper gastrointestinal bleeding. Ann Intern Med 2003;139:843–57.
44. Chavez-Tapia NC, Barrientos-Gutierrez T, Tellez-Avila F, et al. Meta-analysis: antibiotic prophylaxis for cirrhotic patients with upper gastrointestinal bleeding? An updated Cochrane Review. Aliment Pharmacol Ther 2011;34(5):509–18. http://dx.doi.org/10.1111/j.1365-2036.2011.04746.
45. Pauwels A, Mostefa-Kara N, Debenes B, et al. Systemic antibiotic prophylaxis after gastrointestinal hemorrhage in cirrhotic patients with a high risk of infection. Hepatology 1996;24(4):802–6.
46. Sabat M, Kolle L, Soriano G, et al. Parenteral antibiotic prophylaxis of bacterial infections does not improve cost-efficacy of oral norfloxacin in cirrhotic patients with gastrointestinal bleeding. Am J Gastroenterol 1998;93:2457–62.
47. Gulberg V, Deibert P, Ochs A, et al. Prevention of infectious complications after transjugular intrahepatic portosystemic shunt in cirrhotic patients with a single dose of ceftriaxone. Hepatogastroenterology 1999;46:1126–30.
48. Fernandez J, Ruiz del Arbol L, Gomez C, et al. Norfloxacin vs ceftriaxone in the prophylaxis of infections in patients with advanced cirrhosis and hemorrhage. Gastroenterology 2006;131:1049–56.
49. Hébert PC, Wells G, Blajchman MA. A multicenter, randomized, controlled clinical trial of transfusion requirements in critical care. N Engl J Med 1990;340(6):409–17.
50. Villanueva C, Colomo A, Bosch A, et al. Transfusion strategies for acute upper gastrointestinal bleeding. N Engl J Med 2013;368(1):11–21.
51. Pollack CV Jr. Managing bleeding in anticoagulated patients in the emergency care setting. J Emerg Med 2013;45(3):467–77.
52. Lankiewicz M, Hays J, Friedman K, et al. Urgent reversal of warfarin with prothrombin complex concentrate. J Thromb Haemost 2006;4(5):967–70.
53. Hickey M, Gatien M, Taljaard M, et al. Outcomes of urgent warfarin reversal using fresh frozen plasma versus prothrombin complex concentrate in the emergency department. Circulation 2013;128:360–4.
54. Dentali F, Marchesi C, Pierfranceschi MG, et al. Safety of prothrombin complex concentrates for rapid anticoagulation reversal of vitamin K antagonists. Thromb Haemost 2007;98(4):790–7.
55. Eerenberg ES, Kamphuisen PW, Sijpkens MK, et al. Reversal of rivaroxaban and dabigatran by prothrombin complex concentrate a randomized, placebo-controlled, crossover study in healthy subjects. Circulation 2011;124(14):1573–9.
56. Jaramillo JL, de la Mata M, Miño G, et al. Somatostatin versus sengstaken balloon tamponade for primary haemostasia of bleeding esophageal varices: a randomized pilot study. J Hepatol 1991;12(1):100–5.
57. Terblanche J, Yakoob HI, Bornman PC, et al. Acute bleeding varices: a five-year prospective evaluation of tamponade and sclerotherapy. Ann Surg 1981; 194(4):521.

Endoscopic Management of Acute Peptic Ulcer Bleeding

Yidan Lu, MD[a], Yen-I Chen, MD[a], Alan Barkun, MD, MSc[a,b],*

KEYWORDS

- Peptic ulcer bleeding • Upper gastrointestinal bleeding • Endoscopy • Gastric ulcer
- Duodenal ulcer • Nonvariceal upper gastrointestinal hemorrhage

KEY POINTS

- Endoscopy should be performed within 24 hours of presentation in patients with upper gastrointestinal bleeding.
- Pre-endoscopic prokinetics should be considered in patients who are suspected of having a significant amount of blood in the upper gastrointestinal tract, such as those with positive nasogastric aspirate or active hematemesis, to improve the endoscopic view and decrease the need for repeat endoscopy.
- Endoscopic therapy should be performed in lesions with high-risk stigmata (Forrest classification I–IIB) with combination therapy or monotherapy using current endoscopic hemostatic agents except for epinephrine, which should not be used alone as definitive therapy.
- Postendoscopic care includes testing and eradication of *Helicobacter pylori*, avoidance of nonsteroidal anti-inflammatory drugs whenever possible, and the use of proper gastroprotective strategies in patients requiring ongoing antiplatelet and anticoagulant therapy.

INTRODUCTION

Peptic ulcers are the most frequently encountered cause of upper gastrointestinal bleeding (UGIB), with an annual incidence of 19.4 to 57.0 per 100,000 individuals.[1] Ulcers account for one-third to half of all presentations of acute UGIB.[1–3] A large United States inpatient database reveals declining trends in the incidence of both UGIB and peptic ulcer bleeding.[1] Similarly, the mortality from UGIB has also

Disclosure: No conflicts of interest to disclose.
Yidan Lu and Yen-I Chen are co-authors.
[a] Division of Gastroenterology, McGill University Health Center, McGill University, 1650 Cedar Avenue, Montréal H3G 1A4, Canada; [b] Division of Clinical Epidemiology, McGill University Health Center, McGill University, 687 Pine Avenue West, Montréal H3A 1A1, Canada
* Corresponding author. Division of Gastroenterology, McGill University Health Center, Montreal General Hospital Site, 1650 Cedar Avenue, Room D7-185, Montréal H3G 1A4, Canada.
E-mail address: alan.barkun@muhc.mcgill.ca

Gastroenterol Clin N Am 43 (2014) 677–705
http://dx.doi.org/10.1016/j.gtc.2014.08.003
0889-8553/14/$ – see front matter © 2014 Elsevier Inc. All rights reserved.

decreased from 2.95% to 2.45%.[1] In the management of UGIB, the use of endoscopy plays a fundamental role in the diagnosis, treatment, and prognostication of UGIB. Pre-endoscopic considerations such as the use of prokinetics and timing of endoscopy are reviewed, with a focus on the endoscopic management of peptic ulcer bleeding. Such management includes the use of the available hemostatic modalities, including emerging therapies, which will be reviewed along with their comparative effectiveness. Proton-pump inhibitors (PPIs) after endoscopy, indications for second-look endoscopy, and the use of secondary pharmacologic prophylaxis are also discussed. Issues of risk stratification and initial resuscitation are discussed in an article elsewhere in this issue by Meltzer and Klein.

PROKINETICS

Prokinetic agents such as erythromycin and metoclopramide can be administered before endoscopy to improve endoscopic yield and reduce the need for a repeat endoscopy. Erythromycin, a motilin agonist, can be given at a dose of 250 mg intravenously, and metoclopramide 10 mg intravenously 30 to 60 minutes before endoscopy. The use of erythromycin is favored based on current data. Doses used in the literature range from 3 to 4 mg/kg of erythromycin administered 20 to 90 minutes before endoscopy. Furthermore, the QT-interval–prolonging effect of erythromycin should be taken into consideration, and an electrocardiogram first performed.

The use of prokinetics should be considered in acute UGIB, particularly when targeting patients with active bleeding and/or evidence of blood in the stomach.[4] A meta-analysis comprising 3 randomized controlled trials (RCTs) with erythromycin and 2 abstracts with metoclopramide included a total of 162 patients, all showing evidence of active bleeding with blood in the stomach,[5] showed that a prokinetic agent, in comparison with placebo or no treatment, led to a significant reduction in the need for repeat endoscopy (odds ratio [OR] 0.55; 95% confidence interval [CI] 0.32–0.94). This effect was not preserved when analyzing metoclopramide alone (OR 1.22; 95% CI 0.35–4.25).[5] No differences were noted for blood transfusions or need for surgery, while mortality was not analyzed. A more recent meta-analysis solely looking at erythromycin showed similar results, with improvement in the visualization of the gastric mucosa (OR 3.43; 95% CI 1.81–6.50), and a decrease in the need for a second-look endoscopy (OR 0.47; 95% CI 0.26–0.83).[6] Of note, the effect of erythromycin in decreasing units of blood transfused and length of stay in hospital reached significance[7] when an additional trial that only included patients with variceal bleeding[8] was added to the meta-analysis.[7,9]

Pre-endoscopic intravenous PPI administration and nasogastric lavage can also be considered before endoscopy; these details are discussed elsewhere.

TIMING OF ENDOSCOPY

The performance of early endoscopy within 24 hours of patient presentation is warranted for most patients.[4,10] This practice has been shown to be safe for all patients at risk, allows for earlier discharge of low-risk patients,[11] and improves outcomes in those at high risk.[4] Lower costs are also associated with early discharge after endoscopy of low-risk patients.[12]

Several RCTs and retrospective cohort studies have examined very early endoscopy at less than 2 to 3, less than 6, less than 8, and less than 12 hours, compared with less than 24 to 48 hours.[13] Faster time to endoscopy yielded higher rates of finding high-risk stigmata of bleeding at endoscopy,[14–16] and similarly higher rates of hemostasis being performed[16,17] without demonstrable effects on outcomes of rebleeding, need for surgery, or duration of hospitalization. This finding contrasts with those of studies looking at early endoscopy (<24 hours) showing a significant decreased length of stay in hospital.[18] Moreover, decreased rebleeding and need for surgery[19] were also observed, particularly among high-risk patients (ulcer with active bleeding or visible vessel, or varices).[18]

In higher-risk patients, one study randomizing patients to endoscopy at less than 12 hours versus greater than 12 hours from patient presentation detected a significantly reduced need for blood transfusions, and shorter hospitalization (4 vs 14.5 days) in the subgroup of patients with coffee grounds or bloody nasogastric aspirate.[20] In parallel, one observational study demonstrated, using a receiver-operating curve analysis, that a longer time to endoscopy (>13 hours) predicted all-cause in-hospital mortality in patients with a Blatchford score of 12 or higher.[21] The robustness of the results is limited by the lack of randomization and adjustment for possible confounders that can influence mortality. As a result, the American College of Gastroenterology guidelines on ulcer bleeding suggest that endoscopy within 12 hours may be considered in high-risk patients. Similarly, the United Kingdom UGIB toolkit produced by the Academy of Royal Medical Colleges recommends endoscopy at less than 6 to 12 hours in "urgent-risk" patients,[22] a practice that is currently not supported by high-quality evidence for nonvariceal UGIB (NVUGIB),[23] though appropriate in the context of suspected variceal bleeding, in which case endoscopy within 12 hours is suggested.[24]

Data from bleeding registries show that a significant proportion of patients have a delay greater than 24 hours before undergoing upper endoscopy. Though variable, rates of early endoscopy range from 50% in a United Kingdom bleeding audit[25] up to 82% in a large Danish registry.[26] Reasons behind such delays are likely multifactorial; however, several reports from administrative databases relay a "weekend effect" whereby patients presenting on weekends are less likely to undergo early endoscopy, and have higher mortality, which may[27–29] or may not result from longer endoscopy delays.[30] Nevertheless, endoscopy within 24 hours of patient presentation should be targeted as a stand-alone quality indicator when managing patients with acute UGIB.[31]

ENDOSCOPIC DIAGNOSIS AND RISK STRATIFICATION

The endoscopic findings of a bleeding ulcer have prognostic implications in terms of rebleeding, need for surgery, and mortality. As a result, they are integrated in risk assessment scores such as the complete Rockall score, and are further used to determine the need for endoscopic hemostasis. The stigmata of recent bleeding are used to characterize the endoscopic appearance at the base of the bleeding ulcer, and are commonly categorized according to the Forrest classification into high-risk stigmata (HRS) and low-risk stigmata (LRS) (**Table 1**). HRS comprise active spurting bleeding

Table 1
Forrest classification of stigmata of recent bleeding

Stigmata of Recent Hemorrhage		Forrest Classification
Active spurting bleeding	High-risk stigmata	IA
Active oozing bleeding		IB
Nonbleeding visible vessel		IIA
Adherent clot		IIB
Flat pigmented spot	Low-risk stigmata	IIC
Clean base		III

(Forrest IA), active oozing bleeding (Forrest IB), nonbleeding visible vessel (Forrest IIA), and adherent clot (Forrest IIB). Low-risk lesions that include flat pigmented spots (Forrest IIC) and clean base ulcers (Forrest III) are more prevalent, reaching a prevalence of more than 50%.[3,32,33] Older data predating the routine use of endoscopic hemostasis reveal a natural history with rebleeding rates of 55% (17%–100%) (Forrest IA and IB), 43% (0%–81%) (Forrest IIA), 22% (14%–36%) (Forrest IIB), 10% (0%–13%) (Forrest IIC), and 5% (0%–10%) (Forrest III).[34] Significant interobserver variability has been reported in the identification of endoscopic stigmata.[35] Nonetheless, when ulcer bleeding stigmata are surveyed with sequential endoscopic evaluations, an evolution of stigmata is noted, suggesting various phases of healing whereby a bleeding vessel progressively evolves after endoscopic therapy into a clean base ulcer.[32] Furthermore, most rebleeding episodes were noted within the first 72 hours, consistent with the natural history of ulcer healing.[32]

In patients with LRS ulcers, endoscopic hemostasis has not been shown to alter outcomes.[36,37] The treatment of patients with pigmented spots or clean base ulcers therefore consists of oral acid suppressive pharmacotherapy alone. In contradistinction, endoscopic therapy in ulcer bleeding has been well established to decrease continued or recurrent bleeding, surgery, and mortality, particularly in patients with active bleeding and nonbleeding visible vessel.[36,37] For such patients, the magnitude of improvement in outcome measures from an earlier meta-analysis of 30 RCTs is as follows: further bleeding (OR 0.38; 95% CI 0.32–0.45), surgery (OR 0.36; 95% CI 0.28–0.45), and mortality (OR 0.55; 95% CI 0.40–0.6).[37] The benefits of endoscopic therapy for patients with HRS were confirmed in a more recent meta-analysis demonstrating the superiority of any endoscopic method over pharmacotherapy (which included one trial using high-dose intravenous PPI) for rebleeding (OR 0.35; 95% CI 0.27–0.46), surgery (OR 0.57; 95% CI 0.41–0.81), and mortality (OR 0.57; 95% CI 0.37–0.89).[38] Similarly, Laine and McQuaid[39] found decreased rebleeding and surgery with endoscopic therapy in comparison with no endoscopic therapy for active bleeding and nonbleeding visible vessel. However, they did not detect statistically significant benefits with regard to mortality, or in any outcomes among patients with adherent clots. Endoscopic hemostasis is therefore indicated in all patients with HRS, whereas ulcers with LRS can be managed with pharmacotherapy only, and do not warrant therapy. The more detailed management of lesions with adherent clots is somewhat controversial (see later discussion).

ENDOSCOPIC THERAPY

Endoscopic therapy is indicated in patients presenting with NVUGIB and HRS on endoscopy (see **Table 1**). Meta-analyses have found that endoscopic therapy for ulcers with these features significantly decreased rebleeding, surgery, and mortality.[36,37] In contradistinction, low-risk lesions such as ulcers with flat, pigmented spot (Forrest IIC) or clean based (Forrest III) are associated with lower incidences of rebleeding, and endoscopic therapy has not been shown to be beneficial.[32,34] In terms of endoscopic modalities, there are several techniques that have been developed including injection, thermal, and mechanical therapies and, more recently, hemostatic powders. In addition, several ancillary methods to improve endoscopic risk stratification of bleeding lesions and hemostasis such as Doppler ultrasonography, magnification endoscopy, and chromoendoscopy,[40] have also emerged. The following is an overview of the different endoscopic therapies, with a specific focus on the techniques involved in their successful deployment.

Injection Therapy

Different injectates have been developed, including epinephrine, hypertonic saline, sclerosants (polidocanol, ethanolamine, absolute alcohol, sodium tetradecyl sulfate), and tissue adhesives (cyanoacrylate, thrombin, fibrin). Injection therapy has been widely performed most likely because of its ease of use, availability, and extensive experience with its application by most endoscopists. Injections are delivered through a 25-gauge retractable catheter (**Fig. 1**A). Epinephrine (1:10,000 or 1:20,000 dilution) is the most common injectate used in the control of NVUGIB, and should be performed in increments of 0.5 to 1.5 mL in all 4 quadrants around the ulcer base with or without injections into the center of the ulcerated lesion itself (see **Fig. 1**B).[41] It is important that the main mechanism responsible for successful hemostasis is likely due to the tamponade effect from the volume of the injection rather than the vasoconstrictive mechanism of the epinephrine or resulting platelet aggregation.[34,42] In fact, randomized controlled data suggest that higher total volumes (13–45 mL) per bleeding lesion may decrease rebleeding rates, presumably because of the greater tamponade effect.[43–45] The application of epinephrine is simple and requires little skill, such that its application can be easily performed with both tangential and en-face positioning, and may be the initial agent of choice in massive gastrointestinal (GI) hemorrhage where rapid control of the bleeding field with other modalities can be difficult to achieve because of the obscured view. However injection therapies have been shown to be inferior to monotherapies with both thermal or mechanical modalities and combination therapies.[4,39,46] Pooled data for injection therapy (including trials on epinephrine monotherapy, alcohol monotherapy, and a combination of other injectates) reveals a reduction in rebleeding (OR 0.43; 95% CI 0.24–0.78) compared with pharmacotherapy[38] in patients with HRS. Despite evidence of comparable initial hemostasis success,[39] epinephrine injection is inferior to other monotherapies (thermal, fibrin glue, and clip), as already discussed, with a higher incidence of rebleeding (OR 1.72; 95% CI 1.08–2.78) and surgery (OR 2.27; 95% CI 1.02–5.00) when used alone.[39] In a meta-analysis of 16 RCTs, Calvet and colleagues[46] demonstrated that epinephrine injection, followed by a second modality, provides additional benefits with regard to reducing

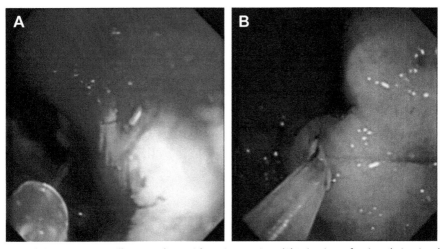

Fig. 1. (*A*) Injection needle near ulcer with active oozing. (*B*) Injection of epinephrine in ulcer resulting in mucosal blanching.

rebleeding (OR 0.53; 95% CI 0.40–0.69), surgery (OR 0.64; 95% CI 0.46–0.90), and mortality (OR 0.51; 95% CI 0.31–0.84) when compared with epinephrine monotherapy. Mortality benefits were not reproduced in more recent analyses.[38,39,47] In summary, there is strong evidence suggesting that epinephrine injection should not be used alone for the treatment of ulcer bleeding with HRS.

The role of other injectates, such as sclerosants and tissue adhesives, in the management of NVUGIB are less well defined. Sclerosants including polidocanol, ethanolamine, absolute alcohol, and sodium tetradecyl sulfate are associated with a risk of tissue necrosis, perforation, and vessel thrombosis.[48–53] Sclerosant therapy has nonetheless been associated with significant benefits in reducing rebleeding, surgery, and mortality in comparison with no therapy,[39] and can be considered in the management algorithm of NVUGIB.[4] Tissue adhesives such as cyanoacrylate, thrombin, and fibrin, on the other hand, have not been evaluated as extensively, and are often limited by their high acquisition costs and lack of availability.[54] In comparison with epinephrine, these agents are rarely used in the routine treatment of patients with NVUGIB.

Thermal Therapy

Thermal therapy applies heat or electric current to bleeding lesions, which can lead to coagulation of vessels and successful hemostasis. Thermal treatment can be divided into contact (electrocoagulation or heater probe) and noncontact techniques.

Contact electrocoagulation

Endoscopic contact electrocoagulation is available as monopolar, bipolar (BEC), or multipolar (MEC) electrocautery. Unlike the monopolar modality, the electric circuit with BEC or MEC terminates locally at the tip of the probe and decreases in intensity as the target tissue desiccates with electrocautery, thereby limiting the depth of penetration and decreasing the risk for perforation.[55] Optimal BEC/MEC is best performed using a large-diameter (10F, 3.2 mm) probe with firm, constant pressure on the high-risk lesion and application of low energy (15 W) electrocoagulation for 10 to 12 seconds until flattening of vessels or adequate coagulation of the stigmata (**Fig. 2**).[56] In other words, the goal is to achieve coaptive coagulation, with hemostasis occurring from physical occlusion and tamponade of the vessels in the bed of the bleeding lesion,

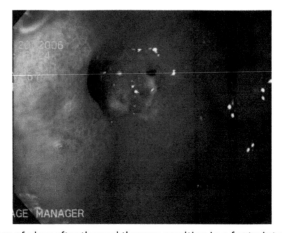

Fig. 2. Appearance of ulcer after thermal therapy, resulting in a footprint with achievement of hemostasis.

followed by thermal coagulation. Data from porcine models suggest that longer dura-tion of electrocoagulation (tamponade station) increases the energy and coagulation, whereas increasing the watt setting does not improve the transfer of coagulation owing to the rapid increase in impedance.[56] Therefore, long-duration (10–12 seconds) and low-energy (15 W) electrocoagulation are preferred for optimal coaptive coagula-tion.[57,58] In terms of delivery, contact electrocoagulation is easy to use, allows for simultaneous, foot pedal–controlled water irrigation, and is effective in both bleeding and nonbleeding HRS. However, MEC/BEC may be difficult to use in the tangential position given that electric current occurs at the tip of the catheter.

Contact heater probe
The heater probe dissipates heat at the tip and sides of the probe, leading to coagu-lation of high-risk lesions in both the en-face and tangential position. Similarly to con-tact electrocoagulation, the application is best performed using a large-diameter probe (10F, 3.2 mm) and requires firm constant pressure with the target lesion; how-ever, unlike BEC or MEC, coagulation is provided in the form of heat energy (25–30 J) and is delivered in a pulsatile fashion (4–5 pulses).[58–60] The main advantage of the heater or gold probe over contact electrocoagulation is its ability to provide coagula-tion through the tip and sides of the probe, therefore allowing for ease of application in both the tangential and en-face position. The heater probe also allows for foot pedal–controlled water irrigation, and is effective in both bleeding and nonbleeding HRS.[38]

The use of contact thermal therapy, namely heater probe and electrocoagulation, is beneficial in achieving hemostasis in patients with high-risk lesions, as evidenced by reduced rebleeding (OR 0.44; 95% CI 0.36–0.54), surgery (OR 0.39; 95% CI 0.27–0.55), and mortality rates (OR 0.58; 95% CI 0.34–0.98) when compared with no endo-scopic treatment,[39] although the impact on mortality was not reproduced in a separate meta-analysis (OR 0.64; 95% CI 0.25–1.65).[38] Aside from the previously discussed benefits over epinephrine monotherapy, comparison of contact thermal therapy with other modalities, alone or in combination, have not yielded consistent results to favor the use of one approach over another.[38,61] It is worth mentioning that although pooled meta-analytical data comparing the combination of injection and thermal therapy with thermal monotherapy did not show any significant differences in rebleeding, subgroup analysis favored combination therapy after the removal of 2 less generalizable trials, resulting in decreased risks of rebleeding (OR 0.37; 95% CI 0.14–0.97).[38] Overall, as data to confidently support the use of one modality over another are lacking, technical considerations may better dictate the use of thermal therapy. In addition, thermocoa-gulation can be used either alone or in combination with injection therapy.[4]

Noncontact thermal therapy
Argon plasma coagulation (APC) is unique in its ability to deliver electrocautery in a noncontact fashion through the delivery of monopolar, alternating current through ionized argon gas. Electrical current is delivered to the target tissue via electrically charged argon gas that is propelled from the catheter tip. Coagulation is mostly super-ficial (up to 2.4 mm according to in vitro studies[62]), given that the argon plasma beam shifts away from coagulated tissue, which loses its conduction ability because of in-creases in electrical resistance with desiccation, therefore preventing further tissue damage and perforation.[57,63,64] In terms of application, the optimal distance between probe and target tissue is estimated to be 2 to 8 mm. Direct contact between the probe and the target lesion should be avoided to prevent submucosal dissection and submucosal argon gas insufflation, which causes significant pain, pneumatosis, and risk of perforation.[65] APC seems to be ideal for shallow and broadly defined

bleeding lesions such as angiodysplasia, radiation telangiectasia, and gastric antral vascular ectasia, also known as watermelon stomach.[62,66–69]

The use of APC in ulcer bleeding has been evaluated in several trials that compared this approach with a variety of other modalities including heater probe,[70] sclerotherapy,[71,72] epinephrine in combination with heater probe,[73] endoclips,[74] or polidocanol, with no differences in patient outcomes.[39] However, decreased rebleeding was seen when compared with distilled water injection.[72] A single small randomized trial using epinephrine plus APC versus heater probe in patients with high-risk ulcer bleeding showed improved initial hemostasis in the APC arm.[75]

Endoclips

A wide variety of hemostatic mechanical therapies have been developed over the years; however, the endoscopic deployment of endoclips remains the most extensively studied and widely available technique in the management of NVUGIB. It achieves hemostasis through direct compression or tamponade of vessels and tissue approximation of bleeding stigmata (**Fig. 3**). Moreover, unlike most other endoscopic devices, the use of endoclips is usually associated with minimal to no tissue damage, therefore leading potentially to faster ulcer healing.[76] However, its deployment requires precision, en-face positioning, and may be inadequate in fibrotic ulcer beds given its weak tensile strength.[76] It is also noteworthy that endoclips come in many different sizes, lengths, and shapes, grasping and rotational abilities, and deployment mechanisms. Therefore, familiarity with locally available endoclips should be acquired before their use in emergency situations.

The use of endoclips is effective for ulcer bleeding and can be used alone or in combination with epinephrine, or as an alternative to thermal coagulation.[4] Although endoclips have not been compared with pharmacotherapy alone, several RCTs have assessed the benefit of endoclips with or without epinephrine injection, and in comparison with injection and thermal therapy. Again, benefits in rebleeding (OR 0.22; 95% CI 0.09–0.55) and need for surgery (OR 0.22; 95% CI 0.06–0.83) are significant only when endoclips are compared with epinephrine alone.[39] A meta-analysis evaluating 15 studies including 1156 patients highlighted the important heterogeneity across trials that have compared endoclips with thermocoagulation, with or without injection.[77] Individual trials have reported disparate results regarding the superiority or inferiority of endoclips in comparison with thermal therapy.[39] Furthermore, one meta-analysis demonstrated a benefit of endoclips over thermal therapy for rebleeding (OR 0.24;

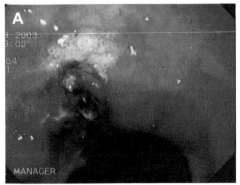 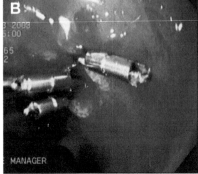

Fig. 3. (A) Ulcer with nonbleeding visible vessel. (B) Appearance of ulcer after the application of endoclips.

95% CI 0.06–0.95),[38] though statistically less robust. Additional considerations such as ulcer location can help direct the decision to use endoclips rather than another hemostatic modality, as higher endoclip failure is seen for ulcers situated in the posterior wall of the duodenum and gastric body, and along the lesser gastric curvature.[77]

In addition to the general recommendation to avoid epinephrine monotherapy,[4] some organizations have recently suggested that thermal or combination therapy may be favored over endoclips or sclerosants when managing actively bleeding lesions,[78] and that thermal therapy should be used with epinephrine[10] based on lower-quality evidence.

Endoscopic hemostatic powders

Recently, novel endoscopic topical hemostatic powders such as the Ankaferd Blood Stopper (ABS), EndoClot, and TC-325 have been adapted to digestive endoscopy and the management of gastrointestinal bleeding (GIB). ABS (Ankaferd Health Products Ltd, Istanbul, Turkey) is a herbal extract derived from 5 different plants that achieves hemostasis by promoting the formation of a protein network behaving as an anchor for erythrocyte aggregation.[79] This agent, however, is not available in North America.

The EndoClot Polysaccharide Hemostatic System (EndoClot-PHS; EndoClot Plus, Inc, Santa Clara, CA, USA) is another emerging hemostatic powder composed of a biocompatible, nonpyogenic, starch-derived compound. It achieves hemostasis by effecting mechanical tamponade and rapid absorption of water from serum, leading to concentration of platelets and clotting factors and thereby accelerating the clotting cascade.[80] At present, the literature on EndoClot is limited to 1 abstract reporting its successful use as an adjuvant therapy in UGIB in 6 patients.[81] Therefore more data are needed with regard to GIB, and the EndoClot is currently not approved for use in North America. TC-325 (Hemospray; Cook Medical, Winston-Salem, NC, USA) is composed of a proprietary inorganic biologically inert powder that, when put in contact with moisture in the GI tract, becomes coherent, thus serving as a mechanical barrier for hemostasis.[82] In addition, it may provide a scaffold, enhancing platelet aggregation and possibly activating clotting factors.[83] However, the powder only adheres to actively bleeding lesions, so its use in high-risk lesions without active spurting or oozing is likely ineffective in providing appropriate hemostasis. The endoscopic powder is propelled from a canister under CO_2 pressure and is delivered through a catheter onto the bleeding lesion (**Fig. 4**A, B). The TC-325 catheter should be maintained 1 to 2 cm from the high-risk lesion, and application should be performed in a noncontact fashion (see **Fig. 4**C). The endoscopic powder will aggregate immediately when it comes into contact with moisture; therefore, efforts should be made to keep the tip of the catheter dry and to avoid suctioning while it is in use or while the powder is settling. Flushing the accessory channel of the endoscope with a 60-mL syringe of air before TC-325 application is also recommended to ensure that the tip of the catheter does not come into contact with moisture during insertion. With the current second-generation Hemospray delivery system, application of the powder occurs by engaging the trigger button, which results in an initial burst of CO_2 gas followed by the release of the hemostatic powder. The accumulation of CO_2 gas may become uncomfortable for the patient. Advantages associated with TC-325 use include ease of application with a lack of need for precise targeting (although the powder needs to reach the actively bleeding site), noncontact and nontraumatic hemostasis, and ability to cover large surfaces of bleeding. As such it may be the ideal modality for massive NVUGIB where rapid control of the bleeding field is critical, and in hemorrhage arising from GI malignancies where bleeding often stems from friable, irregular, and diffusely bleeding surfaces.

Sung and colleagues[1] first described the use of TC-325 in GIB in a prospective pilot study involving 20 patients with NVUGIB treated with Hemospray, resulting in an

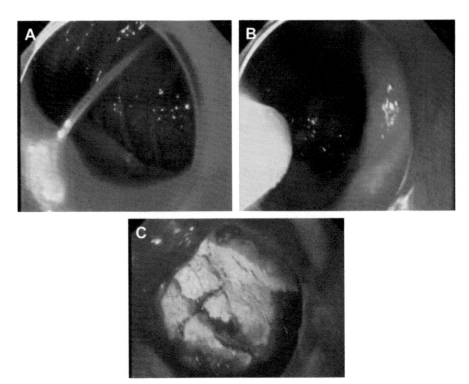

Fig. 4. (*A*) Ulcer with spurting vessel. (*B*) Hemospray catheter advanced near target lesion. (*C*) Appearance of ulcer following the application of Hemospray, resulting in hemostasis.

immediate hemostasis of 95%. Subsequently a multicenter, retrospective study including 63 patients with NVUGIB demonstrated a rate of immediate hemostasis and of 7-day rebleeding with TC-325 therapy for 85% (95% CI 76%–94%) and 15% (95% CI 5%–25%), respectively.[84] More specifically, this study included 25 patients with peptic ulcer bleeding who received TC-325 monotherapy, which resulted in an immediate hemostasis of 76% (95% CI 59%–93%) and a 7-day rebleeding rate of 16% (95% CI 0%–32%). Retrospective data at a single institution recently demonstrated the versatility and effectiveness of TC-325 in both the upper and lower GI tracts in 67 cases of TC-325 therapy in patients with a variety of bleeding disorders including 21 cases of NVUGIB of nonmalignant etiology.[85] The rate of immediate hemostasis and early rebleeding (within 72 hours of TC-325 application) for NVUGIB were 95.2% and 29.4%, respectively. In addition, the powder residency time on the bleeding lesions was demonstrated to be less than 24 hours. Therefore, the current thinking is that TC-325 should not be used as the sole modality in lesions at high risk of rebleeding following the first 24 hours, such as peptic ulcer bleeding with HRS; indeed other modalities, namely thermal or mechanical therapies, should be added to ensure sustained hemostasis. In terms of safety, no major complications, including intestinal obstruction or vascular embolization, have been observed in more than 150 patients treated with TC-325 for GIB.[84–87]

ADHERENT CLOTS

The approach to ulcers with an overlying clot is to irrigate the lesion in an attempt to dislodge the blood clot and reveal the underlying stigma. Vigorous washing for up to

5 minutes is effective in removing the clot in about 40% of lesions.[88] Ulcers with clots resistant to such manipulation are defined as adherent clots (Forrest IIB). These lesions can be further managed by mechanical clot removal without disrupting the pedicle to expose the ulcer base (after preliminary dilute epinephrine injection around the ulcer), followed by endoscopic therapy according to the stigmata of recent bleeding.[4]

The optimal management algorithm for adherent clots remains controversial, as RCTs comparing medical with endoscopic therapy have yielded diverging results. Indeed, some trials have shown that endoscopic therapy decreases rebleeding in adherent clots,[89,90] whereas others,[91,92] including one trial using contemporary high-dose intravenous PPI,[93] have demonstrated low rebleeding rates with acid suppression alone. A previous meta-analysis combining 6 studies with 240 patients suggested a significant reduction in rebleeding with endoscopic hemostasis.[94] However, this work was criticized because of statistical shortcomings and marked heterogeneity of the combined trials, namely differing PPI regimens used in the control arms of the included studies.[95] A more recent meta-analysis failed to detect significant benefits of endoscopic therapy over no endoscopic therapy for adherent clots in terms of rebleeding, need for surgery, or mortality.[39] Consensus guidelines state that endoscopic therapy can be considered while acknowledging that intensive PPI therapy alone may be adequate.[4]

PROTON-PUMP INHIBITORS POSTENDOSCOPIC THERAPY

PPI use in ulcer bleeding improves outcomes. A Cochrane analysis of 31 trials with 5792 patients revealed that PPI use decreases rebleeding (OR 0.45; 95% CI 0.36–0.57), the need for surgery (OR 0.56; 95% CI 0.45–0.70), or repeat endoscopy (OR 0.40; 95% CI 0.30–0.53) regardless of endoscopic hemostasis. A reduction in mortality was achieved only in trials conducted in Asian patients, and more importantly, in patients with active bleeding or nonbleeding visible vessel who had first undergone successful endoscopic hemostasis and who received high-dose intravenous PPIs (80 mg bolus and 8 mg/h infusion for 72 hours).

Another meta-analysis assessing high-dose intravenous PPI as an adjunct to endoscopic hemostasis further supports the observed decrease in rebleeding (OR 0.40; 95% CI 0.28–0.59), surgery (OR 0.43; 95% CI 0.24–0.76), and mortality (OR 0.41; 95% CI 0.20–0.84).[39] Alternative dosing and oral routes have not yielded consistent results to allow for confident routine recommendations of such regimens.[96] All patients with HRS should be treated with high-dose intravenous PPI after endoscopic hemostasis for 72 hours, a period during which most rebleeding occurs.[32] This practice also appears to be cost-effective.[97–99]

SECOND-LOOK ENDOSCOPY

A second-look endoscopy refers to the performance of a preplanned repeat endoscopy 16 to 24 hours following the initial endoscopy, aimed at assessing the need for further endoscopic therapy directed toward any remaining HRS, if present. This practice has previously shown rebleeding benefits,[100,101] although many of the trials did not include concomitant PPI use and used epinephrine monotherapy, a technique now shown to be suboptimal. In fact, in the setting of high-dose intravenous PPI, second-look endoscopy did not provide added benefits.[102] A recent meta-analysis acknowledges the decreased rebleeding conferred by second-look endoscopy in certain high-risk patients with active bleeding, in the absence of high-dose PPI, but discourages against its routine practice in all patients.[103] Consequently, consensus guidelines have concluded that contemporary data do not favor such practice.[4] While further studies are needed to delineate high-risk groups that may benefit from routine second-look endoscopy,[78] the added cost it would entail also needs to be considered.[97] A rebleeding rate exceeding 31% may be needed to offset the cost of a second endoscopy.[104]

In settings where the primary hemostasis is uncertain, and where the initial evaluation was incomplete because of blood clots, repeat endoscopy may be warranted.[105]

PREDICTORS OF FAILURE OF ENDOSCOPIC THERAPY

Rebleeding after endoscopy occurs in 10% to 15% patients presenting with NVU-GIB,[106] although reported values vary in the literature. Data specific to ulcer bleeding vary between 6.3% and 25.2%.[107] Several independent predictors of endoscopic failure have been identified based on both pre-endoscopic and endoscopic features. These predictors include hemodynamic instability (OR 3.30; 95% CI 2.57–4.24), transfusion requirement, and hemoglobin less than 10 g/dL (OR 1.73; 95% CI 1.14–2.62).[107] Active bleeding at endoscopy (OR 1.70; 95% CI 1.31–2.22), the location of bleeding ulcer in either the posterior duodenal wall (OR 3.83; 95% CI 1.38–10.66) or gastric high lesser curvature (OR 2.86; 95% CI 1.69–4.86), in addition to greater ulcer size, particularly larger than 2 cm, also contribute to higher rebleeding rates.[107]

In patients with clinical evidence of rebleeding, a second endoscopy should be attempted to achieve hemostasis. Indeed, comparing endoscopic retreatment with surgery, rates of successful hemostasis in the endoscopy arm reached 73% (35 of 48 patients), with overall lower complication rates, but comparable mortality and length of stay.[108] Failure of repeat endoscopy should be treated with transcatheter arterial embolization or surgery.[109] Details pertaining to such therapies are discussed in articles elsewhere in this issue.

HELICOBACTER PYLORI TESTING

Helicobacter pylori eradication has been demonstrated in a meta-analysis to be significantly more effective than PPI therapy alone in preventing rebleeding from peptic ulcer disease.[110] As such, consensus guidelines have recommended that all patients with peptic ulcer bleeding undergo *H pylori* evaluation, with subsequent eradication if tested positive.[4,111,112] It is important that if the evaluation for *H pylori* is negative in the acute setting, repeat testing is indicated. Indeed, a systematic review of 23 studies showed that diagnostic tests for *H pylori* infection (including serology, histology, urea breath test, rapid urease test, stool antigen, and culture) are associated with high positive predictive values (0.85–0.99) but low negative predictive values (0.45–0.75) in the setting of acute GIB, with 25% to 55% of *H pylori*–infected patients yielding false-negative results.[113,114] This high false-negative rate in acute bleeding may be related, at least in part, to an alkaline milieu imparted by the presence of blood in the gastric lumen, resulting in proximal migration of the bacterium.[115]

MANAGEMENT OF NONSTEROIDAL ANTI-INFLAMMATORY DRUGS IN PATIENTS WITH PEPTIC ULCER BLEEDING

In patients with previous ulcer bleeding, nonsteroidal anti-inflammatory drugs (NSAIDs) should be discontinued. If absolutely needed, a combination of cyclooxygenase-2 (COX-2) inhibitor with a PPI is recommended.[116,117] Adding a PPI to a traditional NSAID or using a COX-2 inhibitor alone reduces the risk of upper gastrointestinal complications; however, the combination of COX-2 inhibitor with

PPI has been shown to be associated with the greatest reductions in risk.[115,116] RCTs have demonstrated that administration of a COX-2 inhibitor plus a PPI when compared with COX-2 inhibitor alone further decreases the risk of rebleeding following an episode of acute peptic ulcer hemorrhage.[118–120] However, there may be an increased risk of cardiovascular events with the use of COX-2 inhibitors, as demonstrated by 2 meta-analyses.[121,122] As such, when reinstituting NSAID therapy following NVUGIB, the risk of cardiovascular events must be balanced with the risk of GI complications on an individual basis. Following an episode of NVUGIB an alternative to NSAID therapy should first be sought and, if necessary, use of a COX-2 inhibitor with a PPI should be favored.[116]

ACUTE MANAGEMENT OF ANTIPLATELET AND ANTICOAGULATION THERAPY IN PATIENTS WITH PEPTIC ULCER BLEEDING

In the event of acute NVUGIB, ongoing aspirin (acetylsalicylic acid; ASA) intake should be held; however, prolonged discontinuation should be avoided. In a meta-analysis, ASA nonadherence or withdrawal was associated with a 3-fold increase in major cardiac events.[123] Moreover, a recent retrospective cohort study from Sweden demonstrated that prolonged discontinuation of ASA, in the context of secondary cardiovascular prophylaxis following acute GIB, led to a 7-fold increase in cardiovascular events or death.[124] The observed thrombosis time is usually between 7 and 30 days, which is in keeping with the ASA-inhibited platelet circulation time of about 10 days.[125,126] In addition, data from one randomized controlled trial suggest that the cardiovascular protection associated with early reinstitution of ASA outweighs the gastrointestinal bleeding risks.[127] Based on these results, consensus recommendations suggest that ASA therapy should be held in acute peptic ulcer bleeding, and restarted as soon as the risk for cardiovascular complication is thought to outweigh the risk for GIB.[4] Practically the authors recommend that ASA be reintroduced within 3 to 5 days of the index bleed after appropriate endoscopic and pharmacologic therapy, with appropriate discussions among the multidisciplinary treatment team that can include general practitioners, internists, cardiologists, neurologists, gastroenterologists, and intensivists. Data on the optimal management of clopidogrel and dual antiplatelet therapy (DAPT) in the acute context of bleeding are lacking.

Vitamin K antagonists such as warfarin should also be held during the setting of an acute GI bleed, and efforts should be made to correct the coagulopathy. In the Canadian Registry on Non-Variceal Upper Gastrointestinal Bleeding and Endoscopy (RUGBE) cohort of 1869 patients, a presenting international normalized ratio (INR) of greater than 1.5 was associated with an almost 2-fold increased risk of mortality (OR 1.95; 95% CI 1.13–3.41), without any increased risk of rebleeding.[128] Data using a historical cohort comparison showed that correcting an INR to less than 1.8, as part of intensive resuscitation, led to lower mortality and fewer myocardial infarctions.[129] Therefore, current guidelines on NVUGIB support the correction of a coagulopathy; however, this should not delay endoscopy.[4] This recent consensus recommendation is based on the recognition of the benefits of early endoscopic intervention coupled with the decreased tissue damage associated with newer ligation hemostatic techniques such as endoscopic clips or hemostatic powders. Moreover, limited observational data also suggest that endoscopic hemostasis can be safely performed in patients with an elevated INR less than 2.5.[130] Although fresh frozen plasma (FFP) may be administered for the reversal of warfarin-induced coagulopathy in patients presenting with life-threatening hemorrhage, prothrombin complex concentrate (PCC) may be a better adapted blood product in this setting. Contrary to FFP, PCC does not need to be frozen during storage, and therefore can be administered more rapidly without the need for thawing. Furthermore, PCC is associated with more effective warfarin reversal, faster infusion rates, lower volumes of administration, and fewer adverse events including thrombotic complications.[131,132] In addition, the use of PCC may be more cost-effective than FFP in the setting of urgent warfarin reversal.[133]

Lastly, the emergence of direct thrombin and factor Xa inhibitors may present a new challenge in acute GIB, given that neither FFP nor PCC have been found to be effective in reversing these agents[134]; however, PCC may still be considered in severe hemorrhage, based on its variable success in animal and in vitro studies as well as in healthy nonbleeding human volunteers.[135,136] Developments of specific reversal agents for these novel oral anticoagulants (nOAC) are currently under way.

MANAGEMENT OF LONG-TERM ANTIPLATELET THERAPY FOLLOWING PEPTIC ULCER HEMORRHAGE

Peptic ulcer disease (PUD) with or without bleeding is a common complication of long-term ASA administration for cardiothrombotic prophylaxis.[137,138] Both H2 receptor antagonists (H2RA) and PPIs have been used in peptic ulcer prophylaxis. The efficacy of H2RA was demonstrated in an RCT showing that famotidine, 20 mg twice daily, can reduce the incidence of peptic ulcer and erosive esophagitis while on ASA in comparison with placebo-based endoscopic assessment at 12 weeks.[139] Clinical outcomes, however, were not assessed in this study, which only assessed patients at low risk of a GI complication. More recently, an RCT by Ng and colleagues,[140] comparing famotidine 40 mg twice daily with pantoprazole 20 mg daily, demonstrated the superiority of the PPI over H2RA in terms of reducing dyspepsia and upper GIB in patients on long-term ASA and a history of PUD with or without bleeding (these patients are at highest risk of bleeding recurrence). Therefore, current consensus guidelines recommend PPI prophylaxis in patients on ASA and high-risk features for gastrointestinal complications such as a history of PUD with or without bleeding.[4]

In addition to PPI prophylaxis, patients who require long-term ASA following acute peptic ulcer bleeding should undergo testing and eradication of H pylori.[4] Data from an RCT demonstrated similar effectiveness in bleeding prophylaxis between H pylori eradication and PPI administration following ulcer bleeding in patients requiring chronic ASA over a 6-month period.[141] However, discrepant results, from Lai and colleagues,[142] demonstrated a high rebleeding rate with ASA following an attempt at H pylori eradication. This result may be due, at least in part, to the fact that many of the subjects in this group failed eradication therapy. Therefore, H pylori testing with eradication coupled with the use of long-term PPI in patients requiring chronic ASA use following an ulcer bleed is recommended.[4] The long-term benefits of sole H pylori eradication in patients having bled while on ASA has been shown, in a retrospective cohort study, to be associated with very low rebleeding rates even after a period of 10 years.[143]

Clopidogrel administration following peptic ulcer bleeding is also associated with high rebleeding rates of 9% to 14%,[144,145] and PPI prophylaxis should be considered. RCT data reported by Hsu and colleagues[146] comparing PPI with placebo in patients on clopidogrel and a history of PUD showed a decreased incidence of recurrent PUD when endoscopy was performed at 6-month follow-up. In terms of DAPT, data on PPI gastroprotection, in a patient population at no particularly high risk for bleeding based on history, has been well described in the COGENT trial,[147] showing a significant reduction in GIB (hazard ratio 0.34; 95% CI 0.18–0.63). Therefore, the authors suggest PPI gastroprotection for patients on clopidogrel monotherapy and a history of PUD, whereas societies have suggested that all patients on DAPT should receive PPI routinely, irrespective of previous history of PUD with or without bleeding.[137,138,148]

Pharmacokinetic and platelet ex vivo assay studies have suggested that PPIs may reduce the antiplatelet effects of clopidogrel,[149–151] as have several clinical observational data. However, these findings are confounded by methodological limitations, covariate imbalances in patient characteristics, and the absence of correction for statistical heterogeneity. In fact, following multivariate adjustment, any attenuating effect of PPI on the beneficial clinical effect of clopidogrel seems to be very limited or nonexistent.[152,153] In addition, the COGENT trial comparing DAPT (ASA + clopidogrel) and PPI with DAPT and placebo showed no significant differences in the incidence of major cardiovascular events.[147] However, this trial was terminated prematurely, with a median follow-up time of 133 days, and before the planned full enrollment number was achieved. Lastly, 3 systematic reviews using the best-quality observational studies did not show any significant increase in cardiovascular events with the use of PPI with clopidogrel.[153–155] In summary, high-quality evidence supporting a clinically significant interaction between PPI and clopidogrel is presently lacking. Consequently, most consensus guidelines, including those from the American College of Cardiology, American Heart Association, American College of Gastroenterology (ACG), Canadian Association of Gastroenterology, and the most recent ACG guidelines in the management of gastroesophageal reflux disease,[156] all recommend that patients currently receiving these agents should continue without changing their treatment regimen unless advised by their health care providers.

MANAGEMENT OF LONG-TERM ANTICOAGULATION FOLLOWING PEPTIC ULCER BLEEDING

Warfarin therapy, a vitamin K antagonist, is associated with a significant risk of bleeding, which is accentuated by its narrow therapeutic window. In fact, systematic reviews show that in community practice the therapeutic target (INR 2.0–3.0) is only achieved in 63.6% of patients, with a rate of major hemorrhage (from any source) ranging from 1% to 7.4% per year.[157–159] Controlled data on the benefit of PPI therapy in preventing GIB in patients on warfarin is currently lacking. A population-based, nested case-control study evaluating PPI in patients using antiplatelet therapies and/or oral anticoagulants showed an overall decrease in GIB; however, although there was a trend toward less bleeding in the subgroup analysis of patients on warfarin, it did not reach statistical significance (OR 0.48; 95% CI 0.22–1.04).[160] Nevertheless, the authors recommend that patients on warfarin therapy receive PPI prophylaxis in the presence of previous PUD with or without bleeding.

Triple therapy (ie, DAPT and an oral anticoagulant) is indicated in patients who are at high risk for cardiothrombotic and cardioembolic events. Warfarin combined with DAPT increases the risk of GIB substantially, with one study showing a hazard ratio of 5.0 (95% CI 1.4–17.8) compared with DAPT alone.[161] A randomized controlled trial by Ng and colleagues,[162] comparing PPI with H2RA as gastroprotective agents in patients who presented with acute coronary syndrome and treated with DAPT and enoxaparin or thrombolytics, demonstrated significant reduction in GIB with the use of esomeprazole versus famotidine. More recently, Dewilde and colleagues[163] compared the risk of hemorrhage (from all sources) in an RCT with triple therapy (ASA, clopidogrel, and warfarin/heparin) versus double therapy (anticoagulation and clopidogrel) in patients with high cardioembolic risk factors who underwent percutaneous coronary intervention (PCI). Double therapy was shown to be associated with lower all-cause bleeding except for intracranial hemorrhage. More specifically, in terms of GIB, double therapy was also accompanied by lower bleeding risks when compared with triple therapy, with bleeding rates of 2.9% versus 8.8%, respectively. In addition, withholding ASA was not associated with higher thrombotic events, which is consistent with previous RCTs suggesting similar antithrombotic effectiveness between ASA and warfarin.[164,165] However, the study was underpowered to detect a significant difference in thrombotic complications. In addition, PPI use was unregimented in this study and could have been a major confounder. Overall, the authors recommend that all patients on triple therapy receive PPI prophylaxis regardless of a history of peptic ulcer or GIB. Given a lack of high-level evidence, in patients with previous history of peptic ulcer bleeding a decision to withhold ASA must include consideration of the patient's cardiovascular risks, and appropriate discussions with other appropriate professionals (such as the treating cardiologist) and the patient.

MANAGEMENT OF LONG-TERM NOVEL ANTICOAGULANTS FOLLOWING PEPTIC ULCER BLEEDING

Unlike warfarin, novel anticoagulants, including direct thrombin and factor Xa inhibitors, are not limited by a narrow therapeutic window and do not require routine monitoring of the therapeutic target. Agents such as dabigatran, rivaroxaban, apixaban, and edoxaban are currently used or are undergoing large-scale evaluation in patients with atrial fibrillation, deep vein thrombosis (DVT)/pulmonary embolism, and DVT prophylaxis. However, data from RCTs have shown concerning association with increased risk for GI hemorrhage.[166,167] A recent systematic review of 43 trials showed a modest but significant increase risk for GIB (OR 1.45; 95% CI 1.07–1.97) with the use of nOAC when compared with standard of care (warfarin and/or unfractionated

Table 2
Antiplatelets and oral anticoagulants (OAC) bleeding risks and recommended gastroprotection

	Risk of GIB: OR (95% CI)	Routine PPI	PPI Post PUD ± Bleeding
Low-dose ASA	2.07 (1.61–2.66) vs placebo[169]		+[4,78,148]
Clopidogrel	1.67 (1.27–2.20) vs no treatment[170]		+[148]
DAPT	3.90 (2.78–5.47) vs no treatment[170]	+[a,147]	
Warfarin	1.94 (1.61–2.34) vs no treatment[170]		+[148]
Triple therapy: ASA/ clopidogrel/OAC	5.0 (1.4–17.8) vs DAPT[161]	+[a,162]	
Novel OAC	1.45 (1.07–1.97) vs warfarin and/or UFH/LMWH[168]		+[b]

Recommendations based on expert consensus guidelines.
All patients should undergo *H pylori* testing/eradication post PUD complicated or not, regardless of antiplatelet/OAC use.[4,78,111,112,137,147]
Abbreviations: ASA, aspirin; CI, confidence interval; DAPT, dual antiplatelet therapy; GIB, gastrointestinal bleeding; LMWH, low molecular weight heparin; OAC, oral anticoagulant; OR, odds ratio; PPI, proton-pump inhibitor; PUD, peptic ulcer disease; UFH, unfractionated heparin.
[a] No guideline; refers to the highest-level evidence available.
[b] Recommendations by the authors based on existing evidence discussed in the text.
Data from Refs.[4,78,111,112,137,147]

heparin/low molecular weight heparin).[168] Furthermore, the pooled OR for dabigatran was 1.58 (95% CI 1.29–193) with a number needed to harm of 83, whereas the pooled OR for rivaroxaban was 1.48 (95% CI 1.21–1.82). Neither apixaban nor edoxaban were associated with increased GIB. Of note, no head-to-head evaluations have been completed between these nOACs; therefore, it is premature to conclude which nOAC is associated with the lowest risk for GIB.

With the ongoing large-scale implementation of nOAC, GIB associated with these agents will gain importance in the practice of gastroenterologists. Of note, the nOAC trials to date do not include patients at high risk of GI complications, such as those with a history of GIB or PUD. Moreover, the severity of GIB with nOAC when compared with warfarin is largely unknown, which is especially pertinent considering the lack of effective reversal agents. In terms of GI prophylaxis, the concomitant use of PPI with nOAC has not been evaluated. However, given the benefits of PPI use with ASA, clopidogrel, DAPT, and triple therapy–related GIB, the authors recommend its use in patients on nOAC with a history of PUD, complicated or not, until further data are available (**Table 2**).

SUMMARY

Endoscopic evaluation with hemostasis, if indicated, represents the mainstay in the management of peptic ulcer bleeding. It should be performed within 24 hours of patient presentation, following hemodynamic resuscitation. Endoscopic risk stratification into HRS and LRS further dictates management with the use of either monotherapy or combination endoscopic therapy to achieve hemostasis in patients with high-risk lesions. The choice between injection, thermal, and mechanical modalities, and the use of hemostatic powders, depends on individual preferences, availability, and ulcer characteristics. Epinephrine injection monotherapy should, however, be avoided. All patients with HRS should receive 72 hours of high-dose intravenous PPI after endoscopic hemostasis to further significantly decrease rebleeding, need for surgery, and mortality in high-risk patients. Secondary prophylaxis with regard to *H pylori* testing and eradication, appropriate continued acid suppression, and the optimal management of NSAIDs, ASA, antiplatelets, and anticoagulant agents according to current guidelines is needed to decrease bleeding recurrence.

REFERENCES

1. Laine L, Yang H, Chang SC, et al. Trends for incidence of hospitalization and death due to GI complications in the United States from 2001 to 2009. Am J Gastroenterol 2012;107(8):1190–5. http://dx.doi.org/10.1038/ajg.2012.168 [quiz: 6]. pii:ajg2012168.
2. Hearnshaw SA, Logan RF, Lowe D, et al. Acute upper gastrointestinal bleeding in the UK: patient characteristics, diagnoses and outcomes in the 2007 UK audit. Gut 2011;60(10):1327–35. http://dx.doi.org/10.1136/gut.2010.228437. pii:gut.2010.228437.
3. Enestvedt BK, Gralnek IM, Mattek N, et al. An evaluation of endoscopic indications and findings related to nonvariceal upper-GI hemorrhage in a large multicenter consortium. Gastrointest Endosc 2008;67(3):422–9. http://dx.doi.org/10.1016/j.gie.2007.09.024. pii:S0016-5107(07)02688-0.
4. Barkun AN, Bardou M, Kuipers EJ, et al. International consensus recommendations on the management of patients with nonvariceal upper gastrointestinal bleeding. Ann Intern Med 2010;152(2):101–13. http://dx.doi.org/10.1059/0003-4819-152-2-201001190-00009. pii:152/2/101.

5. Barkun AN, Bardou M, Martel M, et al. Prokinetics in acute upper GI bleeding: a meta-analysis [Systematic reviews and meta-analyses]. Gastrointest Endosc 2010;72(6):1138–45. http://dx.doi.org/10.1016/j.gie.2010.08. 011. pii:S0016-5107(10)01967-X.

6. Szary NM, Gupta R, Choudhary A, et al. Erythromycin prior to endoscopy in acute upper gastrointestinal bleeding: a meta-analysis [Systematic reviews and meta-analyses]. Scand J Gastroenterol 2011;46(7–8):920–4. http://dx.doi.org/10.3109/00365521.2011.568520.

7. Bai Y, Guo JF, Li ZS. Meta-analysis: erythromycin before endoscopy for acute upper gastrointestinal bleeding [Systematic reviews and meta-analyses]. Aliment Pharmacol Ther 2011;34(2):166–71. http://dx.doi.org/10.1111/j.1365-2036.2011.04708.x.

8. Altraif I, Handoo FA, Aljumah A, et al. Effect of erythromycin before endoscopy in patients presenting with variceal bleeding: a prospective, randomized, double-blind, placebo-controlled trial. Gastrointest Endosc 2011;73(2):245–50. http://dx.doi.org/10.1016/j.gie.2010.09.043. pii:S0016-5107(10)02181-4.

9. Theivanayagam S, Lim RG, Cobell WJ, et al. Administration of erythromycin before endoscopy in upper gastrointestinal bleeding: a meta-analysis of randomized controlled trials [Systematic reviews and meta-analyses]. Saudi J Gastroenterol 2013;19(5):205–10. http://dx.doi.org/10.4103/1319-3767.118120.

10. NICE. Acute upper gastrointestinal bleeding: management: NHS National Institute for Health and Clinical Excellence. 2012 [cited February 25, 2013]. Available at: http://www.nice.org.uk/nicemedia/live/13762/59549/59549.pdf. Accessed September 9, 2014.

11. Spiegel BM, Vakil NB, Ofman JJ. Endoscopy for acute nonvariceal upper gastrointestinal tract hemorrhage: is sooner better? A systematic review [Systematic reviews and meta-analyses]. Arch Intern Med 2001;161(11):1393–404. pii:ira00052.

12. Cipolletta L, Bianco MA, Rotondano G, et al. Outpatient management for low-risk nonvariceal upper GI bleeding: a randomized controlled trial. Gastrointest Endosc 2002;55(1):1–5. http://dx.doi.org/10.1067/mge.2002.119219.

13. Tsoi KK, Ma TK, Sung JJ. Endoscopy for upper gastrointestinal bleeding: how urgent is it? Nat Rev Gastroenterol Hepatol 2009;6(8):463–9. http://dx.doi.org/10.1038/nrgastro.2009.108. pii:nrgastro.2009.108.

14. Schacher GM, Lesbros-Pantoflickova D, Ortner MA, et al. Is early endoscopy in the emergency room beneficial in patients with bleeding peptic ulcer? A "fortuitously controlled" study. Endoscopy 2005;37(4):324–8. http://dx.doi.org/10.1055/s-2004-826237.

15. Bjorkman DJ, Zaman A, Fennerty MB, et al. Urgent vs. elective endoscopy for acute non-variceal upper-GI bleeding: an effectiveness study. Gastrointest Endosc 2004;60(1):1–8.

16. Targownik LE, Murthy S, Keyvani L, et al. The role of rapid endoscopy for high-risk patients with acute nonvariceal upper gastrointestinal bleeding. Can J Gastroenterol 2007;21(7):425–9.

17. Tai CM, Huang SP, Wang HP, et al. High-risk ED patients with nonvariceal upper gastrointestinal hemorrhage undergoing emergency or urgent endoscopy: a retrospective analysis. Am J Emerg Med 2007;25(3):273–8. http://dx.doi.org/10.1016/j.ajem.2006.07.014.

18. Cooper GS, Chak A, Way LE, et al. Early endoscopy in upper gastrointestinal hemorrhage: associations with recurrent bleeding, surgery, and length of hospital stay. Gastrointest Endosc 1999;49(2):145–52.

19. Cooper GS, Chak A, Connors AF Jr, et al. The effectiveness of early endoscopy for upper gastrointestinal hemorrhage: a community-based analysis. Med Care 1998;36(4):462–74.
20. Lin HJ, Wang K, Perng CL, et al. Early or delayed endoscopy for patients with peptic ulcer bleeding. A prospective randomized study. J Clin Gastroenterol 1996;22(4):267–71.
21. Lim LG, Ho KY, Chan YH, et al. Urgent endoscopy is associated with lower mortality in high-risk but not low-risk nonvariceal upper gastrointestinal bleeding. Endoscopy 2011;43(4):300–6. http://dx.doi.org/10.1055/s-0030-1256110.
22. Academy of Medical Royal Colleges. Upper gastrointestinal bleeding toolkit. 2011 [cited December 15, 2013]. Available at: http://www.aomrc.org.uk/projects/item/upper-gastrointestinal-bleeding-toolkit.html. Accessed September 9, 2014.
23. Barkun AN, Bardou M, Kuipers EJ, et al. How early should endoscopy be performed in suspected upper gastrointestinal bleeding? Am J Gastroenterol 2012;107(2):328–9. http://dx.doi.org/10.1038/ajg.2011.363.
24. Garcia-Tsao G, Sanyal AJ, Grace ND, et al. Prevention and management of gastroesophageal varices and variceal hemorrhage in cirrhosis. Hepatology 2007;46(3):922–38. http://dx.doi.org/10.1002/hep.21907.
25. Hearnshaw SA, Logan RF, Lowe D, et al. Use of endoscopy for management of acute upper gastrointestinal bleeding in the UK: results of a nationwide audit. Gut 2010;59(8):1022–9. http://dx.doi.org/10.1136/gut.2008.174599. pii: gut.2008.174599.
26. Rosenstock SJ, Moller MH, Larsson H, et al. Improving quality of care in peptic ulcer bleeding: nationwide cohort study of 13,498 consecutive patients in the Danish Clinical Register of Emergency Surgery. Am J Gastroenterol 2013; 108(9):1449–57. http://dx.doi.org/10.1038/ajg.2013.162.
27. Jairath V, Kahan BC, Logan RF, et al. Mortality from acute upper gastrointestinal bleeding in the United Kingdom: does it display a "weekend effect"? Am J Gastroenterol 2011;106(9):1621–8. http://dx.doi.org/10.1038/ajg.2011.172.
28. Ananthakrishnan AN, McGinley EL, Saeian K. Outcomes of weekend admissions for upper gastrointestinal hemorrhage: a nationwide analysis. Clin Gastroenterol Hepatol 2009;7(3):296–302.e1. http://dx.doi.org/10.1016/j.cgh.2008.08.013.
29. Shaheen AA, Kaplan GG, Myers RP. Weekend versus weekday admission and mortality from gastrointestinal hemorrhage caused by peptic ulcer disease. Clin Gastroenterol Hepatol 2009;7(3):303–10. http://dx.doi.org/10.1016/j.cgh.2008.08.033.
30. Tsoi KK, Chiu PW, Chan FK, et al. The risk of peptic ulcer bleeding mortality in relation to hospital admission on holidays: a cohort study on 8,222 cases of peptic ulcer bleeding. Am J Gastroenterol 2012;107(3):405–10. http://dx.doi.org/10.1038/ajg.2011.409.
31. Kanwal F, Barkun A, Gralnek IM, et al. Measuring quality of care in patients with nonvariceal upper gastrointestinal hemorrhage: development of an explicit quality indicator set. Am J Gastroenterol 2010;105(8):1710–8. http://dx.doi.org/10.1038/ajg.2010.180.
32. Lau JY, Chung SC, Leung JW, et al. The evolution of stigmata of hemorrhage in bleeding peptic ulcers: a sequential endoscopic study. Endoscopy 1998;30(6):513–8. http://dx.doi.org/10.1055/s-2007-1001336.
33. Marmo R, Koch M, Cipolletta L, et al. Predictive factors of mortality from nonvariceal upper gastrointestinal hemorrhage: a multicenter study. Am J Gastroenterol

2008;103(7):1639–47. http://dx.doi.org/10.1111/j.1572-0241.2008.01865.x [quiz: 48]. pii:AJG1865.

34. Laine L, Peterson WL. Bleeding peptic ulcer. N Engl J Med 1994;331(11): 717–27. http://dx.doi.org/10.1056/NEJM199409153311107.

35. Laine L, Freeman M, Cohen H. Lack of uniformity in evaluation of endoscopic prognostic features of bleeding ulcers. Gastrointest Endosc 1994;40(4):411–7 pii:S0016510794000374.

36. Sacks HS, Chalmers TC, Blum AL, et al. Endoscopic hemostasis. An effective therapy for bleeding peptic ulcers. JAMA 1990;264(4):494–9.

37. Cook DJ, Guyatt GH, Salena BJ, et al. Endoscopic therapy for acute nonvariceal upper gastrointestinal hemorrhage: a meta-analysis [Systematic reviews and meta-analyses]. Gastroenterology 1992;102(1):139–48. pii:S001650859 200009X.

38. Barkun AN, Martel M, Toubouti Y, et al. Endoscopic hemostasis in peptic ulcer bleeding for patients with high-risk lesions: a series of meta-analyses. Gastrointest Endosc 2009;69(4):786–99. http://dx.doi.org/10.1016/j.gie.2008.05.031. pii: S0016-5107(08)01854-3.

39. Laine L, McQuaid KR. Endoscopic therapy for bleeding ulcers: an evidence-based approach based on meta-analyses of randomized controlled trials. Clin Gastroenterol Hepatol 2009;7(1):33–47. http://dx.doi.org/10.1016/j.cgh.2008. 08.016 [quiz: 1–2]. pii:S1542-3565(08)00842-2.

40. Cipolletta L, Bianco MA, Salerno R, et al. Improved characterization of visible vessels in bleeding ulcers by using magnification endoscopy: results of a pilot study. Gastrointest Endosc 2010;72:413–8.

41. Chung SC, Leung JW, Steele RJ, et al. Endoscopic injection of adrenaline for actively bleeding ulcers: a randomised trial. Br Med J (Clin Res Ed) 1988; 296(6637):1631–3.

42. O'Brien JR. Some effects of adrenaline and anti-adrenaline compounds on platelets in vitro and in vivo. Nature 1963;200:763–4.

43. Lin HJ, Hsieh YH, Tseng GY, et al. A prospective, randomized trial of large-versus small-volume endoscopic injection of epinephrine for peptic ulcer bleeding. Gastrointest Endosc 2002;55(6):615–9. pii:S0016510702086480.

44. Liou TC, Lin SC, Wang HY, et al. Optimal injection volume of epinephrine for endoscopic treatment of peptic ulcer bleeding. World J Gastroenterol 2006; 12(19):3108–13.

45. Park CH, Lee SJ, Park JH, et al. Optimal injection volume of epinephrine for endoscopic prevention of recurrent peptic ulcer bleeding. Gastrointest Endosc 2004;60(6):875–80.

46. Calvet X, Vergara M, Brullet E, et al. Addition of a second endoscopic treatment following epinephrine injection improves outcome in high-risk bleeding ulcers. Gastroenterology 2004;126(2):441–50. pii:S0016508503017876.

47. Vergara M, Calvet X, Gisbert JP. Epinephrine injection versus epinephrine injection and a second endoscopic method in high risk bleeding ulcers. Cochrane Database Syst Rev 2007;(2):CD005584. http://dx.doi.org/10.1002/14651858. CD005584.pub2.

48. Benedetti G, Sablich R, Lacchin T. Endoscopic injection sclerotherapy in nonvariceal upper gastrointestinal bleeding. A comparative study of polidocanol and thrombin. Surg Endosc 1991;5(1):28–30.

49. Chester JF, Hurley PR. Gastric necrosis: a complication of endoscopic sclerosis for bleeding peptic ulcer. Endoscopy 1990;22(6):287. http://dx.doi.org/10.1055/s-2007-1012873.

50. Levy J, Khakoo S, Barton R, et al. Fatal injection sclerotherapy of a bleeding peptic ulcer. Lancet 1991;337(8739):504.
51. Loperfido S, Patelli G, La Torre L. Extensive necrosis of gastric mucosa following injection therapy of bleeding peptic ulcer. Endoscopy 1990;22(6):285–6. http://dx.doi.org/10.1055/s-2007-1010728.
52. Randall GM, Jensen DM, Hirabayashi K, et al. Controlled study of different sclerosing agents for coagulation of canine gut arteries. Gastroenterology 1989;96(5 Pt 1):1274–81.
53. Rutgeerts P, Geboes K, Vantrappen G. Experimental studies of injection therapy for severe nonvariceal bleeding in dogs. Gastroenterology 1989;97(3):610–21.
54. Bhat YM, Banerjee S, Barth BA, et al. Tissue adhesives: cyanoacrylate glue and fibrin sealant. Gastrointest Endosc 2013;78(2):209–15. http://dx.doi.org/10.1016/j.gie.2013.04.166.
55. Laine L. Therapeutic endoscopy and bleeding ulcers. Bipolar/multipolar electrocoagulation. Gastrointest Endosc 1990;36(5 Suppl):S38–41.
56. Laine L, Long GL, Bakos GJ, et al. Optimizing bipolar electrocoagulation for endoscopic hemostasis: assessment of factors influencing energy delivery and coagulation. Gastrointest Endosc 2008;67(3):502–8. http://dx.doi.org/10.1016/j.gie.2007.09.025. pii:S0016-5107(07)02689-2.
57. Conway JD, Adler DG, Diehl DL, et al. Endoscopic hemostatic devices. Gastrointest Endosc 2009;69(6):987–96. http://dx.doi.org/10.1016/j.gie.2008.12.251.
58. Kovacs TO, Jensen DM. Endoscopic therapy for severe ulcer bleeding. Gastrointest Endosc Clin N Am 2011;21(4):681–96. http://dx.doi.org/10.1016/j.giec.2011.07.012.
59. Fullarton GM, Birnie GG, Macdonald A, et al. Controlled trial of heater probe treatment in bleeding peptic ulcers. Br J Surg 1989;76(6):541–4.
60. Machicado GA, Jensen DM. Thermal probes alone or with epinephrine for the endoscopic haemostasis of ulcer haemorrhage. Baillieres Best Pract Res Clin Gastroenterol 2000;14(3):443–58. http://dx.doi.org/10.1053/bega.2000.0089.
61. Marmo R, Rotondano G, Piscopo R, et al. Dual therapy versus monotherapy in the endoscopic treatment of high-risk bleeding ulcers: a meta-analysis of controlled trials [Systematic reviews and meta-analyses]. Am J Gastroenterol 2007;102(2):279–89. http://dx.doi.org/10.1111/j.1572-0241.2006.01023.x [quiz: 469]. pii:AJG1023.
62. Johanns W, Luis W, Janssen J, et al. Argon plasma coagulation (APC) in gastroenterology: experimental and clinical experiences. Eur J Gastroenterol Hepatol 1997;9(6):581–7.
63. Farin G, Grund KE. Technology of argon plasma coagulation with particular regard to endoscopic applications. Endosc Surg Allied Technol 1994;2(1):71–7.
64. Watson JP, Bennett MK, Griffin SM, et al. The tissue effect of argon plasma coagulation on esophageal and gastric mucosa. Gastrointest Endosc 2000;52(3):342–5. http://dx.doi.org/10.1067/mge.2000.108412.
65. Ginsberg GG, Barkun AN, Bosco JJ, et al. The argon plasma coagulator: February 2002. Gastrointest Endosc 2002;55(7):807–10.
66. Kwan V, Bourke MJ, Williams SJ, et al. Argon plasma coagulation in the management of symptomatic gastrointestinal vascular lesions: experience in 100 consecutive patients with long-term follow-up. Am J Gastroenterol 2006;101(1):58–63. http://dx.doi.org/10.1111/j.1572-0241.2006.00370.x.
67. Rolachon A, Papillon E, Fournet J. Is argon plasma coagulation an efficient treatment for digestive system vascular malformation and radiation proctitis? Gastroenterol Clin Biol 2000;24(12):1205–10 [in English, French].

68. Kwak HW, Lee WJ, Woo SM, et al. Efficacy of argon plasma coagulation in the treatment of radiation-induced hemorrhagic gastroduodenal vascular ectasia. Scand J Gastroenterol 2013. http://dx.doi.org/10.3109/00365521.2013.865783.

69. Chiu YC, Lu LS, Wu KL, et al. Comparison of argon plasma coagulation in management of upper gastrointestinal angiodysplasia and gastric antral vascular ectasia hemorrhage. BMC Gastroenterol 2012;12:67. http://dx.doi.org/10.1186/1471-230X-12-67.

70. Cipolletta L, Bianco MA, Rotondano G, et al. Prospective comparison of argon plasma coagulator and heater probe in the endoscopic treatment of major peptic ulcer bleeding. Gastrointest Endosc 1998;48(2):191–5.

71. Skok P, Krizman I, Skok M. Argon plasma coagulation versus injection sclerotherapy in peptic ulcer hemorrhage–a prospective, controlled study. Hepatogastroenterology 2004;51(55):165–70.

72. Wang HM, Hsu PI, Lo GH, et al. Comparison of hemostatic efficacy for argon plasma coagulation and distilled water injection in treating high-risk bleeding ulcers. J Clin Gastroenterol 2009;43(10):941–5. http://dx.doi.org/10.1097/MCG.0b013e31819c3885.

73. Chau CH, Siu WT, Law BK, et al. Randomized controlled trial comparing epinephrine injection plus heat probe coagulation versus epinephrine injection plus argon plasma coagulation for bleeding peptic ulcers. Gastrointest Endosc 2003;57(4):455–61. http://dx.doi.org/10.1067/mge.2003.125.

74. Taghavi SA, Soleimani SM, Hosseini-Asl SM, et al. Adrenaline injection plus argon plasma coagulation versus adrenaline injection plus hemoclips for treating high-risk bleeding peptic ulcers: a prospective, randomized trial. Can J Gastroenterol 2009;23(10):699–704.

75. Karaman A, Baskol M, Gursoy S, et al. Epinephrine plus argon plasma or heater probe coagulation in ulcer bleeding. World J Gastroenterol 2011;17(36):4109–12. http://dx.doi.org/10.3748/wjg.v17.i36.4109.

76. Chuttani R, Barkun A, Carpenter S, et al. Endoscopic clip application devices. Gastrointest Endosc 2006;63(6):746–50. http://dx.doi.org/10.1016/j.gie.2006.02.042.

77. Sung JJ, Tsoi KK, Lai LH, et al. Endoscopic clipping versus injection and thermocoagulation in the treatment of non-variceal upper gastrointestinal bleeding: a meta-analysis [Systematic reviews and meta-analyses]. Gut 2007;56(10):1364–73. http://dx.doi.org/10.1136/gut.2007.123976. pii:gut.2007.123976.

78. Laine L, Jensen DM. Management of patients with ulcer bleeding. Am J Gastroenterol 2012;107(3):345–60. http://dx.doi.org/10.1038/ajg.2011.480 [quiz: 61]. pii:ajg2011480.

79. Goker H, Haznedaroglu IC, Ercetin S, et al. Haemostatic actions of the folkloric medicinal plant extract Ankaferd Blood Stopper. J Int Med Res 2008;36(1):163–70.

80. Moosavi S, Chen YI, Barkun AN. TC-325 application leading to transient obstruction of a post-sphincterotomy biliary orifice. Endoscopy 2013;45(Suppl 2 UCTN):E130. http://dx.doi.org/10.1055/s-0032-1326370.

81. Halkerston K, Evans J, Ismail D, et al. PWE-046 Early clinical experience of EndoclotTM in the treatment of acute gastro-intestinal bleeding. Gut 2013;52:A149.

82. Barkun AN, Moosavi S, Martel M. Topical hemostatic agents: a systematic review with particular emphasis on endoscopic application in gastrointestinal bleeding [Systematic reviews and meta-analyses]. Gastrointest Endosc 2013;77(5):692–700.

83. Holster IL, De Maat MP, Ducharme R, et al. In vitro examination of the effects of the hemostatic powder (Hemospray) on coagulation and thrombus formation in humans. Gastrointest Endosc 2012;75:AB240.

84. Smith LA, Stanley AJ, Bergman JJ, et al. Hemospray application in nonvariceal upper gastrointestinal bleeding: results of the survey to evaluate the application of Hemospray in the luminal tract. J Clin Gastroenterol 2013. http://dx.doi.org/10.1097/MCG.0000000000000054.

85. Chen YI, Barkun A, Nolan S. TC-325 in the management of upper and lower GI bleeding: a two-year experience at a single institution. Endoscopy, in press.

86. Chen YI, Barkun AN, Soulellis C, et al. Use of the endoscopically applied hemostatic powder TC-325 in cancer-related upper GI hemorrhage: preliminary experience (with video). Gastrointest Endosc 2012;75(6):1278–81. http://dx.doi.org/10.1016/j.gie.2012.02.009.

87. Soulellis CA, Carpentier S, Chen YI, et al. Lower GI hemorrhage controlled with endoscopically applied TC-325 (with videos). Gastrointest Endosc 2013;77(3):504–7. http://dx.doi.org/10.1016/j.gie.2012.10.014.

88. Laine L, Stein C, Sharma V. A prospective outcome study of patients with clot in an ulcer and the effect of irrigation. Gastrointest Endosc 1996;43(2 Pt 1):107–10. pii:S0016510796000478.

89. Jensen DM, Kovacs TO, Jutabha R, et al. Randomized trial of medical or endoscopic therapy to prevent recurrent ulcer hemorrhage in patients with adherent clots. Gastroenterology 2002;123(2):407–13 pii:S001650850200118X.

90. Bleau BL, Gostout CJ, Sherman KE, et al. Recurrent bleeding from peptic ulcer associated with adherent clot: a randomized study comparing endoscopic treatment with medical therapy. Gastrointest Endosc 2002;56(1):1–6. pii:S0016510702000007.

91. Khuroo MS, Yattoo GN, Javid G, et al. A comparison of omeprazole and placebo for bleeding peptic ulcer. N Engl J Med 1997;336(15):1054–8. http://dx.doi.org/10.1056/NEJM199704103361503.

92. Javid G, Masoodi I, Zargar SA, et al. Omeprazole as adjuvant therapy to endoscopic combination injection sclerotherapy for treating bleeding peptic ulcer. Am J Med 2001;111(4):280–4 pii:S0002-9343(01)00812-9.

93. Sung JJ, Chan FK, Lau JY, et al. The effect of endoscopic therapy in patients receiving omeprazole for bleeding ulcers with nonbleeding visible vessels or adherent clots: a randomized comparison. Ann Intern Med 2003;139(4):237–43. pii:139/4/237.

94. Kahi CJ, Jensen DM, Sung JJ, et al. Endoscopic therapy versus medical therapy for bleeding peptic ulcer with adherent clot: a meta-analysis [Systematic reviews and meta-analyses]. Gastroenterology 2005;129(3):855–62. http://dx.doi.org/10.1053/j.gastro.2005.06.070. pii:S0016-5085(05)01358-2.

95. Laine L. Systematic review of endoscopic therapy for ulcers with clots: can a meta-analysis be misleading? [Systematic reviews and meta-analyses]. Gastroenterology 2005;129(6):2127. http://dx.doi.org/10.1053/j.gastro.2005.10.039 [author reply: 2127–8]. pii:S0016-5085(05)02199-2.

96. Neumann I, Letelier LM, Rada G, et al. Comparison of different regimens of proton pump inhibitors for acute peptic ulcer bleeding. Cochrane Database Syst Rev 2013;(6):CD007999. http://dx.doi.org/10.1002/14651858.CD007999.pub2.

97. Spiegel BM, Ofman JJ, Woods K, et al. Minimizing recurrent peptic ulcer hemorrhage after endoscopic hemostasis: the cost-effectiveness of competing strategies. Am J Gastroenterol 2003;98(1):86–97. http://dx.doi.org/10.1111/j.1572-0241.2003.07163.x. pii:S0002927002058318.

98. Tsoi KK, Lau JY, Sung JJ. Cost-effectiveness analysis of high-dose omeprazole infusion before endoscopy for patients with upper-GI bleeding. Gastrointest Endosc 2008;67(7):1056–63. http://dx.doi.org/10.1016/j.gie.2007.11.056. pii: S0016-5107(07)03199-9.

99. Barkun AN, Herba K, Adam V, et al. High-dose intravenous proton pump inhibition following endoscopic therapy in the acute management of patients with bleeding peptic ulcers in the USA and Canada: a cost-effectiveness analysis. Aliment Pharmacol Ther 2004;19(5):591–600.

100. Marmo R, Rotondano G, Bianco MA, et al. Outcome of endoscopic treatment for peptic ulcer bleeding: is a second look necessary? A meta-analysis [Systematic reviews and meta-analyses]. Gastrointest Endosc 2003;57(1):62–7. http://dx.doi.org/10.1067/mge.2003.48. pii:S0016510703500141.

101. Tsoi KK, Chan HC, Chiu PW, et al. Second-look endoscopy with thermal coagulation or injections for peptic ulcer bleeding: a meta-analysis [Systematic reviews and meta-analyses]. J Gastroenterol Hepatol 2010;25(1):8–13. http://dx.doi.org/10.1111/j.1440-1746.2009.06129.x.

102. Chiu P, Joeng H, Choi C, et al. The effect of scheduled second endoscopy against intravenous high dose omeprazole infusion as an adjunct to therapeutic endoscopy in prevention of peptic ulcer rebleeding-a prospective randomized study. Gastroenterology 2006;130:A121.

103. El Ouali S, Barkun AN, Wyse J, et al. Is routine second-look endoscopy effective after endoscopic hemostasis in acute peptic ulcer bleeding? A meta-analysis [Systematic reviews and meta-analyses]. Gastrointest Endosc 2012;76(2): 283–92. http://dx.doi.org/10.1016/j.gie.2012.04.441. pii:S0016-5107(12)02156-6.

104. Imperiale TF, Kong N. Second-look endoscopy for bleeding peptic ulcer disease: a decision-effectiveness and cost-effectiveness analysis. J Clin Gastroenterol 2012;46(9):e71–5. http://dx.doi.org/10.1097/MCG.0b013e3182410351.

105. Chiu PW, Sung JJ. High risk ulcer bleeding: when is second-look endoscopy recommended? Clin Gastroenterol Hepatol 2010;8(8):651–4. http://dx.doi.org/10.1016/j.cgh.2010.01.008 [quiz: e87].

106. Jairath V, Barkun AN. Improving outcomes from acute upper gastrointestinal bleeding. Gut 2012;61(9):1246–9. http://dx.doi.org/10.1136/gutjnl-2011-300019.

107. Garcia-Iglesias P, Villoria A, Suarez D, et al. Meta-analysis: predictors of rebleeding after endoscopic treatment for bleeding peptic ulcer [Systematic reviews and meta-analyses]. Aliment Pharmacol Ther 2011;34(8):888–900. http://dx.doi.org/10.1111/j.1365-2036.2011.04830.x.

108. Lau JY, Sung JJ, Lam YH, et al. Endoscopic retreatment compared with surgery in patients with recurrent bleeding after initial endoscopic control of bleeding ulcers. N Engl J Med 1999;340(10):751–6. http://dx.doi.org/10.1056/NEJM199903113401002.

109. Lu Y, Loffroy R, Lau JY, et al. Multidisciplinary management strategies for acute non-variceal upper gastrointestinal bleeding. Br J Surg 2014;101(1):e34–50. http://dx.doi.org/10.1002/bjs.9351.

110. Gisbert JP, Khorrami S, Carballo F, et al. H. pylori eradication therapy vs. antisecretory non-eradication therapy (with or without long-term maintenance antisecretory therapy) for the prevention of recurrent bleeding from peptic ulcer. Cochrane Database Syst Rev 2004;(2):CD004062. http://dx.doi.org/10.1002/14651858.CD004062.pub2.

111. Malfertheiner P, Megraud F, O'Morain CA, et al. Management of Helicobacter pylori infection–the Maastricht IV/Florence Consensus Report. Gut 2012;61(5): 646–64. http://dx.doi.org/10.1136/gutjnl-2012-302084.

112. Sung JJ, Chan FK, Chen M, et al. Asia-Pacific Working Group consensus on non-variceal upper gastrointestinal bleeding. Gut 2011;60(9):1170–7. http://dx. doi.org/10.1136/gut.2010.230292.

113. Calvet X, Barkun A, Kuipers EJ, et al. Is *H. pylori* testing clinically useful in the acute setting of upper gastrointestinal bleeding? A systematic review [abstract]. [Systematic reviews and meta-analyses]. Gastroenterology 2009; 136(5):A-605.

114. Gisbert JP, Abraira V. Accuracy of *Helicobacter pylori* diagnostic tests in patients with bleeding peptic ulcer: a systematic review and meta-analysis [Systematic reviews and meta-analyses]. Am J Gastroenterol 2006;101(4):848–63. http://dx.doi.org/10.1111/j.1572-0241.2006.00528.x.

115. McColl KE. Clinical practice. *Helicobacter pylori* infection. N Engl J Med 2010; 362(17):1597–604. http://dx.doi.org/10.1056/NEJMcp1001110.

116. Rostom A, Moayyedi P, Hunt R, Canadian Association of Gastroenterology Consensus Group. Canadian consensus guidelines on long-term nonsteroidal anti-inflammatory drug therapy and the need for gastroprotection: benefits versus risks. Aliment Pharmacol Ther 2009;29(5):481–96. http://dx.doi.org/10. 1111/j.1365-2036.2008.03905.x.

117. Abraham NS, Hlatky MA, Antman EM, et al. ACCF/ACG/AHA 2010 expert consensus document on the concomitant use of proton pump inhibitors and thienopyridines: a focused update of the ACCF/ACG/AHA 2008 expert consensus document on reducing the gastrointestinal risks of antiplatelet therapy and NSAID use. Am J Gastroenterol 2010;105(12):2533–49. http://dx.doi. org/10.1038/ajg.2010.445.

118. Chan FK, Wong VW, Suen BY, et al. Combination of a cyclo-oxygenase-2 inhibitor and a proton-pump inhibitor for prevention of recurrent ulcer bleeding in patients at very high risk: a double-blind, randomised trial. Lancet 2007;369(9573): 1621–6. http://dx.doi.org/10.1016/S0140-6736(07)60749-1.

119. Laine L, Curtis SP, Cryer B, et al. Assessment of upper gastrointestinal safety of etoricoxib and diclofenac in patients with osteoarthritis and rheumatoid arthritis in the Multinational Etoricoxib and Diclofenac Arthritis Long-term (MEDAL) programme: a randomised comparison. Lancet 2007;369(9560):465–73. http://dx. doi.org/10.1016/S0140-6736(07)60234-7.

120. Scheiman JM, Yeomans ND, Talley NJ, et al. Prevention of ulcers by esomeprazole in at-risk patients using non-selective NSAIDs and COX-2 inhibitors. Am J Gastroenterol 2006;101(4):701–10. http://dx.doi.org/10.1111/j.1572-0241.2006. 00499.x.

121. Kearney PM, Baigent C, Godwin J, et al. Do selective cyclo-oxygenase-2 inhibitors and traditional non-steroidal anti-inflammatory drugs increase the risk of atherothrombosis? Meta-analysis of randomised trials [Systematic reviews and meta-analyses]. BMJ 2006;332(7553):1302–8. http://dx.doi.org/10.1136/bmj. 332.7553.1302.

122. Rostom A, Dube C, Lewin G, et al. Nonsteroidal anti-inflammatory drugs and cyclooxygenase-2 inhibitors for primary prevention of colorectal cancer: a systematic review prepared for the U.S. Preventive Services Task Force [Systematic reviews and meta-analyses]. Ann Intern Med 2007;146(5):376–89.

123. Biondi-Zoccai GG, Lotrionte M, Agostoni P, et al. A systematic review and meta-analysis on the hazards of discontinuing or not adhering to aspirin among 50,279 patients at risk for coronary artery disease [Systematic reviews and meta-analyses]. Eur Heart J 2006;27(22):2667–74. http://dx.doi.org/10.1093/ eurheartj/ehl334. pii:ehl334.

124. Derogar M, Sandblom G, Lundell L, et al. Discontinuation of low-dose aspirin therapy after peptic ulcer bleeding increases risk of death and acute cardiovascular events. Clin Gastroenterol Hepatol 2013;11(1):38–42. http://dx.doi.org/10.1016/j.cgh.2012.08.034.

125. Aguejouf O, Eizayaga F, Desplat V, et al. Prothrombotic and hemorrhagic effects of aspirin. Clin Appl Thromb Hemost 2009;15(5):523–8. http://dx.doi.org/10.1177/1076029608319945.

126. Sibon I, Orgogozo JM. Antiplatelet drug discontinuation is a risk factor for ischemic stroke. Neurology 2004;62(7):1187–9.

127. Sung JJ, Lau JY, Ching JY, et al. Continuation of low-dose aspirin therapy in peptic ulcer bleeding: a randomized trial. Ann Intern Med 2010;152(1):1–9. http://dx.doi.org/10.7326/0003-4819-152-1-201001050-00179.   pii:0003-4819-152-1-201001050-00179.

128. Shingina A, Barkun AN, Razzaghi A, et al. Systematic review: the presenting international normalised ratio (INR) as a predictor of outcome in patients with upper nonvariceal gastrointestinal bleeding [Systematic reviews and meta-analyses]. Aliment Pharmacol Ther 2011;33(9):1010–8. http://dx.doi.org/10.1111/j.1365-2036.2011.04618.x.

129. Baradarian R, Ramdhaney S, Chapalamadugu R, et al. Early intensive resuscitation of patients with upper gastrointestinal bleeding decreases mortality. Am J Gastroenterol 2004;99(4):619–22. http://dx.doi.org/10.1111/j.1572-0241.2004.04073.x.

130. Choudari CP, Rajgopal C, Palmer KR. Acute gastrointestinal haemorrhage in anticoagulated patients: diagnoses and response to endoscopic treatment. Gut 1994;35(4):464–6.

131. Ogawa S, Szlam F, Ohnishi T, et al. A comparative study of prothrombin complex concentrates and fresh-frozen plasma for warfarin reversal under static and flow conditions. Thromb Haemost 2011;106(6):1215–23. http://dx.doi.org/10.1160/TH11-04-0240.

132. Hickey M, Gatien M, Taljaard M, et al. Outcomes of urgent warfarin reversal with frozen plasma versus prothrombin complex concentrate in the emergency department. Circulation 2013;128(4):360–4. http://dx.doi.org/10.1161/CIRCULATIONAHA.113.001875.

133. Guest JF, Watson HG, Limaye S. Modeling the cost-effectiveness of prothrombin complex concentrate compared with fresh frozen plasma in emergency warfarin reversal in the United Kingdom. Clin Ther 2010;32(14):2478–93. http://dx.doi.org/10.1016/j.clinthera.2011.01.011.

134. Baron TH, Kamath PS, McBane RD. Management of antithrombotic therapy in patients undergoing invasive procedures. N Engl J Med 2013;368(22):2113–24. http://dx.doi.org/10.1056/NEJMra1206531.

135. Siegal DM, Cuker A. Reversal of novel oral anticoagulants in patients with major bleeding. J Thromb Thrombolysis 2013. http://dx.doi.org/10.1007/s11239-013-0885-0.

136. Alikhan R, Rayment R, Keeling D, et al. The acute management of haemorrhage, surgery and overdose in patients receiving dabigatran. Emerg Med J 2013. http://dx.doi.org/10.1136/emermed-2012-201976.

137. Chan FK. Anti-platelet therapy and managing ulcer risk. J Gastroenterol Hepatol 2012;27(2):195–9. http://dx.doi.org/10.1111/j.1440-1746.2011.07029.x.

138. Almadi MA, Barkun A, Brophy J. Antiplatelet and anticoagulant therapy in patients with gastrointestinal bleeding: an 86-year-old woman with peptic ulcer disease. JAMA 2011;306(21):2367–74. http://dx.doi.org/10.1001/jama.2011.1653.

139. Taha AS, McCloskey C, Prasad R, et al. Famotidine for the prevention of peptic ulcers and oesophagitis in patients taking low-dose aspirin (FAMOUS): a phase III, randomised, double-blind, placebo-controlled trial. Lancet 2009;374(9684): 119–25. http://dx.doi.org/10.1016/S0140-6736(09)61246-0.

140. Ng FH, Wong SY, Lam KF, et al. Famotidine is inferior to pantoprazole in preventing recurrence of aspirin-related peptic ulcers or erosions. Gastroenterology 2010;138(1):82–8. http://dx.doi.org/10.1053/j.gastro.2009.09.063.

141. Chan FK, Chung SC, Suen BY, et al. Preventing recurrent upper gastrointestinal bleeding in patients with *Helicobacter pylori* infection who are taking low-dose aspirin or naproxen. N Engl J Med 2001;344(13):967–73. http://dx.doi.org/10.1056/NEJM200103293441304.

142. Lai KC, Lam SK, Chu KM, et al. Lansoprazole for the prevention of recurrences of ulcer complications from long-term low-dose aspirin use. N Engl J Med 2002; 346(26):2033–8. http://dx.doi.org/10.1056/NEJMoa012877.

143. Chan FK, Ching JY, Suen BY, et al. Effects of *Helicobacter pylori* infection on long-term risk of peptic ulcer bleeding in low-dose aspirin users. Gastroenterology 2013;144(3):528–35. http://dx.doi.org/10.1053/j.gastro.2012.12.038 pii: S0016-5085(13)00072-3.

144. Chan FK, Ching JY, Hung LC, et al. Clopidogrel versus aspirin and esomeprazole to prevent recurrent ulcer bleeding. N Engl J Med 2005;352(3):238–44. http://dx.doi.org/10.1056/NEJMoa042087.

145. Lai KC, Chu KM, Hui WM, et al. Esomeprazole with aspirin versus clopidogrel for prevention of recurrent gastrointestinal ulcer complications. Clin Gastroenterol Hepatol 2006;4(7):860–5. http://dx.doi.org/10.1016/j.cgh.2006.04.019.

146. Hsu PI, Lai KH, Liu CP. Esomeprazole with clopidogrel reduces peptic ulcer recurrence, compared with clopidogrel alone, in patients with atherosclerosis. Gastroenterology 2011;140(3):791–8. http://dx.doi.org/10.1053/j.gastro.2010.11.056.

147. Bhatt DL, Cryer BL, Contant CF, et al. Clopidogrel with or without omeprazole in coronary artery disease. N Engl J Med 2010;363(20):1909–17. http://dx.doi.org/10.1056/NEJMoa1007964.

148. Bhatt DL, Scheiman J, Abraham NS, et al. ACCF/ACG/AHA 2008 expert consensus document on reducing the gastrointestinal risks of antiplatelet therapy and NSAID use: a report of the American College of Cardiology Foundation Task Force on Clinical Expert Consensus Documents. J Am Coll Cardiol 2008; 52(18):1502–17. http://dx.doi.org/10.1016/j.jacc.2008.08.002.

149. Small DS, Farid NA, Payne CD, et al. Effects of the proton pump inhibitor lansoprazole on the pharmacokinetics and pharmacodynamics of prasugrel and clopidogrel. J Clin Pharmacol 2008;48(4):475–84. http://dx.doi.org/10.1177/0091270008315310.

150. Gilard M, Arnaud B, Cornily JC, et al. Influence of omeprazole on the antiplatelet action of clopidogrel associated with aspirin: the randomized, double-blind OCLA (Omeprazole CLopidogrel Aspirin) study. J Am Coll Cardiol 2008;51(3): 256–60. http://dx.doi.org/10.1016/j.jacc.2007.06.064.

151. O'Donoghue ML, Braunwald E, Antman EM, et al. Pharmacodynamic effect and clinical efficacy of clopidogrel and prasugrel with or without a proton-pump inhibitor: an analysis of two randomised trials. Lancet 2009;374(9694):989–97. http://dx.doi.org/10.1016/S0140-6736(09)61525-7.

152. Kwok CS, Loke YK. Meta-analysis: the effects of proton pump inhibitors on cardiovascular events and mortality in patients receiving clopidogrel [Systematic reviews and meta-analyses]. Aliment Pharmacol Ther 2010;31(8):810–23. http://dx.doi.org/10.1111/j.1365-2036.2010.04247.x.

153. Siller-Matula JM, Jilma B, Schror K, et al. Effect of proton pump inhibitors on clinical outcome in patients treated with clopidogrel: a systematic review and meta-analysis [Systematic reviews and meta-analyses]. J Thromb Haemost 2010;8(12):2624–41. http://dx.doi.org/10.1111/j.1538-7836.2010.04049.x.

154. Lima JP, Brophy JM. The potential interaction between clopidogrel and proton pump inhibitors: a systematic review [Systematic reviews and meta-analyses]. BMC Med 2010;8:81. http://dx.doi.org/10.1186/1741-7015-8-81.

155. Kwok CS, Jeevanantham V, Dawn B, et al. No consistent evidence of differential cardiovascular risk amongst proton-pump inhibitors when used with clopidogrel: meta-analysis [Systematic reviews and meta-analyses]. Int J Cardiol 2012. http://dx.doi.org/10.1016/j.ijcard.2012.03.085.

156. Katz PO, Gerson LB, Vela MF. Guidelines for the diagnosis and management of gastroesophageal reflux disease. Am J Gastroenterol 2013;108(3):308–28. http://dx.doi.org/10.1038/ajg.2012.444 [quiz: 29].

157. van Walraven C, Jennings A, Oake N, et al. Effect of study setting on anticoagulation control: a systematic review and metaregression [Systematic reviews and meta-analyses]. Chest 2006;129(5):1155–66. http://dx.doi.org/10.1378/chest.129.5.1155.

158. Wiedermann CJ, Stockner I. Warfarin-induced bleeding complications - clinical presentation and therapeutic options. Thromb Res 2008;122(Suppl 2):S13–8. http://dx.doi.org/10.1016/S0049-3848(08)70004-5.

159. Levine MN, Raskob G, Beyth RJ, et al. Hemorrhagic complications of anticoagulant treatment: the Seventh ACCP Conference on Antithrombotic and Thrombolytic Therapy. Chest 2004;126(3 Suppl):287S–310S. http://dx.doi.org/10.1378/chest.126.3_suppl.287S.

160. Lin KJ, Hernandez-Diaz S, Garcia Rodriguez LA. Acid suppressants reduce risk of gastrointestinal bleeding in patients on antithrombotic or anti-inflammatory therapy. Gastroenterology 2011;141(1):71–9. http://dx.doi.org/10.1053/j.gastro.2011.03.049.

161. DeEugenio D, Kolman L, DeCaro M, et al. Risk of major bleeding with concomitant dual antiplatelet therapy after percutaneous coronary intervention in patients receiving long-term warfarin therapy. Pharmacotherapy 2007;27(5):691–6. http://dx.doi.org/10.1592/phco.27.5.691.

162. Ng FH, Tunggal P, Chu WM, et al. Esomeprazole compared with famotidine in the prevention of upper gastrointestinal bleeding in patients with acute coronary syndrome or myocardial infarction. Am J Gastroenterol 2012;107(3):389–96. http://dx.doi.org/10.1038/ajg.2011.385.

163. Dewilde WJ, Oirbans T, Verheugt FW, et al. Use of clopidogrel with or without aspirin in patients taking oral anticoagulant therapy and undergoing percutaneous coronary intervention: an open-label, randomised, controlled trial. Lancet 2013;381(9872):1107–15. http://dx.doi.org/10.1016/S0140-6736(12)62177-1.

164. van Es RF, Jonker JJ, Verheugt FW, et al, Antithrombotics in the Secondary Prevention of Events in Coronary Thrombosis-2 Research Group. Aspirin and coumadin after acute coronary syndromes (the ASPECT-2 study): a randomised controlled trial. Lancet 2002;360(9327):109–13. http://dx.doi.org/10.1016/S0140-6736(02)09409-6.

165. Hurlen M, Abdelnoor M, Smith P, et al. Warfarin, aspirin, or both after myocardial infarction. N Engl J Med 2002;347(13):969–74. http://dx.doi.org/10.1056/NEJMoa020496.

166. Patel MR, Mahaffey KW, Garg J, et al. Rivaroxaban versus warfarin in nonvalvular atrial fibrillation. N Engl J Med 2011;365(10):883–91. http://dx.doi.org/10.1056/NEJMoa1009638.
167. Connolly SJ, Ezekowitz MD, Yusuf S, et al. Dabigatran versus warfarin in patients with atrial fibrillation. N Engl J Med 2009;361(12):1139–51. http://dx.doi.org/10.1056/NEJMoa0905561.
168. Holster IL, Valkhoff VE, Kuipers EJ, et al. New oral anticoagulants increase risk for gastrointestinal bleeding: a systematic review and meta-analysis [Systematic reviews and meta-analyses]. Gastroenterology 2013;145(1):105–12.e15. http://dx.doi.org/10.1053/j.gastro.2013.02.041 pii:S0016-5085(13)00290-4.
169. Laine L. Review article: gastrointestinal bleeding with low-dose aspirin - what's the risk? Aliment Pharmacol Ther 2006;24(6):897–908. http://dx.doi.org/10.1111/j.1365-2036.2006.03077.x.
170. Delaney JA, Opatrny L, Brophy JM, et al. Drug drug interactions between antithrombotic medications and the risk of gastrointestinal bleeding. Can Med Assoc J 2007;177(4):347–51. http://dx.doi.org/10.1503/cmaj.070186.

Endoscopic Management of Nonvariceal, Nonulcer Upper Gastrointestinal Bleeding

CrossMark

Eric T.T.L. Tjwa, MD, PhD*, I. Lisanne Holster, MD, PhD,
Ernst J. Kuipers, MD, PhD

KEYWORDS

- UGIB • Angiodysplasia • Dieulafoy • GAVE • Gastric cancer • Hemospray • OTSC

KEY POINTS

- Although peptic ulcer and esophagogastric varices remain the most common causes of upper gastrointestinal bleeding, a quarter to half of these events is due to a range of other conditions.
- Endoscopy is the mainstay for diagnosis of these bleeds, as well as the management of the largest proportion of them.
- Endoscopic treatment makes use of the same modalities as used for peptic ulcer and varices.
- Evidence for specific endoscopic therapy per specific cause is mounting.
- The use of novel modalities such as hemostatic powder, self-expandable metal stents, and over-the-scope-clips have expanded and may replace other treatment methods.

INTRODUCTION

The endoscopic management of gastrointestinal (GI) hemorrhage consists of injection therapy (with epinephrine or cyanoacrylate and other sclerosing agents), endoscopic thermal therapy, mechanical modalities such as hemoclips and over-the-scope-clips, and more recently, topical hemostatic sprays.[1,2] Solid evidence exists on how these modalities can be used in peptic ulcer and variceal bleeds, but it is less clear for other causes. This article deals with the endoscopic management of nonvariceal, nonulcer upper gastrointestinal bleeding (UGIB).[3–6]

Financial disclosures: E.T.T.L. Tjwa has received an unrestricted educational grant from Cook Medical Ireland.
Department of Gastroenterology and Hepatology, Erasmus MC University Medical Centre, PO box 2040, 3000 CA, Rotterdam, The Netherlands
* Corresponding author. Erasmus MC University Medical Centre, Room Hs-312, 's Gravendijkwal 230, Rotterdam 3015 CE, The Netherlands.
E-mail address: E.tjwa@erasmusmc.nl

Gastroenterol Clin N Am 43 (2014) 707–719
http://dx.doi.org/10.1016/j.gtc.2014.08.004
0889-8553/14/$ – see front matter © 2014 Elsevier Inc. All rights reserved.

gastro.theclinics.com

EROSIVE CAUSES OF UGIB

Nonsteroidal antiinflammatory drugs are the principal cause for drug-induced erosions. They can be responsible for intramucosal petechial hemorrhage, superficial hemorrhagic erosions, gastroduodenitis, and ulceration.[7] In an endoscopic study of 187 patients using low-dose aspirin for at least 3 months with and without gastroprotective agents, erosions were observed in 34% and 63% of subjects, respectively.[8,9]

Other classes of drugs that can lead to erosions and ulceration are selective serotonin reuptake inhibitors, corticosteroids, nitrogen-containing bisphosphonates, potassium tablets, some antibiotics (eg, erythromycin, nalidixic acid, sulfonamides, and derivatives), and various chemotherapeutic agents.[7]

Larger hiatal hernia can result in linear erosions and ulcers or so-called *Cameron lesions* within the stomach at the impression of the diaphragm.[10] They predominantly occur along the lesser curvature. They most likely occur as a result of the combination of chronic mechanical trauma (eg, rubbing of the mucosal folds at the level of the diaphragm during respiratory excursions) and acid injury. Local ischemia may also play a role. Cameron lesions are found in about 5% of patients with hiatal hernia undergoing upper endoscopy; two-thirds of these patients have multiple lesions.[11] They may occur in 10% to 20% of patients with a hernia greater than or equal to 5 cm.[12]

Erosive esophago-gastro-duodenitis has many possible causes such as excessive alcohol consumption, use of mucosal erosion–causing drugs (see earlier discussion),[13] gastroesophageal reflux, and *Helicobacter pylori* infection.[14–16] Gastroduodenal erosions infrequently cause clinically significant blood loss.[3,5,14,17–20]

Endoscopic Management of Erosive Causes of UGIB

Endoscopy has only a marginal role in the treatment of hemorrhage caused by erosions. The treatment of choice is acid suppression, leading to healing of erosions and normalization of hemoglobin levels. The outcome is generally excellent. Acute bleeds sometimes require endoscopic treatment such as of a visible vessel, for which the treatment is similar to the approach of gastroduodenal ulcers. A different approach may be the control of bleeding by a topical hemostatic spray. Hemospray (Cook Medical, Winston Salem, NC, USA) is a novel proprietary powder specifically developed for the treatment of UGIB.[21,22] It is a nonorganic mineral blended powder that is thought to work via absorption of liquids at the bleeding site, forming an adhesive and cohesive mechanical barrier over the bleeding site. In a large European observational study in 63 patients with UGIB due to various causes, the application of Hemospray as primary monotreatment led to immediate hemostasis in 85% of patients with a 7-day rebleeding rate of 15%. When used as salvage therapy, after failure of conventional endoscopic treatment modalities, initial hemostasis was 100% and rebleeding 25%, reflecting the refractory nature of these lesions. Causes of nonvariceal, nonulcer UGIB included erosive esophagitis, gastritis, and/or duodenitis (n = 7), as well as Dieulafoy lesions, gastric antral vascular ectasia (GAVE), and Mallory-Weiss lesions.[23] Concomitant use of antithrombotics, mostly causative for erosive UGIB, do not appear to influence the success rates of Hemospray.[22]

UGIB CAUSED BY VASCULAR ANOMALIES

Vascular anomalies that most commonly cause UGIB include angiodysplasia, Dieulafoy lesions, and GAVE. Although not a true anomaly, but rather the result of congestion, portal hypertensive gastropathy is also ranked in this same category of vascular lesions.

Angiodysplasia

Angiodysplasia is defined as a sharply delineated vascular lesion within the mucosa, with a typical red appearance, with flat or slightly raised surface. Angiodysplasia is generally believed to be acquired, but the exact causes are unknown.[24–26] These lesions are often multiple and frequently seen in the colon, but may also involve the stomach and small bowel, including the duodenum. Patients with angiodysplasia can present with chronic iron-deficiency anemia, as well as with acute GI bleeding with melena and seldom hematemesis.[27]

Dieulafoy Lesion

Dieulafoy lesions most commonly occur in the proximal stomach along the lesser curve, but they are incidentally seen in the esophagus,[28] small intestine, and colon.[29] A Dieulafoy lesion consists of a dilated tortuous artery with a diameter up to 3 mm that protrudes through the mucosa and may cause massive GI hemorrhage by erosion of the artery. It is thought that this is due to a combination of factors such as straining of the vascular wall during peristalsis and peptic digestion.[30,31] Bleeding due to Dieulafoy lesions account for 1% to 6% of cases of acute nonvariceal UGIB.[30]

Gastric Antral Vascular Ectasia

GAVE is endoscopically recognized as a pattern of linear red stripes in the antrum separated by normal mucosa. GAVE has been associated with several autoimmune conditions, renal failure, and bone marrow transplantation.[32–35]

GAVE or so-called *watermelon stomach* is often confused with portal hypertensive gastropathy. Although GAVE is closely related to portal hypertension, it can also appear in the absence of portal hypertension, and GAVE generally does not respond to treatments that reduce portal pressure.

Portal Hypertensive Gastropathy

Portal hypertensive gastropathy or congestive gastropathy corresponds to dilated gastric mucosal capillaries without inflammation.[36] It is exclusively observed in patients with portal hypertension. When present in the small intestine or colon, it is termed portal hypertensive enteropathy[37] and portal hypertensive colopathy.[38] The degree of portal hypertension needed for development of portal hypertensive gastropathy remains controversial.[39] Bleeding from these conditions usually occurs as slow, diffusely oozing, but it may also be acute (and even) massive.

Endoscopic Management of Vascular Anomalies and Portal Hypertensive Gastropathy

The current standard of endoscopic treatment of bleeding angiodysplasia consists of coagulation therapy. Although high success rates are achieved for treatment of individual lesions, patients may experience recurrent anemia or overt bleeding. Banding of angiodysplasia has also been demonstrated in a small study of 11 subjects.[40] In case of bleeding angiodysplasia in the small intestines, (repeated) argon plasma coagulation (APC) via enteroscopy has been proved feasible and successful.[41]

Endoscopic treatment is also the first choice in bleeding Dieulafoy lesions[42] and is able to achieve hemostasis in more than 90% of cases.[30] Treatment is usually performed with clipping or band ligation of the lesion.

The first-line treatment of actively bleeding GAVE as well as recurrent bleeding from GAVE has for a long time consisted of repetitive sessions of APC.[43] In case of recurrence, patients have been successfully retreated with APC.[44] More recent publications show that band ligation of bleeding GAVE resulted in fewer treatment sessions for control of bleeding and higher rates of cessation of further bleeding than APC treat-ment.[45–48] Whether this also pertains to persistently decreased recurrence rates remains to be demonstrated (**Fig. 1**).

Endoscopic management has no place in treating portal hypertensive gastro-pathy.[43] Successful treatment should aim at reducing portal venous pressure by means of nonselective β-blockers, vasoactive drugs, and/or transjugular intrahepatic portosystemic shunts.

NEOPLASTIC BLEEDING LESIONS

Neoplastic lesions (both primary and metastatic) of the upper GI tract account for 2% to 8% of the cases of UGIB.[3,5,17–19] Gastric adenocarcinoma is the most prevalent among patients presenting with UGIB.

Endoscopic Management of Neoplastic Bleeding

Conventional endoscopic therapy for bleeding GI tumors is generally not very successful, because most tumors are beyond the reach of thermal or mechanical modalities due to their complex neoangiogenesis.[49] Endoscopic management was assessed in a study of 42 patients with primary upper GI cancer. In approximately half of these patients, severe UGIB was the first presentation of their malignancy, most of which were at an advanced stage with larger ulcerating tumor masses. Endo-scopic hemostasis was only achieved in the lesser advanced, nondiffusely bleeding cancers. Severe bleeding correlated with a poor 1-year survival irrespective of initial hemostasis.[50] Against this background, radiotherapy and/or transarterial embolization (TAE) were for a long time the only alternative treatments for management of bleeding. Radiotherapy has a delayed effect, and the effect of both radiotherapy and emboliza-tion may be transient. In a retrospective study of 30 patients with UGIB from gastric cancer, almost 75% responded to radiotherapy, but rebled within 3 months. Patients who received concurrent chemoradiotherapy had a significant lower rebleeding rate (18%).[51] In a retrospective study of 23 patients with neoplastic UGIB treated with TAE, the overall treatment success was only 50%.[52]

Hemostatic powders are increasingly advocated as an endoscopic treatment of neoplastic bleeding because of its ability to stop diffuse bleeding. Two case series from Canada and France, including a total of 10 patients, showed promising short-term results in the use of Hemospray in bleeding esophageal, gastric, and pancreatic

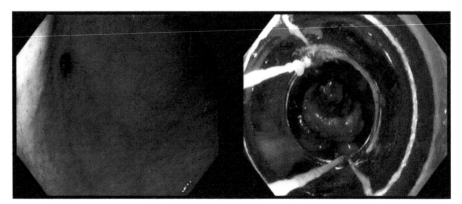

Fig. 1. Dieulafoy lesion in the fundus before and after band ligation.

cancers. In both reports, immediate hemostasis was reached in 100% of the patients and the rebleeding rate after 3 days was 20%.[53,54] Because powder can be endoscopically delivered during the index endoscopy, it provides a rapid and effective treatment modality in the bleeding oncology patient in the acute setting (**Fig. 2**).

UGIB CAUSED BY TRAUMA
Mallory-Weiss Tear

A Mallory-Weiss tear is a common cause of UGIB and typically presents as hematemesis after an initial episode of vomiting without blood. It is defined as a mucosal laceration at the gastroesophageal junction or gastric cardia, usually caused by retching or forceful vomiting.[55] Many factors have been associated with the development of Mallory-Weiss lesions, including alcohol use, use of aspirin and coumarins, paroxysms of coughing, pregnancy, heavy lifting, straining, seizure, blunt abdominal trauma, colonic lavage, and cardiopulmonary resuscitation.[56,57] The amount of blood loss is usually mild. Several epidemiologic studies reported these lesions as the bleeding source in 2% to 8% of patients presenting with acute UGIB.[3,17,18,58,59] In a large UK audit of 5004 patients who underwent endoscopy for UGIB, Mallory-Weiss lesions were the only bleeding source identified in 2.1% of cases and were present in a total 4.3% of cases.[59]

Boerhaave Syndrome and Other Causes of Transmural Perforation

Boerhaave syndrome is a rupture of the esophagus caused by a rapid increase in intraluminal pressure in the distal esophagus combined with negative intrathoracic pressure caused by straining or vomiting. Other causes of benign esophageal perforation include endoscopic and surgical handling and foreign body impaction.[60] In some cases, bleeding may be an accompanying symptom.

Caustic Injury and Foreign Body Ingestion

Ingestion of foreign bodies and toxic substances can be accidental or intentional. The ingestion of strong alkali results in liquefactive necrosis, which is associated with deep tissue penetration and may result in perforation accompanied by bleeding.[61] Acidic agents cause more superficial coagulation necrosis with scarring that may limit the

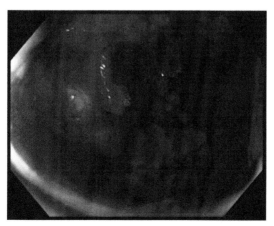

Fig. 2. Hemorrhagic gastric adenocarcinoma of the corpus after hemostasis with Hemospray.

extent of the injury.[62] Bleeding may occur as a result of widespread ulceration. More severe bleeding is however rare.

UGIB is also seen after foreign body ingestion. Most noteworthy in this respect is the ingestion of batteries and magnets leading to leakage and pressure adhesion, which can lead to local ulceration and perforation.[63] Hemorrhage is a frequent complication after foreign body ingestion[64] and results from local pressure or puncture of the mucosa with sometimes fistula formation to an underlying vessel.[65]

Endoscopic Management for Traumatic Bleeding

Most of the Mallory-Weiss lesions stop bleeding spontaneously.[58,66] A minority of cases require endoscopic treatment. In a French series of 218 patients with Mallory-Weiss bleeding, 56 (26%) had active bleeding on endoscopy. In other series, this prevalence ranged from 5% to 44%.[58,67] Various studies have looked at optimal endoscopic treatment. In a trial that randomized 63 patients to either supportive treatment or endoscopic therapy, rebleeding rates after only supportive therapy were higher than that after endoscopic epinephrine injection (25% vs 6%).[67] Endoscopic epinephrine injection, hemoclip placement, and band ligation were equivalent for primary hemostasis, all achieving 100% primary hemostasis.[67–71] Rebleeding rates after band ligation and hemoclip placement were similar in a randomized Korean trial (6%–10%),[70] but significantly lower after band ligation in a French trial (0% vs 18%).[71] It is unknown whether prescription of a proton pump inhibitor accelerates healing.

The "bear-claw" or over-the-scope-clip system (Ovesco Endoscopy, Tübingen, Germany) is a new clipping device developed for closure of large luminal GI defects.[72] These defects may be spontaneous like Boerhaave syndrome or iatrogenic (post-endoscopic submucosal dissection[73] or dehiscence after surgical anastomosis[74]) and include both perforated and bleeding lesions. Until now, evidence regarding the effectiveness of the device only came from case series,[75] but it is expected that over-the-scope-clip system may become an alternative to conventional surgical therapy for traumatic lesions. Endoscopic placement of a self-expandable metal stent (SEMS) can also be considered for Boerhaave syndrome.[60] The authors reported a series of 33 patients with nonmalignant esophageal perforation treated with SEMS placement. Initial sealing of the perforation was achieved in 97% of patients, long-term success without the need for surgical repair in 88%. Treatment was complicated in one-third of patients by stent migration, managed by SEMS repositioning or restenting. In their center, this has now become the initial endoscopic treatment of choice for esophageal perforations that require intervention. Stents need to be removed within 6 weeks after placement, because a longer time in situ often impairs the ease of removal. When a persistent perforation is observed after stent removal, placement of another stent should be considered.

Endoscopy often has little to offer in terms of treatment of bleeding caused by caustic injury. Early prophylactic esophageal stenting preventing stricture formation is currently under investigation.[76]

BLEEDING FROM THE HEPATOPANCREATICOBILIARY TRACT
Hemobilia

Hemobilia or bleeding from the hepatobiliary tract is a rare cause of UGIB. The causes include liver biopsy,[77] percutaneous transhepatic cholangiography, cholecystectomy, endoscopic biliary biopsies/stenting, and hepatic or bile duct tumors. In a review of 222 cases of hemobilia, 65% were iatrogenic, whereas accidental trauma accounted for only 6%.[78,79] In rare cases, bleeding may occur due to a fistula to the portal system or the hepatic vein, which can also lead to rapid onset of extreme jaundice.[80] In most cases, these bleeds are self-limiting and do not require intervention other than preventing biliary obstruction due to clots.

Symptoms of hemobilia can be variable. The classic triad of jaundice, biliary colic, and overt UGIB was in the most recent series only observed in 22% of the patients.[79] Endoscopic retrograde cholangiography is helpful to confirm diagnosis and establish the underlying cause. It can also be of help in clearance of the biliary tree, with stenting if necessary to reduce the risk of renewed obstruction. In rare cases, a lesion of the hepatic vein can establish a connection between the hepatic vein and the biliary tract and instead of hemobilia give rise to opposite flow of bile into the vein. Such bilhemia may lead to marked, acute onset of jaundice. In such a case, biliary stenting can reverse the flow, by rapidly reducing jaundice and allow closure of the leak.[80]

Hemosuccus Pancreaticus

Hemosuccus pancreaticus is caused by a bleeding source in the pancreas, pancreatic duct, or adjacent structures, such as the splenic artery connecting to the pancreatic duct.[81] Hemosuccus is most often due to pancreatic pseudoaneurysms resulting from acute or chronic pancreatitis.[82–84] Usually this involves erosion of the splenic artery leading to hemorrhage into the pancreatic duct. It has been estimated to occur in about 1 in 500 to 1500 cases of UGIB.[82,84] In 2 retrospective studies (n = 40 total), the most frequent complaints at presentation were melena, hematochezia, hematemesis, and epigastric pain.[82,84] Patients may also develop symptoms of nausea and vomiting, weight loss, and jaundice (when the bleed also leads to obstruction of the common bile duct). In an observational report including 31 patients with hemosuccus pancreaticus, the presence of duodenal blood was observed during upper GI endoscopy in only half of the patients.[84]

Endoscopic Management of Hemobilia and Hemosuccus Pancreaticus

Because hemobilia is mostly self-limiting, the role of endoscopic treatment is limited to clearance of the biliary system if needed, with occasional stenting to maintain an open biliary tract. Also for hemosuccus pancreaticus, there is no major role for endoscopic treatment. Selective arterial embolization is successful in 50% of the patients, whereas surgery is often necessary in emergency situations or after failure to control the bleeding by TAE.[84]

MISCELLANEOUS CAUSES OF BLEEDING

In rare cases, UGIB is caused by large- or small-vessel vasculitis,[85–89] which may occur throughout the GI tract.[89] Lesions may typically be very topical, affecting sharply demarcated areas, yet arising at multiple sites. Endoscopic biopsy specimens of the affected area may reveal ulceration and inflammation, but are often insufficient to demonstrate the underlying vasculitis. Diagnosis of the underlying disease is nevertheless mandatory. Treatment mostly starts with corticosteroids and immunosuppressive therapy, together with proton pump inhibitors in patients with upper GI lesions.

Acute gastric ischemia is uncommon because of the stomach's rich vascular supply. Nevertheless it is important to recognize, because progression to necrosis can lead to ulceration, including complications such as bleeding, perforation, and sepsis.[90,91] It may also occur if there is stenosis of the celiac trunk with insufficient collateral circulation.[92] UGIB due to ischemia has been described in a few case reports.[93,94]

Table 1
Causes of nonvariceal, nonulcer UGIB and their specific endoscopic management

Type of Bleeding	Subtype	Endoscopic Management
Erosive		None, possible role for hemostatic powder
Vascular	Angiodysplasia	Coagulation
	Dieulafoy lesion	Hemoclips, band ligation
	GAVE	Coagulation, band ligation
	Portal hypertensive gastropathy	None
Traumatic	Mallory-Weiss lesion	Band ligation, hemoclips, epinephrine injection
	Associated with perforation	Over-the-scope-clips, SEMS
	Caustic	None
Neoplastic		Possible role for hemostatic powder
Hepatopancreaticobiliary	Hemobilia, hemosuccus pancreaticus	None, ERCP to prevent obstruction or to treat bilhemia
Miscellaneous	Vasculitis, ischemic	Possible role for hemostatic powder

Endoscopic Management

Bleeding from these miscellaneous causes usually prohibit successful endoscopic therapy because bleeding is often diffuse and/or nonpulsatile hampering targeted therapy such as hemoclips, band ligation, or thermal therapy. Even though some data are available on the successful use of liberally deployed hemostatic powder,[23] the generalizability of this method is under further investigation. Treating the cause of vasculitis, systemic disease of ischemia will remain cornerstone in the treatment of associated bleeding.

SUMMARY

Although peptic ulcer and esophagogastric varices remain the most common causes of UGIB, a quarter to half of these events is due to a range of other conditions.[3,5,17–19] Endoscopy is the mainstay for diagnosis of these bleeds, as well as the management of the largest proportion of them. Endoscopic treatment makes use of the same modalities as used for peptic ulcer and varices. Evidence for specific endoscopic therapy per specific cause is mounting (**Table 1**). The use of novel modalities such as hemostatic powder, SEMS, and over-the-scope-clips have expanded and often replaced other treatment methods.

REFERENCES

1. Committee ASoP, Early DS, Ben-Menachem T, et al. Appropriate use of GI endoscopy. Gastrointest Endosc 2012;75:1127–31.
2. Barkun AN, Moosavi S, Martel M. Topical hemostatic agents: a systematic review with particular emphasis on endoscopic application in GI bleeding. Gastrointest Endosc 2013;77:692–700.
3. Czernichow P, Hochain P, Nousbaum JB, et al. Epidemiology and course of acute upper gastro-intestinal haemorrhage in four French geographical areas. Eur J Gastroenterol Hepatol 2000;12:175–81.

4. Enestvedt BK, Gralnek IM, Mattek N, et al. An evaluation of endoscopic indications and findings related to nonvariceal upper-GI hemorrhage in a large multicenter consortium. Gastrointest Endosc 2008;67:422–9.
5. van Leerdam ME, Vreeburg EM, Rauws EA, et al. Acute upper GI bleeding: did anything change? Time trend analysis of incidence and outcome of acute upper GI bleeding between 1993/1994 and 2000. Am J Gastroenterol 2003; 98:1494–9.
6. Holster IL, Kuipers EJ. Other causes of upper gastrointestinal bleeding. In: Sung JJ, Kuipers EJ, Barkun AN, editors. Gastrointestinal bleeding. 2nd edition. London: Blackwell Publishing Ltd; 2012. p. 135–76.
7. Gore RM, Levine MS, Ghahremani GG. Drug-induced disorders of the stomach and duodenum. Abdom Imaging 1999;24:9–16.
8. Yeomans ND, Lanas AI, Talley NJ, et al. Prevalence and incidence of gastroduodenal ulcers during treatment with vascular protective doses of aspirin. Aliment Pharmacol Ther 2005;22:795–801.
9. Tamura A, Murakami K, Kadota J, Investigators O-GS. Prevalence and independent factors for gastroduodenal ulcers/erosions in asymptomatic patients taking low-dose aspirin and gastroprotective agents: the OITA-GF study. QJM 2011; 104(2):133–9.
10. Cameron AJ, Higgins JA. Linear gastric erosion. A lesion associated with large diaphragmatic hernia and chronic blood loss anemia. Gastroenterology 1986; 91:338–42.
11. Weston AP. Hiatal hernia with cameron ulcers and erosions. Gastrointest Endosc Clin N Am 1996;6:671–9.
12. Maganty K, Smith RL. Cameron lesions: unusual cause of gastrointestinal bleeding and anemia. Digestion 2008;77:214–7.
13. Sugawa C, Lucas CE, Rosenberg BF, et al. Differential topography of acute erosive gastritis due to trauma or sepsis, ethanol and aspirin. Gastrointest Endosc 1973;19:127–30.
14. Toljamo KT, Niemela SE, Karttunen TJ, et al. Clinical significance and outcome of gastric mucosal erosions: a long-term follow-up study. Dig Dis Sci 2006;51:543–7.
15. Morris A, Nicholson G. Ingestion of campylobacter pyloridis causes gastritis and raised fasting gastric pH. Am J Gastroenterol 1987;82:192–9.
16. Kuipers EJ. Review article: exploring the link between Helicobacter pylori and gastric cancer. Aliment Pharmacol Ther 1999;13(Suppl 1):3–11.
17. Di Fiore F, Lecleire S, Merle V, et al. Changes in characteristics and outcome of acute upper gastrointestinal haemorrhage: a comparison of epidemiology and practices between 1996 and 2000 in a multicentre French study. Eur J Gastroenterol Hepatol 2005;17:641–7.
18. Theocharis GJ, Thomopoulos KC, Sakellaropoulos G, et al. Changing trends in the epidemiology and clinical outcome of acute upper gastrointestinal bleeding in a defined geographical area in Greece. J Clin Gastroenterol 2008;42:128–33.
19. Paspatis GA, Matrella E, Kapsoritakis A, et al. An epidemiological study of acute upper gastrointestinal bleeding in Crete, Greece. Eur J Gastroenterol Hepatol 2000;12:1215–20.
20. McQuaid KR, Laine L. Systematic review and meta-analysis of adverse events of low-dose aspirin and clopidogrel in randomized controlled trials. Am J Med 2006;119:624–38.
21. Sung JJ, Luo D, Wu JC, et al. Early clinical experience of the safety and effectiveness of Hemospray in achieving hemostasis in patients with acute peptic ulcer bleeding. Endoscopy 2011;43:291–5.

22. Holster IL, Kuipers EJ, Tjwa ET. Hemospray in the treatment of upper gastrointestinal hemorrhage in patients on antithrombotic therapy. Endoscopy 2013;45: 63–6.

23. Smith LA, Stanley AJ, Bergman JJ, et al. Hemospray application in nonvariceal upper gastrointestinal bleeding: results of the survey to evaluate the application of hemospray in the luminal tract. J Clin Gastroenterol 2013. [Epub ahead of print].

24. Gilmore PR. Angiodysplasia of the upper gastrointestinal tract. J Clin Gastroenterol 1988;10:386–94.

25. Kaaroud H, Fatma LB, Beji S, et al. Gastrointestinal angiodysplasia in chronic renal failure. Saudi J Kidney Dis Transpl 2008;19:809–12.

26. Mishra PK, Kovac J, de Caestecker J, et al. Intestinal angiodysplasia and aortic valve stenosis: let's not close the book on this association. Eur J Cardiothorac Surg 2009;35:628–34.

27. Chalasani N, Cotsonis G, Wilcox CM. Upper gastrointestinal bleeding in patients with chronic renal failure: role of vascular ectasia. Am J Gastroenterol 1996;91: 2329–32.

28. Ertekin C, Barbaros U, Taviloglu K, et al. Dieulafoy's lesion of esophagus. Surg Endosc 2002;16:219.

29. Moreira-Pinto J, Raposo C, Teixeira da Silva V, et al. Jejunal Dieulafoy's lesion: case report and literature review. Pediatr Surg Int 2009;25:641–2.

30. Lee YT, Walmsley RS, Leong RW, et al. Dieulafoy's lesion. Gastrointest Endosc 2003;58:236–43.

31. Lara LF, Sreenarasimhaiah J, Tang SJ, et al. Dieulafoy lesions of the GI tract: localization and therapeutic outcomes. Dig Dis Sci 2010;55:3436–41.

32. Goel A, Christian CL. Gastric antral vascular ectasia (watermelon stomach) in a patient with Sjogren's syndrome. J Rheumatol 2003;30:1090–2.

33. Viiala CH, Kaye JM, Hurley DM, et al. Watermelon stomach arising in association with Addison's disease. J Clin Gastroenterol 2001;33:173.

34. Ingraham KM, O'Brien MS, Shenin M, et al. Gastric antral vascular ectasia in systemic sclerosis: demographics and disease predictors. J Rheumatol 2010; 37:603–7.

35. Burak KW, Lee SS, Beck PL. Portal hypertensive gastropathy and gastric antral vascular ectasia (GAVE) syndrome. Gut 2001;49:866–72.

36. Thuluvath PJ, Yoo HY. Portal hypertensive gastropathy. Am J Gastroenterol 2002;97:2973–8.

37. Higaki N, Matsui H, Imaoka H, et al. Characteristic endoscopic features of portal hypertensive enteropathy. J Gastroenterol 2008;43:327–31.

38. Bini EJ, Lascarides CE, Micale PL, et al. Mucosal abnormalities of the colon in patients with portal hypertension: an endoscopic study. Gastrointest Endosc 2000;52:511–6.

39. Cubillas R, Rockey DC. Portal hypertensive gastropathy: a review. Liver Int 2010;30:1094–102.

40. Ljubicic N. Endoscopic detachable mini-loop ligation for treatment of gastroduodenal angiodysplasia: case study of 11 patients with long-term follow-up. Gastrointest Endosc 2004;59:420–3.

41. Godeschalk MF, Mensink PB, van Buuren HR, et al. Primary balloon-assisted enteroscopy in patients with obscure gastrointestinal bleeding: findings and outcome of therapy. J Clin Gastroenterol 2010;44:e195–200.

42. Yanar H, Dolay K, Ertekin C, et al. An infrequent cause of upper gastrointestinal tract bleeding: "Dieulafoy's lesion". Hepatogastroenterology 2007;54:1013–7.

43. Garcia N, Sanyal AJ. Portal hypertensive gastropathy and gastric antral vascular ectasia. Curr Treat Options Gastroenterol 2001;4:163–71.
44. Fuccio L, Zagari RM, Serrani M, et al. Endoscopic argon plasma coagulation for the treatment of gastric antral vascular ectasia-related bleeding in patients with liver cirrhosis. Digestion 2009;79:143–50.
45. Sato T, Yamazaki K, Akaike J. Endoscopic band ligation versus argon plasma coagulation for gastric antral vascular ectasia associated with liver diseases. Dig Endosc 2012;24:237–42.
46. Chiu YC, Lu LS, Wu KL, et al. Comparison of argon plasma coagulation in management of upper gastrointestinal angiodysplasia and gastric antral vascular ectasia hemorrhage. BMC Gastroenterol 2012;12:67.
47. Wells CD, Harrison ME, Gurudu SR, et al. Treatment of gastric antral vascular ectasia (watermelon stomach) with endoscopic band ligation. Gastrointest Endosc 2008;68:231–6.
48. Kumar R, Mohindra S, Pruthi HS. Endoscopic band ligation: a novel therapy for bleeding gastric antral vascular ectasia. Endoscopy 2007;39(Suppl 1):E56–7.
49. Heller SJ, Tokar JL, Nguyen MT, et al. Management of bleeding GI tumors. Gastrointest Endosc 2010;72:817–24.
50. Savides TJ, Jensen DM, Cohen J, et al. Severe upper gastrointestinal tumor bleeding: endoscopic findings, treatment, and outcome. Endoscopy 1996;28:244–8.
51. Asakura H, Hashimoto T, Harada H, et al. Palliative radiotherapy for bleeding from advanced gastric cancer: is a schedule of 30 Gy in 10 fractions adequate? J Cancer Res Clin Oncol 2010;137:125–30.
52. Lee HJ, Shin JH, Yoon HK, et al. Transcatheter arterial embolization in gastric cancer patients with acute bleeding. Eur Radiol 2009;19:960–5.
53. Chen YI, Barkun AN, Soulellis C, et al. Use of the endoscopically applied hemostatic powder TC-325 in cancer-related upper GI hemorrhage: preliminary experience (with video). Gastrointest Endosc 2012;75:1278–81.
54. Leblanc S, Vienne A, Dhooge M, et al. Early experience with a novel hemostatic powder used to treat upper GI bleeding related to malignancies or after therapeutic interventions (with videos). Gastrointest Endosc 2013;78:169–75.
55. Mallory GK, Weiss SW. Hemorrhages from lacerations of the cardiac orifice of the stomach due to vomiting. Am J Med Sci 1929;178:506–12.
56. Younes Z, Johnson DA. The spectrum of spontaneous and iatrogenic esophageal injury: perforations, Mallory-Weiss tears, and hematomas. J Clin Gastroenterol 1999;29:306–17.
57. Eisen GM, Baron TH, Dominitz JA, et al. Complications of upper GI endoscopy. Gastrointest Endosc 2002;55:784–93.
58. Kim JW, Kim HS, Byun JW, et al. Predictive factors of recurrent bleeding in Mallory-Weiss syndrome. Korean J Gastroenterol 2005;46:447–54.
59. Hearnshaw SA, Logan RF, Lowe D, et al. Use of endoscopy for management of acute upper gastrointestinal bleeding in the UK: results of a nationwide audit. Gut 2010;59:1022–9.
60. van Heel NC, Haringsma J, Spaander MC, et al. Short-term esophageal stenting in the management of benign perforations. Am J Gastroenterol 2010;105:1515–20.
61. Poley JW, Steyerberg EW, Kuipers EJ, et al. Ingestion of acid and alkaline agents: outcome and prognostic value of early upper endoscopy. Gastrointest Endosc 2004;60:372–7.
62. Kay M, Wyllie R. Caustic ingestions in children. Curr Opin Pediatr 2009;21:651–4.

63. Sahin C, Alver D, Gulcin N, et al. A rare cause of intestinal perforation: ingestion of magnet. World J Pediatr 2010;6:369–71.
64. Syrakos T, Zacharakis E, Antonitsis P, et al. Surgical intervention for gastrointestinal foreign bodies in adults: a case series. Med Princ Pract 2008;17:276–9.
65. Huiping Y, Jian Z, Shixi L. Esophageal foreign body as a cause of upper gastrointestinal hemorrhage: case report and review of the literature. Eur Arch Otorhinolaryngol 2008;265:247–9.
66. Kortas DY, Haas LS, Simpson WG, et al. Mallory-Weiss tear: predisposing factors and predictors of a complicated course. Am J Gastroenterol 2001;96:2863–5.
67. Llach J, Elizalde JI, Guevara MC, et al. Endoscopic injection therapy in bleeding Mallory-Weiss syndrome: a randomized controlled trial. Gastrointest Endosc 2001;54:679–81.
68. Huang SP, Wang HP, Lee YC, et al. Endoscopic hemoclip placement and epinephrine injection for Mallory-Weiss syndrome with active bleeding. Gastrointest Endosc 2002;55:842–6.
69. Park CH, Min SW, Sohn YH, et al. A prospective, randomized trial of endoscopic band ligation vs. epinephrine injection for actively bleeding Mallory-Weiss syndrome. Gastrointest Endosc 2004;60:22–7.
70. Cho YS, Chae HS, Kim HK, et al. Endoscopic band ligation and endoscopic hemoclip placement for patients with Mallory-Weiss syndrome and active bleeding. World J Gastroenterol 2008;14:2080–4.
71. Lecleire S, Antonietti M, Iwanicki-Caron I, et al. Endoscopic band ligation could decrease recurrent bleeding in Mallory-Weiss syndrome as compared to haemostasis by hemoclips plus epinephrine. Aliment Pharmacol Ther 2009;30:399–405.
72. Monkemuller K, Peter S, Toshniwal J, et al. Multipurpose use of the 'bear claw' (over-the-scope-clip system) to treat endoluminal gastrointestinal disorders. Dig Endosc 2014;26(3):350–7.
73. Nishiyama N, Mori H, Kobara H, et al. Efficacy and safety of over-the-scope clip: including complications after endoscopic submucosal dissection. World J Gastroenterol 2013;19:2752–60.
74. Weiland T, Fehlker M, Gottwald T, et al. Performance of the OTSC system in the endoscopic closure of iatrogenic gastrointestinal perforations: a systematic review. Surg Endosc 2013;27:2258–74.
75. Singhal S, Changela K, Papafragkakis H, et al. Over the scope clip: technique and expanding clinical applications. J Clin Gastroenterol 2013;47:749–56.
76. Lee M. Caustic ingestion and upper digestive tract injury. Dig Dis Sci 2010;55:1547–9.
77. Prata Martins F, Bonilha DR, Correia LP, et al. Obstructive jaundice caused by hemobilia after liver biopsy. Endoscopy 2008;40(Suppl 2):E265–6.
78. Sandblom P. Hemobilia (biliary tract hemorrhage). History, pathology, diagnosis, treatment. Springfield (IL): Charles C Thomas; 1972.
79. Green MH, Duell RM, Johnson CD, et al. Haemobilia. Br J Surg 2001;88:773–86.
80. Hommes M, Kazemier G, van Dijk LC, et al. Complex liver trauma with bilhemia treated with perihepatic packing and endovascular stent in the vena cava. J Trauma 2009;67:E51–3.
81. Sandblom P. Gastrointestinal hemorrhage through the pancreatic duct. Ann Surg 1970;171:61–6.
82. Etienne S, Pessaux P, Tuech JJ, et al. Hemosuccus pancreaticus: a rare cause of gastrointestinal bleeding. Gastroenterol Clin Biol 2005;29:237–42.

83. Kuganeswaran E, Smith OJ, Goldman ML, et al. Hemosuccus pancreaticus: rare complication of chronic pancreatitis. Gastrointest Endosc 2000;51:464–5.
84. Vimalraj V, Kannan DG, Sukumar R, et al. Haemosuccus pancreaticus: diagnostic and therapeutic challenges. HPB (Oxford) 2009;11:345–50.
85. Pore G. GI lesions in Henoch-Schonlein purpura. Gastrointest Endosc 2002;55: 283–6.
86. Chae EJ, Do KH, Seo JB, et al. Radiologic and clinical findings of Behcet disease: comprehensive review of multisystemic involvement. Radiographics 2008;28:e31.
87. Perez RA, Silver D, Banerjee B. Polyarteritis nodosa presenting as massive upper gastrointestinal hemorrhage. Surg Endosc 2000;14:87.
88. Pagnoux C, Mahr A, Cohen P, et al. Presentation and outcome of gastrointestinal involvement in systemic necrotizing vasculitides: analysis of 62 patients with polyarteritis nodosa, microscopic polyangiitis, Wegener granulomatosis, Churg-Strauss syndrome, or rheumatoid arthritis-associated vasculitis. Medicine (Baltimore) 2005;84:115–28.
89. Kuipers EJ, van Leeuwen MA, Nikkels PG, et al. Hemobilia due to vasculitis of the gall bladder in a patient with mixed connective tissue disease. J Rheumatol 1991;18:617–8.
90. Steen S, Lamont J, Petrey L. Acute gastric dilation and ischemia secondary to small bowel obstruction. Proc (Bayl Univ Med Cent) 2008;21:15–7.
91. Lewis S, Holbrook A, Hersch P. An unusual case of massive gastric distension with catastrophic sequelae. Acta Anaesthesiol Scand 2005;49:95–7.
92. Mensink PB, Moons LM, Kuipers EJ. Chronic gastrointestinal ischaemia: shifting paradigms. Gut 2010;60:722–37.
93. Fiddian-Green RG, Stanley JC, Nostrant T, et al. Chronic gastric ischemia. A cause of abdominal pain or bleeding identified from the presence of gastric mucosal acidosis. J Cardiovasc Surg (Torino) 1989;30:852–9.
94. Sharlow JW, Cone JB, Schaefer RF. Acute gastric necrosis in the postoperative period. South Med J 1989;82:529–30.

Emerging Endoscopic Therapies for Nonvariceal Upper Gastrointestinal Bleeding

Louis M. Wong Kee Song, MD*, Michael J. Levy, MD

KEYWORDS

- Cryotherapy • Endoscopic suturing • EUS-guided angiotherapy • Hemostasis
- Hemostatic spray • Nonvariceal upper gastrointestinal bleeding
- Over-the-scope clip • Radiofrequency ablation

KEY POINTS

- Emerging techniques for endoscopic hemostasis of nonvariceal upper gastrointestinal bleeding include over-the-scope clips, hemostatic sprays, mucosal ablation devices (cryotherapy and radiofrequency ablation), endoscopic suturing, and endoscopic ultrasound–guided angiotherapy.
- These techniques may be used as primary or rescue therapy, depending on the types of lesions targeted and the response to standard hemostatic modalities.
- An understanding of the technical aspects and limitations of these devices as well as proper patient and lesion selection helps optimize the utilization of these techniques in nonvariceal upper gastrointestinal bleeding.

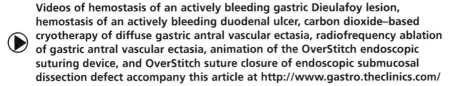

Videos of hemostasis of an actively bleeding gastric Dieulafoy lesion, hemostasis of an actively bleeding duodenal ulcer, carbon dioxide–based cryotherapy of diffuse gastric antral vascular ectasia, radiofrequency ablation of gastric antral vascular ectasia, animation of the OverStitch endoscopic suturing device, and OverStitch suture closure of endoscopic submucosal dissection defect accompany this article at http://www.gastro.theclinics.com/

INTRODUCTION

Injection therapy (eg, epinephrine and sclerosant), thermal coagulation with contact (eg, bipolar) and noncontact (eg, argon plasma coagulation [APC]) probes, and mechanical devices (eg, hemoclips and band ligation) are established modalities for

Disclosures: None.
Division of Gastroenterology and Hepatology, Mayo Clinic, 200 1st Street Southwest, Rochester, MN 55905, USA
* Corresponding author.
E-mail address: wong.louis@mayo.edu

Gastroenterol Clin N Am 43 (2014) 721–737
http://dx.doi.org/10.1016/j.gtc.2014.08.005
0889-8553/14/$ – see front matter © 2014 Elsevier Inc. All rights reserved.

the endoscopic management of nonvariceal upper gastrointestinal bleeding (NVUGIB) lesions.[1] Although these techniques are often effective at achieving hemostasis, the benefit is not always sustained or their application not feasible because of the location, characteristics, and/or extent of the bleeding lesion. The introduction of novel hemostatic devices and innovative use of existing techniques are likely to enhance primary or rescue therapy for NVUGIB lesions that are not amenable, or refractory, to standard therapy. In this article, the techniques and clinical applications of these emerging modalities is highlighted from a device perspective.

OVER-THE-SCOPE CLIPS
Devices and Techniques

Over-the-scope (OTS) clips radically differ in design compared with standard through-the-scope (TTS) clips. In experimental studies, OTS clips provided more secure vascular closure because of the enhanced tissue capture and greater compressive force than TTS clips.[2,3] Two types of OTS clips are currently available. The over-the-scope clip (OTSC, Ovesco Endoscopy AG, Tubingen, Germany) is akin to a bear claw and offers a short learning curve because its setup and deployment are similar to a band ligator. The nitinol-based OTSC is preloaded in a bent state over a clear cap (**Fig. 1**). OTSC caps are available in 3 diameters (11, 12, and 14 mm) and 2 working depths (3 and 6 mm). The clips also come in 3 types of teeth (atraumatic [a], traumatic [t], and gastrostomy closure [gc]) (**Fig. 2**). Both the a (atraumatic or blunt-toothed) and t (traumatic or sharp-toothed) clips have been used for the treatment of focal NVUGIB lesions. The a-type clip is adequate for most pliable bleeding lesions, especially in the thin-walled esophagus. The bite of the t-type clip likely enables more secure anchoring into indurated tissue, such as a fibrotic ulcer base. Similar to band ligation, the OTSC is affixed to the tip of the endoscope; clip deployment is achieved by triggering a string wire connected to a rotating hand wheel that is fastened to the entrance port of the working channel. Suction is applied to engage the target lesion into the cap before release of the clip, which assumes its naturally closed state (Video 1). For indurated lesions (eg, chronic ulcers), a dedicated tripronged anchoring device can assist in retracting the ulcer base into the cap (**Fig. 3**).

The Padlock clip (Aponos Medical Corp, Kingston, NH) is another recently approved OTS clip whose trigger wire is located alongside the shaft of the endoscope. This design, which does not use the working channel, allows more efficient suction of the target lesion into the cap, passage of other accessories, and continued suction of blood and secretions. Deployment of the clip is achieved by squeezing a handheld

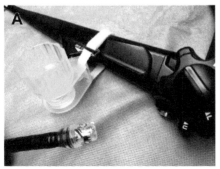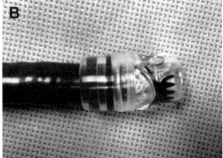

Fig. 1. (A) OTS clip device. (B) OTS clip preloaded onto a clear cap.

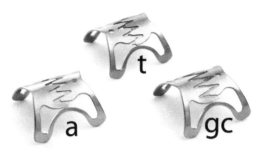

Fig. 2. OTS clips with 3 types of teeth.

device (**Fig. 4**). The Padlock clip has shown reliable closure of defects in a porcine survival study,[4] although clinical usage remains limited. As yet, there are no published data regarding its application in the management of NVUGIB lesions.

Clinical Applications

The reported efficacy and safety of OTSC for the treatment of NVUGIB lesions are limited to a handful of single reports and small case series. The overall success rate ranges from 71% to 100% for the treatment of various bleeding lesions, including Mallory-Weiss tears, peptic ulcers (**Fig. 5**), Dieulafoy lesions (**Fig. 6**), anastomotic ulcers, eroding tumors, and postpolypectomy ulcers (**Fig. 7**).[5–10]

In some studies, OTSC was used primarily as salvage therapy for NVUGIB lesions in which conventional hemostatic therapies had failed. In one retrospective series, OTSC was successful in securing hemostasis in 91% of cases (n = 23), which consisted of duodenal ulcers (n = 12), gastric ulcers (n = 6), Mallory-Weiss tears (n = 2), Dieulafoy lesions (n = 2), and a surgical anastomotic bleed (n = 1). The 2 failures involved peptic ulcers, and there were no adverse events reported.[11] In another series of 9 patients with refractory or major bleeding from nonvariceal upper gastrointestinal (GI) lesions, the technical and clinical success (absence of rebleeding) rates were 100% and 77.8%, respectively. Lesions included gastric ulcers (n = 2), duodenal ulcers (n = 5), a gastric stromal tumor (n = 1), and luminal ulceration secondary to pancreatic

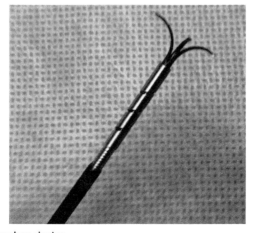

Fig. 3. Tripronged anchor device.

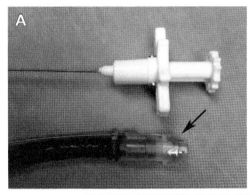

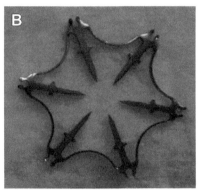

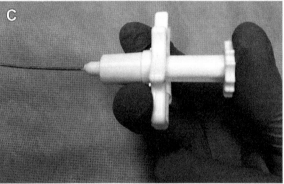

Fig. 4. (A) Padlock clip device mounted on tip of endoscope (*arrow*). (B) Clip configuration after deployment. (C) Squeeze handle for clip deployment.

cancer (n = 1). The 2 failures involved duodenal ulcers. The OTSC retention time was 28 days (range 0–42).[12]

The OTSC seems useful either as a primary modality or as a rescue therapy for NVU-GIB lesions that are refractory to standard therapies. However, disadvantages of the device include the need to withdraw the endoscope to mount the OTSC, potential

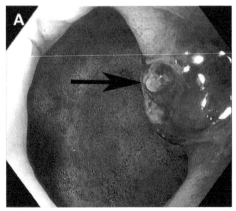

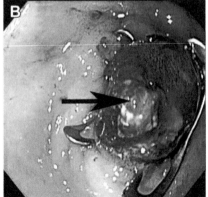

Fig. 5. (A) Pyloric channel ulcer with visible vessel (*arrow*). (B) Appearance following OTS clip placement (*arrow*).

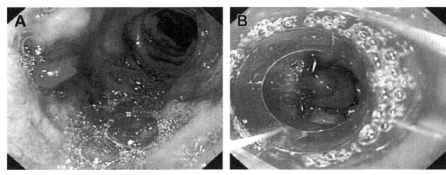

Fig. 6. (A) Duodenal Dieulafoy lesion. (B) Appearance following OTS clip placement.

difficulty in traversing the upper esophageal sphincter or luminal strictures, clip misplacement that interferes with subsequent therapy, and difficulty accessing lesions in certain locations (eg, posterior-inferior wall of duodenum and gastric lesser curve). Its application may also be impaired when attempting to capture firm and/or thick lesions (eg, deeply penetrating fibrotic ulcer) into the OTSC cap despite the assistance of devices for retraction.

Although the cost of a single OTSC device is several-fold higher than that of a conventional TTS clip, the former may be more cost-effective when considering the comparative outcomes, such as the rebleeding rate or number of clips required to achieve hemostasis. Prospective randomized trials and cost-efficacy analyses comparing OTS clip devices with traditional techniques (eg, TTS clips and coaptive coagulation) are anticipated.

HEMOSTATIC SPRAYS
Devices and Techniques

Hemostatic dressings or gauzes are an essential component of the military's first-aid kits for control of external wound bleeding in the battlefield. These dressings incorporate hemostatic agents, derived from chitosan and minerals, in the form of granules and powders.[13]

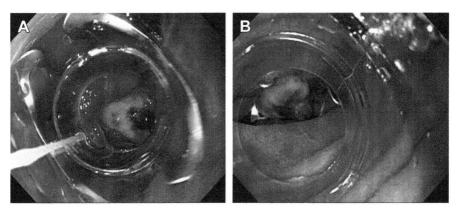

Fig. 7. (A) After duodenal endoscopic mucosal resection with delayed bleeding and visible vessel in ulcer base. (B) Appearance following OTS clip placement.

One such proprietary compound, TC-325, is an inorganic absorbent powder that forms an adherent coagulum at the targeted site; this agent has been integrated into a pressurized carbon dioxide (CO_2) gas–propelled, push-button device for endoscopic hemostasis (**Fig. 8**) (Hemospray, Cook Medical Inc, Bloomington, IN).

The adoption of hemostatic sprays as part of endoscopic therapy has been facilitated by their ease of use. Unlike conventional contact (eg, bipolar probe) and noncontact (eg, APC) thermal modalities, the application of hemostatic sprays requires less precision and can be delivered to poorly accessible anatomic sites, such as the proximal lesser curve of the stomach and posterior wall of the duodenum. Given the mechanism of action, the use of hemostatic sprays is limited to lesions or surface areas that are actively bleeding (**Fig. 9**). The Hemospray powder is delivered in short, 1- to 2-second bursts to the target site via a TTS catheter (Video 2). In one study, up to 150 g of the powder (21 g per cartridge) was allowed per treatment session,[14] although the maximum tolerated dose that can be administered in a single session has not been determined. The coagulum usually sloughs off in a few days and is naturally excreted. Although endoscopic visualization is hampered during Hemospray application, the therapeutic benefit remains because precise targeting is not required. However, the delivery of subsequent therapies, should bleeding persist, is hindered by the cloudy field of view and adherent coagulum. Hemospray is commercially available in several countries but is not yet cleared by the Food and Drug Administration for use in the United States.

Plant-derived hemostatic agents, such as the Ankaferd Blood Stopper (ABS; Ankaferd Health Products Ltd, Istanbul, Turkey), have been described for endoscopic applications. ABS is an herbal extract approved in Turkey for topical treatment of dental and postsurgical external hemorrhage. It induces formation of an encapsulated proteinlike mesh that serves as a scaffold for rapid red blood cell aggregation without significantly interfering with individual coagulation factors or platelets.[15] The ABS solution is sprayed onto the bleeding site until a yellowish-grey adherent coagulum is formed. The amount required (2–25 mL) and the time to hemostasis (seconds to minutes) vary according to bleeding severity and targeted surface area. A polysaccharide-based hemostatic spray agent (EndoClot Plus Inc, Santa Clara, CA) that could be applied endoscopically has been described, although there are no published data regarding its use for nonvariceal upper GI bleeding.[16]

Clinical Applications

In the first prospective pilot study regarding Hemospray, initial hemostasis was achieved in 95% of patients (n = 20) with actively bleeding peptic ulcers. Recurrent

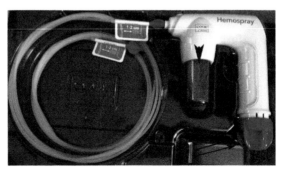

Fig. 8. Handheld Hemospray device with CO_2 gas–propelled canister (*double arrows*) and hemostatic powder cartridge (*arrowhead*). (*Courtesy of* Cook Medical, Winston-Salem, NC; with permission.)

A

B

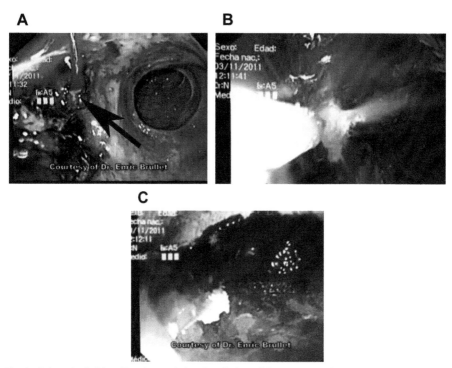

C

Fig. 9. (*A*) Actively bleeding (*arrow*) duodenal ulcer. (*B*) Initiation of Hemospray application. (*C*) Hemostasis achieved following Hemospray application. (*Courtesy of* Dr Enric Brullet, Barcelona, Spain.)

bleeding occurred in 2 patients for an overall success rate of 85%. Clean base ulcers without residual coagulum were noted during second-look endoscopy at 72 hours. No adverse events were reported at the 1-month follow-up.[14] A European multicenter registry study, presented in abstract form, included 71 patients treated with Hemospray as monotherapy (55%), first-line combination therapy (8%), or rescue therapy (34%) for a variety of NVUGIB lesions that included peptic ulcers (58%), esophageal ulcers (4%), tumors (7%), Dieulafoy lesions (4%), after mucosectomy (3%), gastric antral vascular ectasia (GAVE) (3%), and miscellaneous causes (21%). Primary hemostasis was achieved in 85% of patients; adverse events were mostly technical in nature, including occlusion of the spray catheter or instrument channel (n = 5), endoscope adhesion to the mucosa (n = 2), and device failure (n = 1).[17] Hemospray has also been used with variable success for tumor bleeding, an often difficult condition to treat endoscopically.[18,19]

Several single case reports and small case series originating primarily from Turkey have described the hemostatic potential of ABS for various NVUGIB lesions, including Mallory-Weiss tears, Dieulafoy lesions, GAVE, anastomotic ulcers, sphincterotomy sites, postpolypectomy sites, and tumor bleeding.[20,21]

The available evidence supports the use of hemostatic sprays as the primary or bridge therapy, particularly in the management of oozing-type lesions. The efficacy of these agents may be limited in the setting of brisk bleeding because of the rapid wash-away effect of the hemostatic agent[22] and in patients receiving antithrombotic therapy who present with spurting arterial bleeding.[23] Given their mechanism of action, hemostatic agents do not seem to be of value for the management of nonactively bleeding lesions.

CRYOTHERAPY
Devices and Techniques

Cryotherapy causes frostbite injury, which results in superficial mucosal necrosis and ulceration. The treated tissue sloughs within days of therapy, followed by epithelial regeneration over several weeks.[24] Commercially available, catheter-based endoscopic cryotherapy systems use either liquid nitrogen (CSA Medical Inc, Lutherville, MD) or compressed CO_2 gas (Polar Wand, GI Supply, Camp Hill, PA) as cryogens.

The published experience on the application of cryotherapy for NVUGIB lesions is currently limited to the low-cost, portable CO_2 unit. A dedicated spray catheter is extended 1 to 2 cm distal to the tip of the endoscope, and spraying of the compressed CO_2 cryogen is activated by a foot pedal. The technique is based on the principle of the Joule-Thompson effect in which rapid expansion of the CO_2 gas results in freezing to $-78°C$ as it exits the catheter. A high volume of CO_2 gas (~8 L/min) is delivered during the procedure; therefore, a gastric length overtube or a dedicated decompression tube is required to vent the stomach (**Fig. 10**). The cryogenic spray is applied to the targeted mucosal surface until whitening (icing) occurs, which is followed by thawing on termination of spraying (Video 3). The freeze-thaw cycle is typically repeated 3 to 5 times per treatment session.

Clinical Applications

The application of cryotherapy for NVUGIB lesions has focused primarily on GAVE. In a small pilot study (n = 12), the endoscopic appearance and hemoglobin level improved significantly in 50% of transfusion-dependent patients after 3 cryotherapy sessions delivered at 3- to 6-week intervals. A partial response was obtained in the remaining cases. No treatment-related adverse events occurred.[25]

The advantages of cryotherapy include ease of use and the ability to rapidly treat a large surface area. This modality appears suitable for ablation of mucosal vascular lesions, such as GAVE and radiation-induced telangiectasia, particularly when the distribution of these lesions is diffuse and extensive (**Fig. 11**). However, multiple treatment sessions seem necessary before a sustained response is achieved. The optimal treatment protocol based on the type of cryogen used, number of freeze-thaw cycles, duration of cryospray, and time interval between treatment sessions has not been determined.

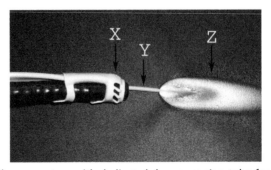

Fig. 10. CO_2 cryotherapy system with dedicated decompression tube for venting (X), cryospray catheter (Y), and icing effect (Z).

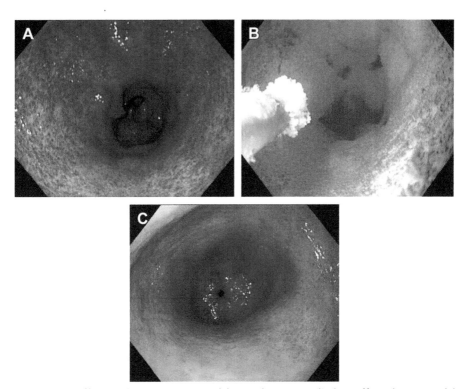

Fig. 11. (*A*) Diffuse and extensive GAVE. (*B*) Cryotherapy applied to affected mucosa. (*C*) Improvement endoscopic appearance of GAVE at 1-month follow-up.

RADIOFREQUENCY ABLATION
Devices and Techniques

Balloon-based and focal catheters for radiofrequency ablation (RFA) (Barrx, Covidien, Mansfield, MA) have been used primarily for the eradication of Barrett esophagus.[26] More recently, OTS focal RFA catheters of various dimensions have been used for the treatment of GAVE.[27–29] A focal RFA catheter consists of a tilting platform containing an array of electrodes that is mounted at the tip of the endoscope (**Fig. 12**). The

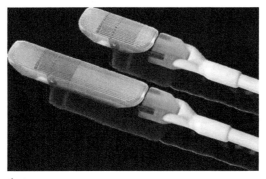

Fig. 12. OTS RFA catheters.

active electrodes range from 15 to 40 mm in length and from 7.5 to 13.0 mm in width. The recently introduced channel RFA catheter has a smaller treatment surface area (15.7 mm × 7.5 mm), but this rotatable TTS device is advantageous in terms of ease of use (**Fig. 13**). It is inserted through an introducer at the entrance port of the working channel and is easily removed for intermittent electrode cleaning, which is often necessary with this device. Following tissue contact, both the focal and channel RFA catheters can provide a uniform superficial depth of thermal injury using a treatment protocol of 2 to 4 energy applications per targeted site at a setting of 12 J/cm^2 (**Fig. 14**). Following the treatment of one area, the catheter is repositioned over an adjacent untreated site for ablation; this process is continued until all affected areas have been ablated (Video 4).

Clinical Applications

As mentioned previously, the application of RFA for NVUGIB has focused primarily on GAVE. In a recent prospective study, 18 of 21 patients (86%) with GAVE refractory to APC became transfusion independent over a 6-month follow-up period after a median of 2 (range 1–3) RFA sessions delivered 4 to 6 weeks apart. Mean hemoglobin increased from 7.8 g/dL to 10.2 g/dL in responders (n = 18). Two adverse events occurred (minor acute bleeding and superficial ulceration), which resolved without intervention.[29]

Although the treated surface area is larger relative to APC, the use of focal RFA catheters is cumbersome and relatively expensive. Technical challenges with the OTS ablation catheters include the potential for difficult esophageal intubation; need for repeated intubations for cleaning the electrode; and difficulty in achieving uniform electrode-tissue contact in some areas, such as the incisura. The advent of the TTS channel RFA device may obviate some of the challenges related to the OTS catheters, although cost may prohibit RFA as the initial therapy for GAVE and for other mucosal-based vascular lesions. Cost-efficacy trials may clarify the position of RFA as the primary therapy for GAVE or as the rescue therapy for refractory cases.

ENDOSCOPIC SUTURING
Devices and Techniques

Among several endoscopic suturing devices that have been evaluated in experimental trials and pilot studies,[30] only one is currently in clinical use (OverStitch, Apollo Endosurgery, Austin, TX) (**Fig. 15**). The OverStitch device requires loading onto a specific double-channel endoscope (GIF 2T160, Olympus Corporation, Tokyo, Japan) and consists of a curved needle with a detachable tip that carries an absorbable or nonabsorbable suture. The handle portion of the system is affixed at the entrance port of the working channel, which activates transfer of the needle tip to enable passage and exit of the suture through tissue (Video 5). A dedicated corkscrewlike retracting device (Helix, Apollo Endosurgery, Austin, TX) or a grasping forceps can be inserted through

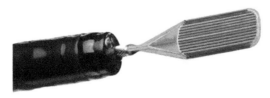

Fig. 13. TTS, rotatable RFA catheter.

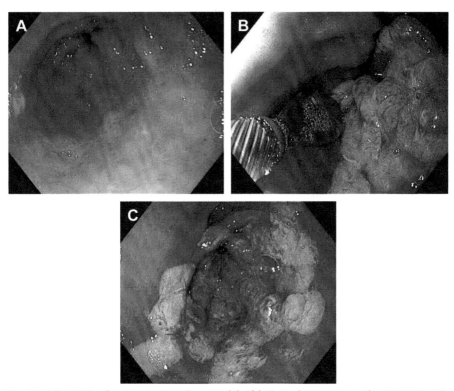

Fig. 14. (*A*) GAVE refractory to APC therapy. (*B*) Ablation of GAVE using the TTS RFA catheter. (*C*) Appearance of treated mucosa following RFA therapy.

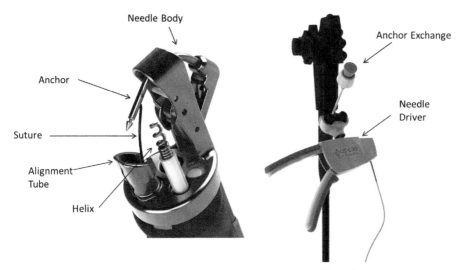

Fig. 15. OverStitch endoscopic suturing system. (*Courtesy of* Apollo Endosurgery, Austin, TX; with permission.)

the second working channel of the endoscope to facilitate tissue approximation for full-thickness suture placement. Stitches can be placed in an interrupted or running fashion without the need for device removal. A cinching catheter is used to tighten and release the suture. The suturing system can be used with or without an esophageal overtube.

Clinical Applications

Data are lacking on the use of the OverStitch suturing device for the acute management of NVUGIB lesions. Although the concept of oversewing a lesion through an endoscope is appealing, device limitations, such as the technical complexity and the need for a specialized double-channel endoscope, impaired visibility in the setting of active bleeding, and restricted maneuverability and access to certain anatomic locations of the upper GI tract, have limited the use of this suturing system in the acute setting. However, the device seems well suited to manage chronic blood loss resulting from anastomotic ulcers[31] and for the prevention of delayed bleeding following endoscopic mucosal resection (EMR) or endoscopic submucosal dissection (ESD) (**Fig. 16** and Video 6).[32]

ENDOSCOPIC ULTRASOUND–GUIDED ANGIOTHERAPY
Devices and Techniques

Endoscopic ultrasound (EUS)–guided angiotherapy with Doppler monitoring of the vascular response is a promising modality for the management of select bleeding

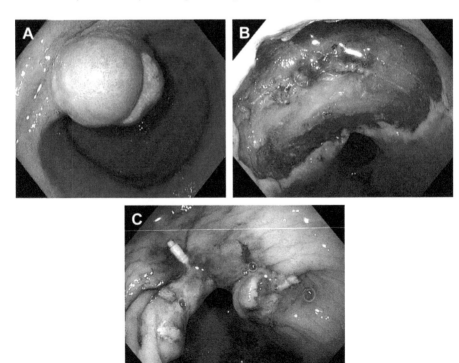

Fig. 16. (A) Large ulcerated antral polypoid lesion. (B) ESD of lesion. (C) Closure of ESD defect for prevention of delayed bleeding.

lesions that are inaccessible or refractory to standard endoscopic and interventional radiologic techniques. EUS may detect culprit vascular lesions in the wall of the GI tract that are not visually apparent at endoscopy[33] and target lesions for fine-needle injection (FNI) of therapeutic agents into feeding vessels (**Fig. 17**).

Standard EUS-guided FNI techniques have been used to inject a variety of agents, including sclerosants, thrombin, and cyanoacrylates, into variceal and nonvariceal lesions.[34–37] Microcoils that were initially developed for percutaneous delivery have been used more recently for EUS-guided angiographic embolization.[38,39]

Clinical Applications

Although most reports on EUS-guided angiotherapy pertain to varices,[38–42] the technique has also been described for the management of NVUGIB lesions. The feasibility of EUS-guided angiotherapy for such lesions was reported in a series of 5 patients, 4 of whom had severe bleeding refractory to standard endoscopic and/or angiographic techniques. EUS-guided injection of absolute alcohol or cyanoacrylate injection into the bleeding vessels of a pancreatic pseudoaneurysm, a duodenal Dieulafoy lesion, a duodenal ulcer, and GI stromal tumors resulted in sustained hemostasis in all cases without adverse events.[43] Other anecdotal reports have demonstrated the successful use of EUS-guided injection of cyanoacrylate or thrombin for hemostasis of a bleeding side branch of the gastroduodenal artery; Dieulafoy lesions; and pseudoaneurysms of viscera, superior mesenteric artery, and splenic artery.[44–49]

A

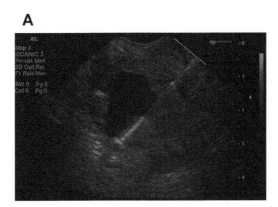

B

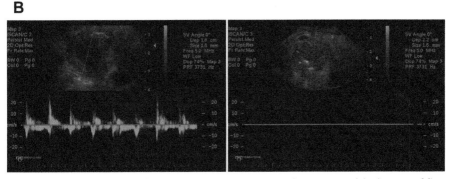

Fig. 17. (*A*) EUS-guided FNI of sclerosant in pancreatic pseudoaneurysm. (*B*) Absence of flow by Doppler following injection therapy.

Although the feasibility and apparent safety of EUS-guided angiotherapy has been demonstrated, broad use among endosonographers has been hampered by a lack of endosonographer training expertise, limited availability of EUS in the acute care setting, precipitation of extraluminal hemorrhage requiring salvage angiographic or surgical therapy, and thromboembolic adverse events. Further studies regarding patient selection criteria, efficacy, and safety of EUS-guided angiotherapy are anticipated.

MISCELLANEOUS

Dedicated stents for esophageal variceal tamponade have been developed as a more appealing alternative to balloon tamponade.[50] Similarly, certain NVUGIB lesions, such as postsphincterotomy and bleeding at cyst-gastrostomy sites, often respond favorably to placement of covered self-expandable metal stents and, thus, should be considered when conventional endoscopic therapies have failed.[51–57]

The injection of tissue glues for various NVUGIB lesions has been described. However, their use should be reserved for bleeding lesions that have failed standard therapy given the potential for serious adverse events, including tissue necrosis, embolization, infection, formation of sinus tracts, and perforation.[58]

SUMMARY

Several new devices and innovative modifications to existing treatment modalities have emerged as effective primary, adjuvant, or rescue therapies for the management of NVUGIB lesions. The indications, efficacy, and safety of these emerging techniques continue to be defined. Such data are eagerly sought to more accurately determine the role of these modalities into the standard clinical treatment algorithm for patients with NVUGIB lesions.

SUPPLEMENTARY DATA

Supplementary data related to this article can be found online at http://dx.doi.org/10.1016/j.gtc.2014.08.005.

REFERENCES

1. ASGE Technology Committee, Conway JD, Adler DG, et al. Endoscopic hemostatic devices. Gastrointest Endosc 2009;69:987–96.
2. Naegel A, Bolz J, Zopf Y, et al. Hemodynamic efficacy of the over-the-scope clip in an established porcine cadaveric model for spurting bleeding. Gastrointest Endosc 2012;75:152–9.
3. Kato M, Jung Y, Gromski MA, et al. Prospective, randomized comparison of 3 different hemoclips for the treatment of acute upper GI hemorrhage in an established experimental setting. Gastrointest Endosc 2012;75:3–10.
4. Guarner-Argente C, Córdova H, Martínez-Pallí G, et al. Yes, we can: reliable colonic closure with the Padlock-G clip in a survival porcine study (with video). Gastrointest Endosc 2010;72:841–4.
5. Kirschniak A, Kratt T, Stüker D, et al. A new endoscopic over-the-scope clip system for treatment of lesions and bleeding in the GI tract: first clinical experiences. Gastrointest Endosc 2007;66:162–7.
6. Kirschniak A, Subotova N, Zieker D, et al. The over-the-scope clip (OTSC) for the treatment of gastrointestinal bleeding, perforations, and fistulas. Surg Endosc 2011;25:2901–5.

7. Albert JG, Friedrich-Rust M, Woeste G, et al. Benefit of a clipping device in use in intestinal bleeding and intestinal leakage. Gastrointest Endosc 2011;74: 389–97.

8. Baron TH, Song LM, Ross A, et al. Use of an over-the-scope clipping device: multicenter retrospective results of the first U.S. experience (with videos). Gastrointest Endosc 2012;76:202–8.

9. Singhal S, Changela K, Papafragkakis H, et al. Over the scope clip: technique and expanding clinical applications. J Clin Gastroenterol 2013;47:749–56.

10. Alcaide N, Peñas-Herrero I, Sancho-Del-Val L, et al. Ovesco system for treatment of postpolypectomy bleeding after failure of conventional treatment. Rev Esp Enferm Dig 2014;106:55–8.

11. Manta R, Galloro G, Mangiavillano B, et al. Over-the-scope clip (OTSC) represents an effective endoscopic treatment for acute GI bleeding after failure of conventional techniques. Surg Endosc 2013;27:3162–4.

12. Chan SM, Chiu PW, Teoh AY, et al. Use of the over-the-scope clip for treatment of refractory upper gastrointestinal bleeding: a case series. Endoscopy 2014;46: 428–31.

13. Gordy SD, Rhee P, Schreiber MA. Military applications of novel hemostatic devices. Expert Rev Med Devices 2011;8:41–7.

14. Sung JJ, Luo D, Wu JC, et al. Early clinical experience of the safety and effectiveness of Hemospray in achieving hemostasis in patients with acute peptic ulcer bleeding. Endoscopy 2011;43:291–5.

15. Goker H, Haznedaroglu IC, Ercetin S, et al. Haemostatic actions of the folkloric medicinal plant extract Ankaferd Blood Stopper. J Int Med Res 2008;36: 163–70.

16. Barkun AN, Moosavi S, Martel M. Topical hemostatic agents: a systematic review with particular emphasis on endoscopic application in GI bleeding. Gastrointest Endosc 2013;7:692–700.

17. Morris AJ, Smith LA, Stanley A, et al. Hemospray for non-variceal upper gastrointestinal bleeding: results of the SEAL dataset (survey to evaluate the application of Hemospray in the luminal tract) [abstract]. Gastrointest Endosc 2012;75: AB133–4.

18. Chen YI, Barkun AN, Soulellis C, et al. Use of the endoscopically applied hemostatic powder TC-325 in cancer-related upper GI hemorrhage: preliminary experience (with video). Gastrointest Endosc 2012;75:1278–81.

19. Leblanc S, Vienne A, Dhooge M, et al. Early experience with a novel hemostatic powder used to treat upper GI bleeding related to malignancies or after therapeutic interventions. Gastrointest Endosc 2013;78:169–74.

20. Beyazit Y, Kekilli M, Haznedaroglu IC, et al. Ankaferd hemostat in the management of gastrointestinal hemorrhages. World J Gastroenterol 2011;17:3962–70.

21. Gungor G, Goktepe MH, Biyik M, et al. Efficacy of Ankaferd Blood Stopper application on nonvariceal upper gastrointestinal bleeding. World J Gastrointest Endosc 2012;4:556–60.

22. Ozaslan E, Purnak T, Haznedaroglu IC. Ankaferd Blood Stopper in GI bleeding: alternative for everything? Gastrointest Endosc 2011;73:185–6.

23. Holster IL, Kuipers EJ, Tjwa ET. Hemospray in the treatment of upper gastrointestinal hemorrhage in patients on antithrombotic therapy. Endoscopy 2013;45: 63–6.

24. Kantsevoy SV, Cruz-Correa MR, Vaughn CA, et al. Endoscopic cryotherapy for the treatment of bleeding mucosal vascular lesions of the GI tract: a pilot study. Gastrointest Endosc 2003;57:403–6.

25. Cho S, Zanati S, Yong E, et al. Endoscopic cryotherapy for the management of gastric antral vascular ectasia. Gastrointest Endosc 2008;68:895–902.

26. Shaheen NJ, Sharma P, Overholt BF, et al. Radiofrequency ablation in Barrett's esophagus with dysplasia. N Engl J Med 2009;360:2277–88.

27. Gross SA, Al-Haddad M, Gill KR, et al. Endoscopic mucosal ablation for the treatment of gastric antral vascular ectasia with the HALO90 system: a pilot study. Gastrointest Endosc 2008;67:324–7.

28. Puri N, Mathur AK, Lopez J, et al. Comparative study of argon plasma coagulation and radiofrequency ablation using Halo90 device for treatment of gastric antral vascular ectasia lesions [abstract]. Gastrointest Endosc 2013;77:AB266.

29. McGorisk T, Krishnan K, Keefer L, et al. Radiofrequency ablation for refractory gastric antral vascular ectasia (with video). Gastrointest Endosc 2013;78:584–8.

30. ASGE Technology Committee, Banerjee S, Barth BA, et al. Endoscopic closure devices. Gastrointest Endosc 2012;76:244–51.

31. Jirapinyo P, Watson RR, Thompson CC. Use of a novel endoscopic suturing device to treat recalcitrant marginal ulceration (with video). Gastrointest Endosc 2012;76:435–9.

32. Kantsevoy SV, Bitner M, Mitrakov AA, et al. Endoscopic suturing closure of large mucosal defects after endoscopic submucosal dissection is technically feasible, fast, and eliminates the need for hospitalization (with videos). Gastrointest Endosc 2014;79:503–7.

33. Fockens P, Meenan J, van Dullemen HM, et al. Dieulafoy's disease: endosonographic detection and endosonography-guided treatment. Gastrointest Endosc 1996;44:437–42.

34. Levy MJ, Chak A, EUS 2008 Working Group. EUS 2008 Working Group document: evaluation of EUS-guided vascular therapy. Gastrointest Endosc 2009; 69(Suppl 2):S37–42.

35. Weilert F, Binmoeller KF. EUS-guided vascular access and therapy. Gastrointest Endosc Clin N Am 2012;22:303–14.

36. Seicean A. Endoscopic ultrasound in the diagnosis and treatment of upper digestive bleeding: a useful tool. J Gastrointestin Liver Dis 2013;22:465–9.

37. Bokun T, Grgurevic I, Kujundzic M, et al. EUS-guided vascular procedures: a literature review. Gastroenterol Res Pract 2013;2013:865945.

38. Binmoeller KF, Weilert F, Shah JN, et al. EUS-guided transesophageal treatment of gastric fundal varices with combined coiling and cyanoacrylate glue injection (with videos). Gastrointest Endosc 2011;74:1019–25.

39. Romero-Castro R, Ellrichmann M, Ortiz-Moyano C, et al. EUS-guided coil versus cyanoacrylate therapy for the treatment of gastric varices: a multicenter study (with videos). Gastrointest Endosc 2013;78:711–21.

40. de Paulo GA, Ardengh JC, Nakao FS, et al. Treatment of esophageal varices: a randomized controlled trial comparing endoscopic sclerotherapy and EUS-guided sclerotherapy of esophageal collateral veins. Gastrointest Endosc 2006;63:396–402 [quiz: 463].

41. Levy MJ, Wong Kee Song LM, Kendrick ML, et al. EUS-guided coil embolization for refractory ectopic variceal bleeding (with videos). Gastrointest Endosc 2008; 67:572–4.

42. Levy MJ, Wong Kee Song LM. EUS-guided angiotherapy for gastric varices: coil, glue, and sticky issues. Gastrointest Endosc 2013;78:722–5.

43. Levy MJ, Wong Kee Song LM, Farnell MB, et al. Endoscopic ultrasound (EUS)-guided angiotherapy of refractory gastrointestinal bleeding. Am J Gastroenterol 2008;103:352–9.

44. Gonzalez JM, Giacino C, Pioche M, et al. Endoscopic ultrasound-guided vascular therapy: is it safe and effective? Endoscopy 2012;44:539–42.
45. Roach H, Roberts SA, Salter R, et al. Endoscopic ultrasound-guided thrombin injection for the treatment of pancreatic pseudoaneurysm. Endoscopy 2005; 37:876–8.
46. Roberts KJ, Jones RG, Forde C, et al. Endoscopic ultrasound-guided treatment of visceral artery pseudoaneurysm. HPB 2012;14:489–90.
47. Chaves DM, Costa FF, Matuguma S, et al. Splenic artery pseudoaneurysm treated with thrombin injection guided by endoscopic ultrasound. Endoscopy 2012;44(Suppl 2):E99–100.
48. Robinson M, Richards D, Carr N. Treatment of a splenic artery pseudoaneurysm by endoscopic ultrasound-guided thrombin injection. Cardiovasc Intervent Radiol 2007;30:515–7.
49. Lameris R, du Plessis J, Nieuwoudt M, et al. A visceral pseudoaneurysm: management by EUS-guided thrombin injection. Gastrointest Endosc 2011;73: 392–5.
50. Wright G, Lewis H, Hogan B, et al. A self-expanding metal stent for complicated variceal hemorrhage: experience at a single center. Gastrointest Endosc 2010; 71:71–8.
51. Itoi T, Yasuda I, Doi S, et al. Endoscopic hemostasis using covered metallic stent placement for uncontrolled post-endoscopic sphincterotomy bleeding. Endoscopy 2011;43:369–72.
52. Shah JN, Marson F, Binmoeller KF. Temporary self-expandable metal stent placement for treatment of post-sphincterotomy bleeding. Gastrointest Endosc 2010;72:1274–8.
53. Aslinia F, Hawkins L, Darwin P, et al. Temporary placement of a fully covered metal stent to tamponade bleeding from endoscopic papillary balloon dilation. Gastrointest Endosc 2012;76:911–3.
54. Canena J, Liberato M, Horta D, et al. Short-term stenting using fully covered self-expandable metal stents for treatment of refractory biliary leaks, post-sphincterotomy bleeding, and perforations. Surg Endosc 2013;27:313–24.
55. DeBenedet AT, Elta GH. Post-sphincterotomy bleeding: fully-covered metal stents for hemostasis. F1000Res 2013;2:171.
56. Săftoiu A, Ciobanu L, Seicean A, et al. Arterial bleeding during EUS-guided pseudocyst drainage stopped by placement of a covered self-expandable metal stent. BMC Gastroenterol 2013;13:93.
57. Iwashita T, Lee JG, Nakai Y, et al. Successful management of arterial bleeding complicating endoscopic ultrasound-guided cystogastrostomy using a covered metallic stent. Endoscopy 2012;44(Suppl 2 UCTN):E370–1.
58. Cameron R, Binmoeller KF. Cyanoacrylate applications in the GI tract. Gastrointest Endosc 2013;77:846–57.

What if Endoscopic Hemostasis Fails?

Alternative Treatment Strategies: Interventional Radiology

Sujal M. Nanavati, MD

KEYWORDS

- Endoscopic hemostasis • Interventional radiology
- Acute upper gastrointestinal bleeding • Treatment • Embolization

KEY POINTS

- Medical and endoscopic therapy has been very successful at diminishing rates of upper gastrointestinal bleeding as well as in its treatment.
- There will be a small but challenging subset of patients for whom endoscopy cannot achieve hemostasis or will not be able to identify the source of bleeding.
- For persistent slow or intermittent bleeding that cannot be localized by esophagogastroduodenoscopy, further diagnostic evaluation with computed tomography angiography or scintigraphy should be considered.
- Individuals with active bleeding that is refractory to endoscopic treatment should undergo transcatheter angiography and intervention (TAI).
- TAI's technical and clinical success rates in most series are more than 90% and 70% for the treatment of upper gastrointestinal bleeding.

INTRODUCTION

Since the 1960s, interventional radiology (IR) has played a role in the management of gastrointestinal (GI) bleeding. What began primarily as a diagnostic modality has evolved into much more of a therapeutic tool. And although the frequency of GI bleeding has diminished thanks to management by pharmacologic and endoscopic methods, the need for additional invasive interventions still exists. Transcatheter angiography and intervention (TAI) is now a fundamental step in the algorithm for the treatment of GI bleeding.

Evolution

- 1963: Selective arteriography for localizing GI bleeding[1,2]
- 1968: Selective arterial infusion of vasopressin to reduce blood flow in superior mesenteric artery (SMA) and to reduce portal venous pressure[3,4]

Interventional Radiology, Department of Radiology and Biomedical Imaging, UCSF, 1001 Potrero Avenue, Rm. 1x55, San Francisco, CA 94110, USA
E-mail address: sujal.nanavati@ucsf.edu

Gastroenterol Clin N Am 43 (2014) 739–752
http://dx.doi.org/10.1016/j.gtc.2014.08.013
0889-8553/14/$ – see front matter © 2014 Elsevier Inc. All rights reserved.

- 1970: Selective embolization of gastroepiploic artery using autologous clot (in conjunction with epinephrine) to stop active bleeding from a gastric ulcer[5]
- 1970s to 1990s: Arterial infusion of vasopressin used to treat GI bleeding[4,6]
- 1990s to the present: Superselective arterial embolization becomes primary endovascular method for treatment of GI bleeding[7,8]

MATERIALS AND METHODS

In 1963, an angiogram was used as a means to help diagnose the presence of, as well as to help localize, a site of GI bleeding. The catheters available at that time allowed access to first-order and some second-order branches of the aorta but often not more distal. Embolic agents existed, but because they could not be deployed superselectively, the affected downstream territory was larger, with greater potential for ischemia. Sometimes, too proximal of an embolization did not treat direct collateral pathways to the bleeding site, resulting in ongoing or promptly recurring hemorrhage. Therefore, safe and effective treatment was somewhat limited.

Given the inability to reach sites of focal bleeding, more regional treatments were applied. Vasoconstrictive medications were administered intra-arterially to limit pressure and blood flow to sites of hemorrhage, facilitating hemostasis by patients' autologous clotting mechanisms. These arterial procedures typically lasted from 12 to 48 hours (**Table 1**).

Although the use of vasoconstrictive medications can be effective, especially for the treatment of diffuse bleeding, it has some clear limitations. Because the medication's effects cannot be confined to its site of administration, it poses significant systemic risks to anyone who has ischemic heart disease or prior stroke by further restricting blood flow to these areas. Additionally, because its effect ends on cessation of infusion, bleeding will resume if a stable clot has not formed. As a result, the rates of recurrence following therapeutic vasoconstriction were reported as high as 71%.[9]

With continued evolution of endovascular tools, however, the treatment options and their safety and efficacy increased significantly.

Probably the most important development that redefined the endovascular world was the development of the microcatheter. Microcatheters are small-diameter catheters (1.7–3.0 F catheters compared with 5–6 F diagnostic catheters) that can be navigated selectively into higher-order branch vessels, thereby allowing the targeting of very focal sites of vascular abnormality (**Figs. 1–3**). The microcatheters serve as a conduit for the instillation of contrast material as well as a variety of embolic agents.

Table 1 Basic procedural tools for TAI in treatment of GI bleeding	
Tool	Use
Access sheaths	Continuous arterial access; conduit through which exchange of catheters can take place without compromising access site; can provide continuous arterial pressure monitoring
Catheters and wires, including microcatheters and microwires	Numerous shapes and sizes allow selective and superselective catheterization to maximize diagnostic evaluation and targeted delivery of therapeutic materials
Embolic agents	Temporary (Gelfoam and autologous clot) and permanent (particulate, coils, liquids[10,11]); to occlude or promote autologous occlusion of target blood vessel
Vasopressin	Vasoconstrictor diminishes pressure and flow to promote autologous hemostasis

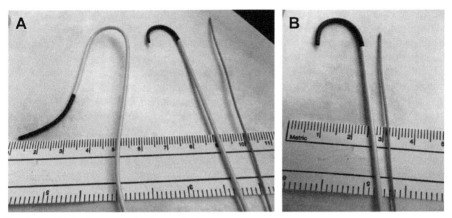

Fig. 1. (A, B) Catheters and microcatheters.

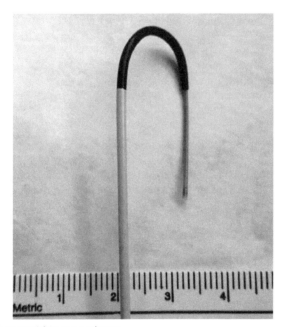

Fig. 2. Microcatheter within 5 F catheter.

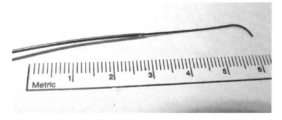

Fig. 3. Microwire within microcatheter

Embolic agents have also evolved significantly over the last few decades. Designed to fill spaces, embolic materials are used to help occlude blood vessels that are or may be supplying the sites of bleeding (**Figs. 4–8**). Preventing blood from reaching the site of vascular defect eliminates the loss of blood through the site.

At the same time, however, embolic agents restrict blood from reaching downstream, which can have ischemic effects on those tissues as well as any nontarget sites of embolization, especially if the collateral vascular supply is limited. This effect is the main risk in performing embolization. Targeted, superselective embolization, however, has helped mitigate the risk.

With improved safety and control, the use of embolization as a therapeutic tool has expanded significantly. This use includes its application in the treatment of upper GI bleeding (UGIB).

Upper Gastrointestinal Bleeding

- Bleeding into the GI tract proximal to the Ligament of Treitz

Cause

- Peptic ulcer disease, duodenal and gastric
- Gastritis and esophagitis
- Mallory-Weiss tear
- Iatrogenic, biopsy, sphincterotomy
- Marginal (postoperative anastomotic) ulcer
- Trauma, including hepatic and pancreatic
- Postpancreatitis pseudoaneurysm
- Dieulafoy lesion

In the realm of GI bleeding, management algorithms are simplified by separating UGIB (sites proximal to the Ligament of Treitz) from lower GI bleeding (sites distal to the Ligament of Treitz). The distinction is important because of both anatomic blood supply considerations as well as accessibility to the various therapeutic modalities.

Typical vascular supply

- *Celiac artery*: distal esophagus, stomach, duodenum, ampulla (pancreaticobiliary) (**Fig. 9**)
- *SMA*: duodenum, ampulla (pancreatic and variant hepatic) (**Fig. 10**)

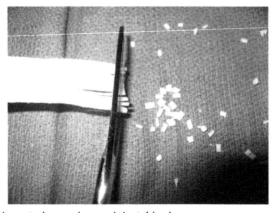

Fig. 4. Gelfoam pieces to be used as an injectable slurry.

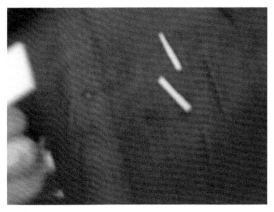

Fig. 5. Gelfoam torpedoes.

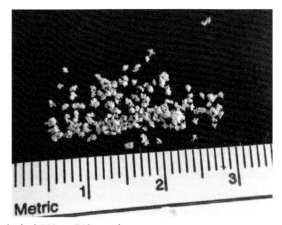

Fig. 6. Polyvinyl alcohol 500 to 710 μm sizes.

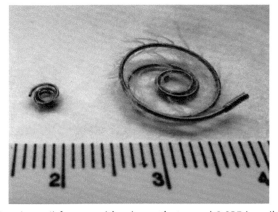

Fig. 7. An 0.018-in microcoil for use with microcatheter and 0.035-in coil.

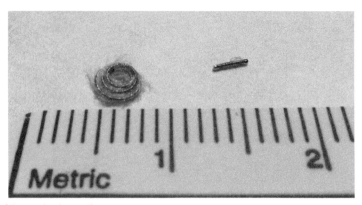

Fig. 8. Additional microcoils.

Upper GI bleeding arises in locations that are normally quite accessible to endoscopy. Additionally, these territories normally have richly overlapping blood supplies that can make hemorrhage difficult to control and recurrence rates higher when treated from intravascular locations, especially when the treatment locations are somewhat removed from the exact site of the vessel defect. For these reasons, endoscopy usually affords the best treatment option for most patients compared with TAI. Surgery is also a key component in the treatment algorithm, though it carries increased morbidity, especially in patients already in a tenuous condition.

For patients with UGIB in whom endoscopic treatment has not been successful, however, or for those who have had prior surgery preventing endoscopic access, TAI should be the next option to consider.

General upper gastrointestinal bleeding treatment considerations

- There is a rich overlap in blood supplies, so *endoscopy is most effective* in both treating and localizing the end sites of bleeding.
- For TAI, the collateral as well as primary blood supply must be evaluated and addressed, often necessitating treatment *proximal and distal* to the site of extravasation.
- Be aware of the patient's surgical *history* and its potential impact on vascular supply.

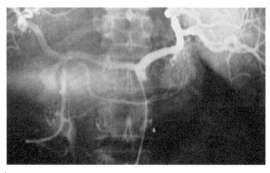

Fig. 9. Celiac arteriogram.

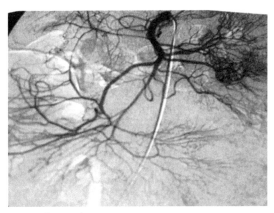

Fig. 10. Superior mesenteric arteriogram.

- *Surgery provides effective treatment*; but carries greater morbidity, especially in already acutely compromised individuals.

Upper gastrointestinal bleeding treatment options

- Watch and wait (most episodes are self-limited[12])
- Endoscopy will be (diagnostic, therapeutic, prognostic)
- Then TAI
- Surgery (endoscopy and TAI will be useful to temporize/optimize before surgery)

Because most episodes of GI bleeding are self-limited, it can sometimes be difficult to decide when to implement invasive treatment. To warrant the potential risk (and maximize the potential therapeutic benefit) of the invasive procedure, the patient's hemodynamic stability can be a primary determinant. Multiple studies have suggested that *hemodynamic instability* correlates with positive findings during catheter angiography, both localization and successful embolization.[13–15] The following parameters can serve as thresholds for the indication for TAI in GI bleeding:

- Systolic blood pressure less than 100 mm Hg
- Heart rate greater than 100 beats per minute
- ≥4 units packed red blood cells (RBCs) transfused in less than 24 hours

It is extremely important to use these parameters as a guide rather than absolute trigger points. They need to be considered in conjunction with each individual's overall clinical condition and comorbidities.

Diagnostic assessment

Endoscopy is usually successful in determining both whether there is active bleeding occurring as well as localizing the site of the bleeding. It should and will almost invariably be the primary diagnostic tool for UGIB. When additional diagnostic assessment is needed (often for difficult to localize or suspected slow or intermittent bleeding), multiple imaging modalities are available. Each one has different sensitivities for minimal bleeding rates and other advantages and disadvantages as well (**Tables 2** and **3**).

Local availability of a particular imaging resource as well as its qualified personnel will certainly affect the selection of diagnostic imaging modality. Otherwise, *factors helping to guide the selection of imaging options* are delineated in the following summary of the American College of Radiology's appropriateness guidelines:

Table 2
Imaging options to assess both UGIB and LGIB

Modality	Potentially Detectable Bleeding Rate (mL/min)
Scintigraphy Tc99 m sulfur colloid and RBCs	0.05–0.1[16–18]
CT angiography	0.35[a,19]
Catheter angiography	0.5[b,1]

Abbreviations: CT, computed tomography; LGIB, lower GI bleeding.
[a] In vitro studies suggest increased sensitivities to as low as 0.05 mL/min.
[b] Based on screen film angiography; studies suggest that digital subtraction angiography (most widely used today) may be 5 to 9 times more sensitive in detecting active bleeding (0.06–0.1 mL/min).[20]

Table 3
Advantages and disadvantages of imaging modalities

Modality	Advantages	Disadvantages
Scintigraphy	Can evaluate up to 24-h period, so greater sensitivity for intermittent or very slow bleeding	Lower accuracy of localization; availability can be limited
CT angiography	Wide availability; rapid acquisition; greater sensitivity compared with catheter angiography; can define pathology and suggest source, even in absence of active bleeding	Nontherapeutic; requires active bleeding at time of contrast instillation to definitively localize bleeding site; potential nephrotoxicity from iodinated contrast
Catheter angiography (TAI)	Therapeutic options; can provide localizing information for surgery	Requires active bleeding at time of image acquisition; invasive procedure with risks of adverse events

Imaging selection
Adapted American College of Radiology's appropriateness criteria on UGIB[21]

- Endoscopy identifies but does not resolve bleeding source:
  - TAI: usually appropriate
  - Computed tomography (CT) or scintigraphy: usually not appropriate
- Undefined source after endoscopy
  - CT: usually appropriate
  - TAI: usually appropriate, especially if brisk, active bleeding
  - Scintigraphy: usually appropriate if slow bleeding
- Undefined source after endoscopy AND history of pancreaticobiliary or aortic lesion or intervention
  - CT: usually appropriate
  - TAI: usually appropriate

Transcatheter Angiography and Intervention

Before using TAI to treat patients with GI bleeding, it will be helpful to perform a few basic tasks that are listed in **Table 4**. Besides aiding in monitoring fluid input and output, having a Foley catheter in place will prevent accumulation of contrast in the

Table 4
Steps to consider in preparation for TAI

Preprocedure	Benefit
Foley catheter	Limits accumulation of contrast in the bladder, which could obscure visualization of foci of contrast extravasation; useful for monitoring resuscitation efforts, fluid inputs and outputs
Oral contrast	If performing a CT to evaluate GI bleeding, avoid use of radiodense contrast agents in the GI tract, as these too can obscure detection of vascular contrast extravasation; water can be used as contrast in GI tract
Antiperistaltic medications	Can aid the benefit of digital subtraction by diminishing misregistration artifacts and stabilizing sites of extravasated contrast pooling; may allow detection of smaller, slower bleeding sites
Coagulopathy/ resuscitation	Continue resuscitation efforts and correction of mild coagulopathy during angiographic procedure, rather than waiting until full correction has been completed; correction might not be possible if significant blood loss is ongoing
Existing diagnostic information/ consultation	Review all diagnostic information already available, imaging and endoscopic; first catheterize the vascular territory that most likely supplies site of bleeding; ideally discuss treatment plan before starting procedure

bladder that may obscure detection of small sites of bleeding in the pelvic area. Similarly, if a CT scan is being performed as part of the diagnostic workup, it is important to avoid the use of radiodense oral contrast agents because they too may obscure the detection of small sites of contrast extravasation during angiography throughout the abdomen and pelvis and especially in the GI tract.

Preprocedural review and intraprocedural considerations

- *Review* all diagnostic imaging findings and surgical history.
- Review endoscopic findings with the gastroenterologist; *clips can help* target treatments, angiographic and surgical.[22]
- Discuss *treatment plans* before starting the procedure, including the possibility of *empiric* embolization (embolization of the vessel even though there is no angiographically demonstrable sign of bleeding; usually based on endoscopic diagnosis or surgical history).
- Administer *antiperistaltic agents* before the procedure.
- *Selective angiography* of celiac artery branches, including the gastroduodenal, proper hepatic, left gastric, and splenic artery may be required for complete diagnostic assessment (**Fig. 11**).
- Evaluate the SMA even if the focus of bleeding has been found and treated in celiac artery territory (**Fig. 12**).
- *Treat both proximal and distal* to the bleeding site, if necessary.
- For endoscopically, but not angiographically, apparent bleeding, there is the option of *empiric embolization*[15,23] to reduce perfusion pressure (gastroduodenal artery for duodenal bleeding; left gastric artery for gastric bleeding).
- Coils, particles, and an absorbable gelatin sponge (Gelfoam) are commonly used (*combination of agents* may be required).[24]
- *Postembolization angiography* is required prior to exam completion.

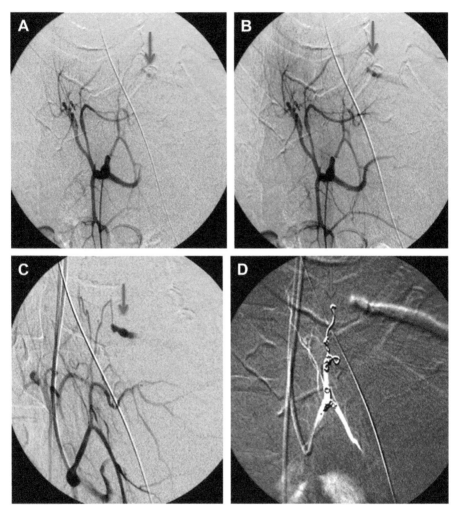

Fig. 11. (*A, B*) Celiac arteriography shows active extravasation (*arrow*) from bleeding ulcer in gastric fundus. (*C*) Left gastric arteriography further delineates extravasation (*arrow*) from superiorly directed branch. (*D*) Successful superselective branch embolization with coils (*arrow*).

RESULTS OF TRANSCATHETER ANGIOGRAPHY AND INTERVENTION IN UPPER GASTROINTESTINAL BLEEDING

Since the beginning of its use in the management of UGIB in the 1960s, TAI has shown increasing technical and clinical success rates. With a goal of hemostasis, most studies since 2000 show technical success rates greater than 90% and clinical success rates greater than 70% (**Tables 5** and **6**).

Additionally, studies suggest comparable clinical results for *empiric (endoscopically, but not angiographically, identified) embolization versus angiographically identified bleeding site embolization.*[15,23,32–35]

And clinical *results are comparable with surgical treatment*, even in patients deemed poor surgical candidates and those with more severe comorbid conditions.[28,29]

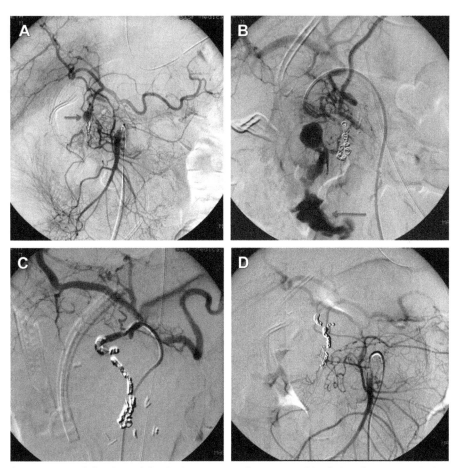

Fig. 12. UGIB following abdominal trauma and surgery with drain placements. Patient had already undergone recent IR embolization of gastroduodenal artery branch but now recurrence of UGIB. (A) Superior mesenteric arteriogram demonstrates large pseudoaneurysm (*straight arrow*) in pancreaticoduodenal branch territory in region of existing coils (*curved arrow*). (B) Selective gastroduodenal arteriography shows pseudoaneurysm and existing coils with extravasation of contrast into duodenum (*arrow*). (C) Selective gastroduodenal arteriography following coil deployment in superior pancreaticoduodenal branch supplying pseudoaneurysm. No filling of pseudoaneurysm is seen. (D) Superior mesenteric arteriography confirms lack of collateral backfilling to pseudoaneurysm from inferior pancreaticoduodenal branches.

Table 5
Technical success (cessation of contrast extravasation)

Study (No. of Patients)	Reported Technical Success (%)
Defreyne et al[25] (29)	97
Larssen et al[26] (36)	92
Loffroy et al[27] (33)	100
Loffroy et al[24] (60)	95
Wong et al[28] (30)	89

Data from Refs.[24–28]

Table 6
Clinical success (no ongoing bleeding or rebleeding, typically measured within 30 d)

Study	Reported Clinical Success (%)
Defreyne et al[25]	79
Ripoll et al[29]	71
Eriksson et al[30]	75
Defreyne et al[31]	88
Larssen et al[26]	72
Loffroy et al[27]	82
Loffroy et al[24]	72
Wong et al[28]	66

Data from Refs.[24–31]

Adverse Events

A 1992 study by Lang[36] reported a postembolization duodenal stricture rate of 16%. Seven of the 9 patients with the strictures had been embolized with a liquid embolic or a very small particle embolic agent to achieve terminal vessel occlusion.

Though this would result in greater likelihood for cessation of bleeding, there would also be a larger region of complete embolization and higher risk of ischemia and infarct. Microcoils and microcatheters now achieve superselective embolization with smaller affected area, and yet more complete, focussed embolization. As a result, more recent studies (since 2000) report major adverse event (those requiring subsequent treatment) rates less than 7%.[15,24,25,29,35,37–39] Most major adverse events seem to occur in individuals with preexisting vascular compromise: prior surgery or radiation treatments.

SUMMARY

Medical and endoscopic therapy has been very successful at diminishing the rates of GI bleeding as well as in its treatment. There will, however, be a small but challenging subset of patients for whom endoscopy cannot achieve hemostasis or will not be able to identify the source of bleeding. For these individuals, additional therapeutic and diagnostic tools will be required.

For persistent slow or intermittent bleeding that cannot be localized by esophagogastroduodenoscopy, further diagnostic evaluation with CT angiography (CTA) or scintigraphy should be considered.

Individuals with brisk, active bleeding that is refractory to endoscopic treatment should undergo TAI. CTA may still be considered but is often unnecessary, especially if the actively bleeding site has been marked with a metallic clip during endoscopy.

With increasing experience and continually evolving technology, TAI's technical and clinical success rates in most series are more than 90% and 70% for treatment of UGIB. Additionally, the rate of complication requiring subsequent treatment has been less than 7% in most studies since the year 2000. Given success rates that are comparable with surgical therapy, which includes the treatment of the sickest patients who are not surgical candidates, TAI should be considered the first option after failure of endoscopic treatment.

In a nutshell, when hemostasis for UGIB cannot be achieved endoscopically, consult the interventional radiologist.

REFERENCES

1. Nusbaum M, Baum S. Radiographic demonstration of unknown sites of gastrointestinal bleeding. Surg Forum 1963;14:374–5.

2. Baum S, Stein G, Nusbaum M, et al. Selective arteriography in the diagnosis of hemorrhage in the gastrointestinal tract. Radiol Clin North Am 1969;7:131–45.
3. Nusbaum M, Baum S, Kuroda K, et al. Control of portal hypertension by selective mesenteric arterial drug infusion. Arch Surg 1968;97:1005–13.
4. Baum S, Nusbaum M. The control of gastrointestinal hemorrhage by selective mesenteric arterial infusion of vasopressin. Radiology 1971;98:497–505.
5. Rösch J, Dotter CT, Brown MJ. Selective arterial embolization. A new method for control of acute gastrointestinal bleeding. Radiology 1972;102:303–6.
6. Baum S, Athanasoulis CA, Waltman AC, et al. Gastrointestinal hemorrhage: angiographic diagnosis and control. Adv Surg 1973;7:149–98.
7. Darcy M. Treatment of lower gastrointestinal bleeding: vasopressin infusion versus embolization. J Vasc Interv Radiol 2003;14(5):535–43.
8. Gordon RL, Ahl KL, Kerlan RK, et al. Selective arterial embolization for the control of lower gastrointestinal bleeding. Am J Surg 1997;174(1):24–8.
9. Waltman AC. Transcatheter embolization versus vasopressin infusion for the control of arteriocapillary gastrointestinal bleeding. Cardiovasc Intervent Radiol 1980;3(4):289–95.
10. Yata S, Ihaya T, Kaminou T, et al. Transcatheter arterial embolization of acute arterial bleeding in the upper and lower gastrointestinal tract with N-butyl-2-cyanoacrylate. J Vasc Interv Radiol 2013;24(3):422–31.
11. Urbano J, Manuel Cabrera J, Franco A, et al. Selective arterial embolization with ethylene-vinyl alcohol copolymer for control of massive lower gastrointestinal bleeding: feasibility and initial experience. J Vasc Interv Radiol 2014;25(6):839–46.
12. Welch CE, Hedberg S. Gastrointestinal hemorrhage. I. General considerations of diagnosis and therapy. Adv Surg 1973;7:95–148.
13. Abbas SM, Bissett IP, Holden A, et al. Clinical variables associated with positive angiographic localization of lower gastrointestinal bleeding. ANZ J Surg 2005;75(11):953–7.
14. Kim JH, Shin JH, Yoon HK, et al. Angiographically negative acute arterial upper and lower gastrointestinal bleeding: incidence, predictive factors, and clinical outcomes. Korean J Radiol 2009;10(4):384–90.
15. Aina R, Oliva VL, Therasse E, et al. Arterial embolotherapy for upper gastrointestinal hemorrhage: outcome assessment. J Vasc Interv Radiol 2001;12:195–200.
16. Alavi A, Dann RW, Baum S, et al. Scintigraphic detection of acute gastrointestinal bleeding. Radiology 1977;124:753–6.
17. Currie G, Towers P, Wheat J. Improved detection and localization of lower gastrointestinal hemorrhage using subtraction scintigraphy: phantom analysis. J Nucl Med Technol 2006;34:160–8.
18. Wu Y, Seto H, Shimizu M, et al. Sequential subtraction scintigraphy with ^{99m}Tc-RBC for the early detection of gastrointestinal bleeding and the calculation of bleeding rates: phantom and animal studies. Nucl Med Commun 1997;18:129–38.
19. Roy-Choudhury SH, Gallacher DJ, Pilmer J, et al. Relative threshold of detection of active arterial bleeding: in vitro comparison of MDCT and digital subtraction angiography. AJR Am J Roentgenol 2007;189:W238–46.
20. Kruger K, Heindel W, Dolken W, et al. Angiographic detection of gastrointestinal bleeding: an experimental comparison of conventional screen-film angiography and digital subtraction angiography. Invest Radiol 1996;31:451–7.
21. Schenker MP, Majdalany BS, Funaki BS, et al. ACR Appropriateness Criteria on upper gastrointestinal bleeding. J Am Coll Radiol 2010;7(11):845–53.
22. Eriksson LG, Sundbom M, Gustavsson S, et al. Endoscopic marking with a metallic clip facilitates transcatheter arterial embolization in upper peptic ulcer bleeding. J Vasc Interv Radiol 2006;17(6):959–64.

23. Lang EV, Picus D, Marx MV, et al. Massive upper gastrointestinal hemorrhage with normal findings on arteriography: value of prophylactic embolization of the left gastric artery. Am J Roentgenol 1992;158(3):547–9.

24. Loffroy R, Guiu B, D'Athis P, et al. Arterial embolotherapy for endoscopically unmanageable acute gastroduodenal hemorrhage: predictors of early rebleeding. Clin Gastroenterol Hepatol 2009;7(5):515–23.

25. Defreyne L, Vanlangenhove P, De Vos M, et al. Embolization as a first approach with endoscopically unmanageable acute nonvariceal gastrointestinal hemorrhage. Radiology 2001;218(3):739–48.

26. Larssen L, Moger T, Bjørnbeth BA, et al. Transcatheter arterial embolization in the management of bleeding duodenal ulcers: a 5.5-year retrospective study of treatment and outcome. Scand J Gastroenterol 2008;43(2):217–22.

27. Loffroy R, Guiu B, Cercueil JP, et al. Refractory bleeding from gastroduodenal ulcers: arterial embolization in high-operative-risk patients. J Clin Gastroenterol 2008;42(4):361–7.

28. Wong TC, Wong KT, Chiu PW, et al. A comparison of angiographic embolization with surgery after failed endoscopic hemostasis to bleeding peptic ulcers. Gastrointest Endosc 2011;73(5):900–8.

29. Ripoll C, Bañares R, Beceiro I, et al. Comparison of transcatheter arterial embolization and surgery for treatment of bleeding peptic ulcer after endoscopic treatment failure. J Vasc Interv Radiol 2004;15(5):447–50.

30. Eriksson LG, Ljungdahl M, Sundbom M, et al. Transcatheter arterial embolization versus surgery in the treatment of upper gastrointestinal bleeding after therapeutic endoscopy failure. J Vasc Interv Radiol 2008;19:1413–8.

31. Defreyne L, De Schrijver I, Decruyenaere J, et al. Therapeutic decision-making in endoscopically unmanageable nonvariceal upper gastrointestinal hemorrhage. Cardiovasc Intervent Radiol 2008;31(5):897–905.

32. Padia SA, Geisinger MA, Newman JS, et al. Effectiveness of coil embolization in angiographically detectable versus non-detectable sources of upper gastrointestinal hemorrhage. J Vasc Interv Radiol 2009;20(4):461–6.

33. Arrayeh E, Fidelman N, Gordon RL, et al. Transcatheter arterial embolization for upper gastrointestinal nonvariceal hemorrhage: is empiric embolization warranted? Cardiovasc Intervent Radiol 2012;35(6):1346–54.

34. Ichiro I, Shushi H, Akihiko I, et al. Empiric transcatheter arterial embolization for massive bleeding from duodenal ulcers: efficacy and complications. J Vasc Interv Radiol 2011;22(7):911–6.

35. Schenker MP, Duszak R Jr, Soulen MC, et al. Upper gastrointestinal hemorrhage and transcatheter embolotherapy: clinical and technical factors impacting success and survival. J Vasc Interv Radiol 2001;12(11):1263–71.

36. Lang EK. Transcatheter embolization in management of hemorrhage from duodenal ulcer: long-term results and complications. Radiology 1992;182:703–7.

37. Poultsides GA, Kim CJ, Orlando R 3rd, et al. Angiographic embolization for gastroduodenal hemorrhage: safety, efficacy, and predictors of outcome. Arch Surg 2008;143(5):457–61.

38. Holme JB, Nielsen DT, Funch-Jensen P, et al. Transcatheter arterial embolization in patients with bleeding duodenal ulcer: an alternative to surgery. Acta Radiol 2006;47(3):244–7.

39. Ljungdahl M, Eriksson LG, Nyman R, et al. Arterial embolisation in management of massive bleeding from gastric and duodenal ulcers. Eur J Surg 2002;168(7): 384–90.

What If Endoscopic Hemostasis Fails?

Alternative Treatment Strategies: Surgery

Philip Wai Yan Chiu, MD, FRCSEd*,
James Yun Wong Lau, MD, FRCSEd

KEYWORDS

- Bleeding peptic ulcer • Surgery • Treatment

KEY POINTS

- With modern advances in therapeutic endoscopy and proton pump inhibitor therapy, the rate of peptic ulcer rebleeding has been significantly reduced and has led to a decline in the need for surgery.
- Patients who develop peptic ulcer rebleeding are usually poor-risk candidates for surgical treatment, with advanced age and multiple comorbidities.
- Before the era of therapeutic endoscopy, early preemptive surgical intervention prevented ulcer rebleeding and achieved lower mortality compared with a more delayed surgical approach; however, the recent reduction in ulcer rebleeding rates now makes preemptive surgical intervention obsolete.
- When ulcer rebleeding does occur, repeat endoscopic hemostasis can achieve similar control of bleeding compared with salvage surgery.
- Endoscopic suturing devices may be able to improve the rate of permanent hemostasis and further reduce the risk of ulcer rebleeding.

INTRODUCTION

In the past decade, numerous studies have attested to the efficacy of endoscopic therapy in controlling ulcer hemorrhage. In 2 separate meta-analyses, endoscopic therapy has been shown to reduce the rate of recurrent bleeding; the need for surgery; and, most importantly, in-hospital deaths.[1,2] In the modern literature, need for surgery is defined as a treatment failure in most trials of endoscopic therapy. In most centers, surgery is reserved for patients with failed endoscopic therapy. A recent study from Denmark that included all hospitals managing acute peptic ulcer bleeding analyzed

Department of Surgery, Institute of Digestive Disease, Prince of Wales Hospital, The Chinese University of Hong Kong, 30–32 Ngan Shing Street, Shatin, NT, Hong Kong, China
* Corresponding author.
E-mail address: philipchiu@surgery.cuhk.edu.hk

Gastroenterol Clin N Am 43 (2014) 753–763
http://dx.doi.org/10.1016/j.gtc.2014.08.006
0889-8553/14/$ – see front matter © 2014 Elsevier Inc. All rights reserved.
gastro.theclinics.com

data on 13,498 patients with peptic ulcer bleeding.[3] Despite improvement in all outcome indicators and a decline in patients requiring surgical intervention, 30-day mortality remained at 11%. Surgery maintains an important gatekeeping role despite its diminished role in the management algorithm of bleeding peptic ulcers. The precise role of surgery in the context of endoscopic hemostasis therapy has not been well studied.

Before endoscopic therapy was widely available, controversies existed as to when was best to apply surgery and which type of surgery should be performed when a patient required it. The goal of surgery was not merely the cessation of hemorrhage but as definitive therapy so as to prevent recurrence of peptic ulcer.[4] In the 1980s, proponents of an aggressive, definitive surgical approach to the management of bleeding peptic ulcer reported an admirable overall mortality of 20%.[5,6] However, there was an increased risk of major adverse events. A minimal surgical approach to achieve primary hemostasis in a significantly shorter surgery time was advocated by other investigators who argued that the minimal surgical approach would result in even lower surgical morbidity and mortality.[4,7,8]

In the modern era of endoscopic management for bleeding peptic ulcer, there are challenges and controversies in the timing and type of surgical procedures to salvage ulcer rebleeding. In this article, the surgical approach to the management of bleeding peptic ulcers is reviewed with a focus on the current evidence and modern surgical techniques to achieve surgical hemostasis.

FACTORS AFFECTING MORTALITY FROM BLEEDING PEPTIC ULCERS

In a population-based United Kingdom audit, a crude mortality figure of 14% was reported among 4185 patients with bleeding peptic ulcer.[9] Mortality was substantially higher among in-patients who developed bleeding (33%) compared with those patients presenting to the emergency department for bleeding (11%). The salient features of the study were that the overall incidence of bleeding was high (103 per 100,000 adults/y) and most patients were elderly. Rockall and colleagues[10] developed a well-known prediction score for mortality from a prospective multicenter population-based study involving 4185 cases of acute upper gastrointestinal (GI) hemorrhage. The Rockall score was subsequently validated in another cohort of 1625 patients. The Rockall score takes into account age, shock, comorbidity, endoscopic diagnosis, and the presence of major stigmata of recent hemorrhage. It has been shown that the risk of mortality increases when the score increases. Our group studied the predictive factors to bleeding peptic ulcer–related mortality after therapeutic endoscopy among 3220 patients.[11] Ulcer rebleeding and need for surgery were identified as significant risk factors for mortality, together with older age, multiple comorbidities, hemodynamic shock, and in-hospital bleeding. In another study, we investigated the causes of mortality among 10,248 cases of upper GI bleeding.[12] Although most patients died secondary to nonbleeding causes, 18.4% died of bleeding-related causes. The most common bleeding-related causes of death included failure to control bleeding during initial endoscopy (primary hemostasis), death within 48 hours of receiving endoscopic therapy, and surgical adverse events. Death was most common among elderly patients with severe comorbidities. Physicians are now faced with an increasing proportion of elderly patients and a further reduction in mortality secondary to improved management is likely to be marginal.

PEPTIC ULCER REBLEEDING AFTER THERAPEUTIC ENDOSCOPY

The current strategies to prevent ulcer rebleeding after therapeutic endoscopy include adjunctive high-dose proton pump inhibitor (PPI) infusion or performance of scheduled second-look endoscopy.[13,14] Prospective randomized trials show that both strategies significantly reduce the rate of peptic ulcer rebleeding. With the consideration of patient discomfort, workload, and costs of scheduled second-look endoscopy, PPI infusion is advocated as the preferred approach after therapeutic endoscopy. The rate of rebleeding after therapeutic endoscopy and PPI infusion is now 5% to 10%. Patients who develop rebleeding are those at high risk for surgical procedures because they are usually elderly with multiple comorbidities.

PREDICTING FAILURE OF ENDOSCOPIC THERAPY

Because rebleeding and need for surgery impose significant patient risk, predicting failure of endoscopic therapy could facilitate intensive monitoring and earlier surgical intervention among these patients. Several studies have defined predictors of rebleeding after endoscopic therapy.[15–18] Of the risk factors evaluated in these studies, the most consistent predictor of rebleeding seems to be the location of the ulcer in the posterior duodenal bulb. Other independent predictors of failure of endoscopic therapy include ulcer size, comorbid illnesses, and older age (**Table 1**). Among 3386 patients who had bleeding peptic ulcers receiving therapeutic endoscopy, our group showed that hypotension, initial hemoglobin level less than 10 g/dL, fresh blood in the stomach, actively bleeding ulcers, and large ulcers were independent factors to predict rebleeding.[19] Parameters identified from these studies are potentially helpful in selecting high-risk patients for planned urgent surgery.

EARLY VERSUS DELAYED SURGERY FOR BLEEDING PEPTIC ULCER

Before the era of therapeutic endoscopy, surgery was the only effective means to stop bleeding in peptic ulcers. The timing for surgery has been a subject of intense debate in the last few decades. Because continued or recurrent bleeding was the single most adverse prognostic factor, surgeons and gastroenterologists aimed to stop the hemorrhage promptly.[8,11] Patients who sustain rebleeding are often elderly with severe comorbid illnesses who poorly tolerate blood loss.[11,12] Early surgery in this subgroup of patients theoretically neutralizes the risk of recurrent bleeding and death. A group from Nottingham, United Kingdom, retrospectively analyzed short-term outcomes of

Table 1
Factors predicting failure of endoscopic therapy in bleeding peptic ulcer

	Saeed et al[17]	Brullet et al[18] N = 106 (DU Only)	Brullet et al[19,a] N = 178 (GU Only)	Villaneuva et al[11]
Age	Yes	No	No	No
Comorbid illnesses	Yes	No	No	Yes
Posterior duodenal bulb	Yes	—	—	Yes
Shock	—	Yes	Yes	—
Ulcer size	—	Yes	Yes	Yes
Stigmata of bleeding	No	—	Yes	No

Abbreviations: DU, duodenal ulcer; GU, gastric ulcer.
  a High lesser curve gastric ulcer.
Data from Refs.[11,17–19]

908 patients with GI bleeding during 1975 to 1980. Twenty-seven percent of patients underwent operations.[20] Comparing the years 1975 to 1977 with 1978 to 1980, the operation rate decreased from about 33% to 21%. The reduction in the rate of operation had no appreciable effect on mortality (13.9% vs 12.9% in gastric ulcers, 9.4% vs 9% in duodenal ulcers). Dronfield and colleagues[21] analyzed data from 2 hospitals in Nottingham with different policies in offering surgery. Of 206 patients from the first hospital, 66 (32%) were operated on compared with 44 (46%) of 96 at another hospital (P = .03). Overall mortality was less in the hospital with a lower rate of operations (12.7% vs 17.7%). The investigators questioned the role of aggressive surgical policy in bleeding peptic ulcer. Rofe and colleagues[22] from Australia reported a series of 86 patients with bleeding gastric and duodenal ulcers in which only 5.1% were operated on. One of 4 patients died after surgery but the overall mortality was only 3.5%. The investigators suggested that a more conservative approach be adopted. Hunt and colleagues[23] advocated aggressive resuscitation in a specialized unit and early surgery in patients with bleeding peptic ulcers. In a decade-long study of 633 patients, 206 patients underwent emergency surgery with an operative mortality of 12%, a decline from the operative mortality of 17.6% that occurred among 142 patients during the previous decade. In a later prospective study over a 6-year period, 376 patients were recruited with bleeding peptic ulcers.[24] Surgery was performed for patients with exsanguinating hemorrhage or shock on admission more than 50 years of age or further bleeding. The operation rate was 21.7% (102 patients). The overall mortality was 7%.

The only prospective randomized study to compare early and delayed surgery in bleeding ulcers came from the Birmingham group.[5] One hundred and four patients were randomized. Criteria for early surgery were 4 units of blood or plasma expander transfused in 24 hours, 1 rebleed, and endoscopic stigmata or 1 previous bleed with 2 years. Criteria for surgery in the delayed group were 8 units of blood or plasma expander in 24 hours, 2 rebleeds, and persistent bleeding requiring 12 units of blood in 48 hours or 16 units in 72 hours. In patients less than 60 years of age, there was no death in either group but the early surgery policy led to an unacceptably high operation rate (52% in the early group and 5% in the delayed group). For patients aged more than 60 years, the operation rate was 62% in the early group and 27% in the delayed group. There were 3 deaths among 48 patients (6%) in the early group compared with 7 deaths among 52 patients (13%) in the delayed group. The difference was not statistically significant on an intention-to-treat analysis. The trial was criticized for the low number of patients in the subgroup analysis and for allowing ongoing exsanguination of patients in the delayed group. In a posttrial 4-year audit from the same group, indications for urgent surgery were modified; patients were operated on if they had exsanguinating hemorrhage or if a spurting vessel was seen at endoscopy.[25] Patients more than 60 years of age were operated on if 1 episode of rebleeding occurred in hospital, and 4 units of blood or colloid for volume replacement or 8 units of blood or colloid were transfused over 48 hours. Of 342 patients, 214 were 60 years of age or older. Fifty-two (24%) of them received surgical hemostasis with an operative mortality of 6%. The evidence for early surgical intervention was inadequate, especially in the modern era in which therapeutic endoscopy has become the primary treatment of bleeding ulcers. However, the trials on timing of surgery clearly show that early intervention was critical in elderly patients. Under a centralized joint medical and surgical unit, early surgical intervention among patients at high risk resulted in a lower overall mortality of 3.7% and surgical mortality of 15.2%.[26]

Planned urgent surgery has been the dogma in the management of bleeding ulcers for many years. Benders and colleagues[27] operated on patients with shock on admission, age greater than 65 years, ulcer size greater than 2 cm, or with stigmata of recent hemorrhage and previous admission for ulcer complication. Sixty-six patients (mean age of 58 years) were included in a 5-year period with no mortality. Mueller and colleagues[28] operated on patients with spurting hemorrhage, nonbleeding visible vessels on posterior duodenal ulcers, blood transfusions greater than 6 units in the first 24 hours, and rebleeding within 48 hours. In a consecutive series of 157 patients, the 30-day mortality was 7%. At present, a planned surgical procedure before ulcer rebleeding is not practically possible with an increasing trend of elderly and high-risk patients, especially when no good selection criteria are available for predicting those who might benefit.

MINIMAL SURGICAL APPROACH FOR BLEEDING PEPTIC ULCER

Besides controversies in the timing of surgery, the type of surgical procedure per-formed to salvage peptic ulcer bleeding after failed therapeutic endoscopy remains debatable. The minimal surgical approach to control bleeding peptic ulcer involves suture plication of the ulcer or ulcerectomy. Ulcer plication is intended to control acute hemorrhage by suture plicating the bleeding vessel, which is commonly applied to bleeding from a posteroinferior duodenal ulcer with plication of branches of the gastroduodenal artery. The recommended strategy is to apply sutures at the 6 and 12 o'clock positions on the posterior duodenal ulcer crater to control the bleeding from the gastroduodenal artery.[29] Berne and Rosoff[30] applied a U configuration of stitches to the center of the ulcer crater after superior and inferior plication. Other surgeons have performed plication over 4 quadrants of the ulcer with figure-eight sutures. The goal is to achieve hemostasis in major arterial branches, including the gastroduodenal artery and the transverse pancreatic artery.[30] Ulcerectomy or excision of the ulcer is generally applied for hemostasis of bleeding gastric ulcer.[31] The advan-tage of excising the bleeding gastric ulcer is to eliminate the risk of rebleeding. More-over, the excised ulcer can be examined by histopathology to identify possible gastric malignancy.

DEFINITIVE SURGICAL APPROACH FOR BLEEDING PEPTIC ULCER

Definitive surgery is intended to stop the acute bleeding and prevent recurrence or further complications from peptic ulcer. Definitive procedures included vagotomy and gastrectomy. Vagotomy can be classified into truncal vagotomy (TV), selective vagotomy, and highly selective vagotomy (HSV). Vagotomy results not only in reduc-tion of acid secretion but also in the loss of coordinated gastric antral-pyloric digestive action.[32,33] Gastrectomy including antrectomy, partial gastrectomy, or total gastrec-tomy is designed to remove the acid-producing parietal cell mass. Antrectomy is the resection of the gastric antrum, which involves distal transaction at the first part of duodenum and proximal transaction 8 to 10 cm above the pylorus along the lesser curvature. Reconstruction after antrectomy can be achieved with Billroth I or Billroth II gastrojejunostomy. In partial gastrectomy, the extent of the resection is proximal to the angular incisura at the level at which the descending branch of the left gastric artery is controlled.

CHOICE OF SURGERY FOR BLEEDING PEPTIC ULCER

Table 2 summarizes the evidence comparing the choice of surgery for treatment of bleeding peptic ulcer. Most studies were conducted before the era of endoscopic therapy for bleeding peptic ulcer. Two randomized trials and 4 case-control studies

Table 2
Summary of trials comparing operative approaches to peptic ulcer bleeding

Author, Year	Type	Number	Operation	Rebleeding (%)	Mortality (%)	Recommendation
Millat et al,[34] 1993	RCT	24	Gastric resection BI + ulcer excision	3	23	Definitive surgery
		36	Gastric resection BII + ulcer excision		22	
		58	Oversewing + vagotomy	17		
Poxon et al,[35] 1991	RCT	25	Partial gastrectomy	0	19	Definitive surgery
		35	Oversewing + vagotomy			
		3	Ulcer excision + vagotomy			
		59	Underrunning	10	26	
		3	Ulcer excision			
Kubba et al,[34] 1996	Case control	24	Underrunning + vagotomy	3	14	Definitive surgery
		3	Ulcer excision + vagotomy			
		9	Partial gastrectomy/antrectomy			
		28	Underrunning	23	23	
		3	Ulcer excision			
Dousset et al,[36] 1995	Case control	10	Antrectomy + vagotomy	0	13	Definitive surgery
		5	Partial gastrectomy			
		29	Oversewing/ulcerectomy	30	24	
		34	Oversewing/ulcerectomy + vagotomy			
Kuttila et al,[37] 1991	Case control	58	GU: partial gastrectomy	10	12	Definitive surgery
		12	GU: ulcerectomy	12	24	
		5	GU: ulcerectomy + vagotomy			
		42	DU: partial gastrectomy ± vagotomy	0	12	
		27	DU: underrunning ± vagotomy	19	22	
Hunt et al,[38] 1990	Case control	81	Partial gastrectomy	10	12	Minimal surgery
		101	Underrunning + vagotomy	17	10	

Definitive surgery refers to vagotomy or antrectomy or gastrectomy; minimal surgery refers to ulcer plication or ulcerectomy.
Abbreviations: BI, Billroth I gastrectomy; BII, Billroth II gastrectomy; RCT, randomized controlled trial.
Data from Refs.[34–38]

showed that definitive surgery outperformed the minimal approach in achieving a lower rate of rebleeding and mortality.[33,35,38-42] TV and drainage procedures were commonly performed to reduce acid for bleeding duodenal ulcer after surgical hemostasis using suture plication at the ulcer base. Madsen[33] investigated 92 patients with bleeding duodenal ulcer treated with emergency oversewing plus selective vagotomy and drainage and reported a perioperative mortality of 8%, with 15% of patients subsequently developing ulcer recurrence and 3 patients sustaining significant postoperative dumping syndrome. This finding indicates that selective vagotomy is not advisable for bleeding duodenal ulcer. HSV has not been widely performed for emergency hemostasis of bleeding peptic ulcer, perhaps because it is more complex and requires longer operative time. Before the era of therapeutic endoscopy, Hunt and McIntyre[39] showed that TV with a drainage procedure was the preferred operation compared with gastrectomy in 201 patients presenting with bleeding peptic ulcer. Gastrectomy was less preferred for large duodenal ulcer because closure of the remnant duodenal stump often resulted in leakage. Poxon and colleagues[40] reported a multicenter prospective randomized trial comparing minimal versus definitive surgery for primary hemostasis of bleeding peptic ulcer. Although there was no difference in overall mortality, incidence of fatal rebleeding was significantly lower in the definitive surgery group. Another study showed that a minimal approach with oversewing of ulcer alone resulted in a lower perioperative mortality of 10% compared with 26% for gastrectomy and 45% for vagotomy and drainage.[43] Kubba and colleagues[41] from the United Kingdom reported on a cohort of 67 patients who failed endoscopic therapy for major peptic ulcer hemorrhage, of whom 31 had simple under-running or excision of ulcers and 36 had more radical surgery. Recurrent bleeding was significantly higher in patients treated by under-running alone (7 vs 1; $P = .01$). There were fewer deaths in the radically treated group (5 vs 7; not significant). The investigators suggested that an aggressive surgical approach should be adopted for severe peptic ulcer hemorrhage after failed endoscopic therapy. Moreover, the performance of partial gastrectomy with gastroduodenal anastomosis may remove the need for closing the duodenal stump and thereby the risk of subsequent duodenal blow-out. However, the results of these studies should be interpreted with caution in the modern era. The role of surgery has changed from initial hemostasis to salvaging endoscopic failures. The choice of surgery is often influenced by the severity of hemorrhage, clinical stability, as well as the physical status of the patient at the time of surgery. Most surgeons opt for minimal surgery in poor-risk patients. In a retrospective series of 101 gastric ulcers that underwent emergency surgery after failed endoscopic therapy over a period of 6 years, patients were analyzed according to their APACHE II scores.[44] Mortality was 5% with a score less than 15. Partial gastrectomy could be performed safely. In 38 patients with scores of 15 or more, mortality was significantly higher at 58%. Partial gastrectomy carried a slightly lower mortality (47% vs 65%) than limited operation (oversewing or ulcer excision alone). Minimal surgery resulted in 22% postoperative bleeding and 12% required reoperation, in which all patients with a score of 15 or more died. The study had inherent limitations. Findings from the study suggested that minimal surgery did not influence outcomes in patients with poor general well-being coming to surgery. Our group conducted a retrospective cohort study on 165 patients with bleeding ulcers who received surgical salvage over a period of 10 years.[34] Patients in the recent 5-year cohort had significantly more comorbidities, higher demand for transfusion, longer hospital stays, as well as higher mortality than the first 5-year cohort. Because most patients treated by salvage surgery in the recent cohort were poor surgical candidates with multiple comorbidities, minimal surgery was performed in 31 of the 42 patients with recurrent bleeding. Definitive surgery will become obsolete when the use of PPIs effectively controls acid secretion and *Helicobacter pylori* eradication serves as a cure for peptic ulcer disease.[16,36]

ENDOSCOPIC RETREATMENT OR SURGERY FOR ULCER REBLEEDING

It is often a dilemma for the managing physician whether at the time of rebleeding to attempt another endoscopic treatment or refer the patient directly to surgery. Repeating endoscopic therapy may not achieve adequate hemostasis but may cause patients to sustain severe effects from the hemorrhage. In a 40-month period during which 3473 patients with bleeding peptic ulcers were admitted, we conducted a randomized trial among patients with rebleeding after endoscopic therapy for bleeding peptic ulcers.[37] Ninety-two subjects (mean age 65 years; 76% men) were randomized, 48 being allocated to endoscopic retreatment and 44 to surgery. On intention-to-treat analysis, endoscopic retreatment and surgery groups did not differ in 30-day mortality (10% vs 18%; $P = .37$), hospital stay (median 10 vs 11 days; $P = .59$), or transfusions (median 8 vs 7 units; $P = .27$). Patients who received surgery sustained a significantly higher rate of complications (7 vs 16; $P = .03$). Endoscopic retreatment was able to control bleeding in three-quarters of patients. In those who failed endoscopic retreatment, salvage surgery carried substantial mortality. In a logistic regression analysis of a small subgroup of patients, ulcers 2 cm in size or larger and hypotension at the time of rebleeding were independent factors predicting failure with endoscopic retreatment.

ALTERNATIVE TO SURGICAL SALVAGE FOR PEPTIC ULCER REBLEEDING

In a 10-year cohort study recruiting 3367 patients with bleeding peptic ulcers, 153 patients sustained rebleeding and required salvage surgery.[34] The 30-day mortality after salvage surgery was 25.5%, which was significantly higher than the mortality reported 20 years earlier. To further reduce the need of surgery, approaches to improve the success of endoscopic hemostasis have been investigated. Swain and colleagues[45] studied the cause of bleeding submucosal arteries among 27 gastrectomy specimens in the management of bleeding peptic ulcers. The larger arteries in the gastrectomy specimens were subserosal, and had a diameter of 0.7 mm. In a lethal ulcer, the bleeding artery measured up to 3.5 mm in diameter. Ulcers located in the posterior wall of the bulbar duodenum and lesser curve of the stomach eroded into major arteries such as the gastroduodenal artery complex and first-generation branches of the left gastric artery. Their sizes exceeded 2 mm, and thus bleeding from these arteries mandates surgical hemostasis. Endoscopic plication is one of the potential novel treatments for bleeding gastric ulcer. A prototype endoscopic suturing device designed to achieve suture plication to the base of a bleeding peptic ulcer has been tested in animal models through a flexible endoscope.[46,47] With the latest development of the Overstitch device, application of overstitch suture plication to bleeding peptic ulcers is now feasible.[48] Endoscopic suturing will also exclude the bleeding ulcer from the intragastric acid and further improve hemostasis and prevent rebleeding.

SUMMARY

Endoscopic hemostasis therapy should be the first-line treatment in bleeding peptic ulcers. Expeditious surgery is indicated in patients with rapid exsanguination and bleeding uncontrolled by endoscopic therapy. Initial endoscopic control creates an opportunity for physicians and surgeons to confer and decide on the optimal treatment strategy. The role of early elective surgery after endoscopic hemostasis remains undefined. It is logical and prudent to select high-risk ulcers based on the severity of index bleeding and large chronic ulcers for early elective surgery. The increasing proportion of elderly patients, often with severe comorbidities, has made most medical providers reluctant to adopt such a strategy. At ulcer rebleeding, controversies abound on the choice of endoscopic retreatment and surgery. In expert centers, endoscopic retreatment can stop bleeding in a high proportion of cases. The success of endoscopic retreatment to a large extent depends on the severity of rebleeding and the ulcer characteristics. In patients with large chronic ulcers and compromised circulatory state, immediate surgery should probably be performed without recourse to endoscopic retreatment. Bleeding ulcers that fail endoscopic therapy are often difficult ulcers, such as ulcers located at the posterior duodenal bulb. These ulcers are technically demanding to most surgeons, underlying the importance of a team approach with experienced GI surgeons. An aggressive approach is often required in these selected ulcers. In future, endoscopic suture plication may serve as an alternative to salvage surgery in the management of bleeding peptic ulcers.

REFERENCES

1. Sacks HS, Chalmers TC, Blum AL, et al. Endoscopic hemostasis: an effective therapy for bleeding peptic ulcers. JAMA 1990;264:494–9.
2. Cook DJ, Guyatt GH, Salena BJ, et al. Endoscopic therapy for acute non-variceal upper gastrointestinal hemorrhage – a meta-analysis. Gastroenterology 1992;102:139.
3. Rosenstock SJ, Møller MH, Larsson H, et al. Improving quality of care in peptic ulcer bleeding: nationwide cohort study of 13,498 consecutive patients in the Danish Clinical Register of Emergency Surgery. Am J Gastroenterol 2013;108(9):1449–57.
4. Boulos PB, Harris J, Wyllie JH, et al. Conservative surgery in 100 patients with bleeding peptic ulcer. Br J Surg 1971;58:817.
5. Morris DL, Hawker PC, Brearley S, et al. Optimal timing of operation for bleeding peptic ulcer: prospective randomized trial. Br Med J (Clin Res Ed) 1984;288:1277–80.
6. Byrne JJ, Guardione VA, Williams LF. Massive gastrointestinal hemorrhage. Am J Surg 1970;120:312.
7. Vogel TT. Critical issues in gastroduodenal hemorrhage: the role of vagotomy and pyloroplasty. Ann Surg 1972;176:144.
8. Weinberg JA. Treatment of the massively bleeding duodenal ulcer by ligation, pyloroplasty and vagotomy. Am J Surg 1961;102:158.
9. Rockall TA, Logan RF, Devlin HB, et al. Incidence and mortality from acute upper gastrointestinal hemorrhage in the United Kingdom. BMJ 1995;311:222–6.
10. Rockall TA, Logan RF, Devlin HB, et al. Risk assessment after acute upper gastrointestinal hemorrhage. Gut 1996;38(3):316–21.
11. Chiu PW, Ng EK, Cheung FK, et al. Predicting mortality in patients with bleeding peptic ulcers after therapeutic endoscopy. Clin Gastroenterol Hepatol 2009;7(3):311–6.
12. Sung JJ, Tsoi KK, Ma TK, et al. Causes of mortality in patients with peptic ulcer bleeding: a prospective cohort study of 10,428 cases. Am J Gastroenterol 2010;105(1):84–9.
13. Chiu PW, Lam CY, Lee SW, et al. Effect of scheduled second therapeutic endoscopy on peptic ulcer rebleeding: a prospective randomized trial. Gut 2003;52:1403–7.

14. Lau JY, Sung JJ, Lee KK, et al. Effect of intravenous omeprazole on recurrent bleeding after endoscopic treatment of bleeding peptic ulcers. N Engl J Med 2000;343(5):310–6.
15. Saeed ZA, Winchester MA, Michaletz PA, et al. A scoring system to predict rebleeding after endoscopic therapy of non-variceal upper gastrointestinal hemorrhage, with a comparison of heat probe and ethanol injection. Am J Gastroenterol 1993;88:1842.
16. Brullet E, Calvet X, Campo R, et al. Factors predicting failure of endoscopic injection therapy in bleeding duodenal ulcer. Gastrointest Endosc 1996;43:111–6.
17. Brullet E, Campo R, Calvet X, et al. Factors related to the failure of endoscopic injection therapy. Gut 1996;39:155–8.
18. Villaneuva C, Balanzo J, Espinos JC, et al. Prediction of therapeutic failure in patients with bleeding peptic ulcer treated with endoscopic injection. Dig Dis Sci 1993;38:2062.
19. Wong SK, Yu LM, Lau JY, et al. Prediction of therapeutic failure after adrenaline injection plus heater probe treatment in patients with bleeding peptic ulcer. Gut 2002;50:322–5.
20. Vellacott KD, Dronfield MW, Atkinson M, et al. Comparison of surgical and medical management of bleeding peptic ulcers. Br Med J (Clin Res Ed) 1982; 284:548–50.
21. Dronfield MW, Atkinson M, Langman MJ. Effect of different operation policies on mortality from bleeding peptic ulcer. Lancet 1979;I:1126–8.
22. Rofe SB, Duggan JM, Smith ER, et al. Conservative treatment of gastrointestinal haemorrhage. Gut 1985;26:481–4.
23. Hunt PS, Hansky J, Korman MG. Mortality in patients with haematemesis and melaena: a prospective study. Br Med J 1979;I:1238–40.
24. Hunt PS. Bleeding gastroduodenal ulcers: selection of patients for surgery. World J Surg 1987;11:289–94.
25. Wheatley KE, Snyman JH, Brearley S, et al. Mortality in patients with bleeding ulcer when those aged 60 or over are operated on early. BMJ 1990;301:272.
26. Holman RA, Davis M, Gough KR, et al. Value of a centralised approach in the management of haematemesis and melaena: experience in a district general hospital. Gut 1990;31:504–8.
27. Benders JS, Bouwman DL, Weaver DW. Bleeding gastroduodenal ulcers: improved outcome from a unified surgical approach. Am Surg 1994;60:313–5.
28. Mueller X, Rothenbuehler JM, Amert A, et al. Outcome of peptic ulcer hemorrhage treated according to a defined approach. World J Surg 1994;18: 406–9.
29. Herrington JL, Davidson J. Bleeding gastroduodenal ulcers: choice of operations. World J Surg 1987;11:304–14.
30. Berne CJ, Rosoff L. Peptic ulcer perforation of the gastroduodenal artery complex. Ann Surg 1969;169:141.
31. Chung SC. Surgery and gastrointestinal bleeding. Gastrointest Endosc Clinics of North America 1997;7(4):687–701.
32. Cheadle WG, Baker PR, Cuschieri A. Pyloric reconstruction for severe vasomotor dumping after vagotomy and pyloroplasty. Ann Surg 1985;202:568.
33. Madsen OG. A follow-up study of patients after treatment for bleeding duodenal ulcers by selective vagotomy and drainage (4–8 years observation time). Acta Chir Scand 1977;143(2):115–9.
34. Chiu PW, Ng EK, Wong SK, et al. Surgical salvage of bleeding peptic ulcers after failed therapeutic endoscopy. Dig Surg 2009;26(3):243–8.

35. Dousset B, Suc B, Boudet MJ, et al. Surgical treatment of severe ulcerous hemorrhages: predictive factors of operative mortality. Gastroenterol Clin Biol 1995;19(3):259–65.
36. Sung JY, Chung SC, Ling TK, et al. Antibacterial treatment of gastric ulcers associated with *Helicobacter pylori*. N Engl J Med 1995;332(3):139–42.
37. Lau JY, Sung JJ, Lam YH, et al. Endoscopic re-treatment compared with surgery in patients with recurrent bleeding after initial endoscopic control of bleeding ulcers. N Engl J Med 1999;340:751–6.
38. Millat B, Hay JM, Valleur P, et al. Emergency surgical treatment for bleeding duodenal ulcer: oversewing plus vagotomy versus gastric resection, a controlled randomized trial. World J Surg 1993;17:568–74.
39. Hunt PS, McIntyre RL. Choice of emergency operative procedure for bleeding duodenal ulcer. Br J Surg 1990;77:1004–6.
40. Poxon VA, Keighley MR, Dykes PW, et al. Comparison of minimal and conventional surgery in patients with bleeding peptic ulcer: a multicenter trial. Br J Surg 1991;78(11):1344–5.
41. Kubba AK, Choudari C, Rajgopal C, et al. The outcome of urgent surgery for major peptic ulcer haemorrhage following failed endoscopic therapy. Eur J Gastroenterol Hepatol 1996;8:1175–8.
42. Kuttila K, Havia T, Pekkala E, et al. Surgery of acute peptic ulcer haemorrhage. Ann Chir Gynaecol 1991;80(1):26–9.
43. Rogers PN, Murray WR, Shaw R, et al. Surgical management of bleeding gastric ulceration. Br J Surg 1988;75(1):16–7.
44. Wang BW, Mok KT, Chang HT, et al. APACHE II score: a useful tool for risk assessment and an aid to decision-making in emergency operation for bleeding gastric ulcer. J Am Coll Surg 1998;187(3):287–94.
45. Swain CP, Storey SW, Bown SG. Nature of the bleeding vessel in recurrently bleeding gastric ulcers. Gastroenterology 1986;19:595.
46. Hu B, Chung SC, Sun LC, et al. Eagle Claw II: A novel endosuture device that uses a curved needle for major arterial bleeding: a bench study. Gastrointest Endosc 2005;62(2):266–70.
47. Chiu PW, Hu B, Lau JY, et al. Endoscopic plication of massively bleeding peptic ulcer by using the Eagle Claw VII device: a feasibility study in a porcine model. Gastrointest Endosc 2006;63(4):681–5.
48. Chiu PW, Phee SJ, Wang Z, et al. Feasibility of full-thickness gastric resection using master and slave transluminal endoscopic robot and closure by Overstitch: a preclinical study. Surg Endosc 2014;28(1):319–24.

Epidemiology, Diagnosis and Early Patient Management of Esophagogastric Hemorrhage

CrossMark

Sumit Kumar, MD, MRCP[a], Sumeet K. Asrani, MD, MSc[b],
Patrick S. Kamath, MD[c],*

KEYWORDS

- Acute variceal bleeding • Esophageal varices • Gastric varices
- Endoscopic variceal ligation

KEY POINTS

- Esophageal and gastric varices are common among persons with cirrhosis.
- Short-term antibiotic prophylaxis, early resuscitation, targeting of conservative goals for blood transfusion, and management of complications such as infection and renal failure are important.
- Combination therapy with vasoactive drugs and endoscopic variceal ligation is the first-line treatment in the management of acute variceal bleeding after adequate hemodynamic resuscitation.
- The MELD score is an important predictor of early mortality after variceal bleeding.

INTRODUCTION
Epidemiology

At the time of initial diagnosis of cirrhosis, approximately half of the patients have esophageal varices, and with the progression of cirrhosis approximately 90% of patients develop esophageal varices.[1-3] Varices are present in approximately 40% of patients with compensated cirrhosis and 60% of patients with ascites.[3,4] Large esophageal varices (>5 mm) are seen in 16% of all patients screened for varices by upper endoscopy.[5] The presence of varices correlates with the severity of liver disease: 20% to 40% of Child-A cirrhosis patients have esophagogastric varices (EGV), compared with up to 85% of Child-C cirrhotics. Patients with primary biliary cirrhosis may develop varices and aute variceal bleeding even in the absence of established cirrhosis.[6]

[a] Department of Internal Medicine, Abington Memorial Hospital, 1200 Old York Road, Abington, PA 19001, USA; [b] Baylor University Medical Center, 3410 Worth Street, Suite 860, Dallas, TX 75246, USA; [c] Division of Gastroenterology and Hepatology, Mayo Clinic College of Medicine, 200 First Street Southwest, Rochester, MN 55905, USA
* Corresponding author.
E-mail address: kamath.patrick@mayo.edu

Gastroenterol Clin N Am 43 (2014) 765–782
http://dx.doi.org/10.1016/j.gtc.2014.08.007
0889-8553/14/$ – see front matter © 2014 Elsevier Inc. All rights reserved.
gastro.theclinics.com

Esophageal Varices

Patients with cirrhosis who do not have varices at the time of initial upper endoscopy develop varices at a rate of 8% per year.[7] The progression of small (<5 mm) to large varices (>5 mm) occurs at a similar rate of 7% to 8% per year.[8] An elevated hepatic venous pressure gradient (HVPG) of greater than >10 mm Hg is an independent predictor of the development of varices.[7] About one-third of patients who have varices develop AVB.[9,10] Patients who are found to have small varices at the time of initial endoscopy have a 5% per year risk of bleeding, compared with 15% per year in those with medium-sized or large varices at diagnosis.[4] Moreover, 40% of patients with AVB spontaneously stop bleeding without any intervention, compared with 80% of those with nonvariceal causes of upper gastrointestinal bleeding.[9] However, patients with severe liver disease (Child C) are less likely to stop bleeding spontaneously. With the current standard of therapy, 80% to 90% of patients have cessation of hemorrhage.[3] Despite treatment, 1 in 4 patients will still show either a failure to control the bleeding or an early recurrence of the hemorrhage in the first 6 weeks after the initial bleeding.[11,12] The risk of rebleeding is highest in the period immediately after the sentinel bleed: 40% of all rebleeding episodes occur within the first 5 days.[13,14] An elevated HVPG of greater than 20 mm Hg, when measured within 24 hours of variceal hemorrhage, is associated with failure to control bleeding and early rebleeding. A Model for End-Stage Liver Disease (MELD) score of 18 or higher is also an independent predictor of early rebleeding.[15,16]

Gastric Varices

Gastric varices (GV) are present in 20% of patients with portal hypertension, and are the source of 5% to 10% of all upper gastrointestinal bleeding episodes in patients with cirrhosis. GV carry a 10% to 16% risk of bleeding in 1 year and 25% risk of bleeding in 2 years.[17] Although the prevalence and bleeding risk of GV are lower, the bleeding is usually more severe, requires more transfusions, and is associated with higher mortality. Even after endoscopic injection of tissue glue, GV bleeding is still associated with high rebleeding rates, ranging from 22% to 37%. The risk of recurrent bleeding depends on the location of the varix: isolated varices in the gastric fundus (53%) bear the highest risk for recurrent bleeding, followed by varices along the greater gastric curvature (19%) and lesser gastric curvature (6%). The annual incidence of bleeding is 4% in patients with Child class A with small varices without red wale signs, and 65% in patients with Child class C with large varices with red wale signs.[18] Large fundal varices may occasionally bleed despite HVPG values of less than 12 mm Hg.[19]

Mortality

Any death occurring in the first 6 weeks after the index bleed is considered a bleeding-related death. Three decades ago, AVB was associated with a mortality of 60% at 6 weeks.[13] With recent developments in pharmacologic and endoscopic treatments, this figure has significantly improved in the present era to 20% or less.[20] Immediate mortality from uncontrolled bleeding is in the range of 4% to 8%.[21] Child class C, MELD score 18 and higher, and failure to control bleeding or early rebleeding predict 6-week mortality.[16,22] Mortality is 0% among patients with Child class A disease and approximately 30% among patients with Child C. Forty percent of deaths are directly related to bleeding and shock, with the remainder being due to renal failure, hepatic encephalopathy (HE), and sepsis.[19] In a recent analysis, MELD greater than 19 predicted 20% or greater mortality, whereas MELD scores of less than 11 predicted less than 5% mortality.[23]

PREDICTIVE MODELS

Multiple studies have identified independent factors that predict the risk of bleeding, rebleeding, and death in AVB (**Table 1**). However, the aggregate conclusions of these studies are discordant, and the predictive value of the combined results is difficult to assess. Predictors of bleeding include presence of decompensated cirrhosis (Child B or C), size of varices, and presence of high-risk stigmata on endoscopy (red wale signs).[10] The risk of further rebleeding, mortality, and complications is highest within the first 6 weeks.[13] In prognostic studies conducted in the current era using standard-of-care interventions (antibiotics, vasoactive drugs, and endoscopic band ligation), the risk of early rebleeding or treatment failure was 15% to 21%, with the

Table 1
Variceal bleeding and predictors of severity, treatment failure, early rebleeding, and mortality

Severity of Variceal Bleed	Treatment Failure	Early Rebleeding	Mortality
	HVPG		
	Alcoholic liver disease		
	Infection		
CTP class/score			CTP class/score
PRBC transfusion			PRBC transfusion
Size and morphology of varices			
Ascites			
Portal Vein Thrombosis			
Hematocrit/Hb at presentation			
Platelet Count		Platelet Count	
Degree of Liver Failure			
		Active bleeding at endoscopy	
	Shock		Shock
	AST		
	First bleed		
			MELD >18
			Encephalopathy
			Hepatocellular carcinoma
			Short interval to admission
			Urea
		Hematemesis	
			Creatinine
			Albumin
			Age
			Early rebleeding
			Prothrombin Time
			Treatment failure
			Bilirubin

Abbreviations: AST, aspartate aminotransferase; CTP, Child-Turcotte-Pugh score; Hb, hemoglobin; HVPG, hepatic venous pressure gradient; MELD, model for end-stage liver disease; PRBC, packed red blood cells.

Adapted from Sarin SK, Kumar A, Angus PW, et al. Diagnosis and management of acute variceal bleeding: Asian Pacific Association for Study of the Liver recommendations. Hepatol Int 2011;5(2):607–24.

risk of early mortality being 6% to 24%.[24] Predictors of rebleeding or treatment failure include MELD score, Child-Turcotte-Pugh (CTP) score, elevated HVPG ($\geq$20 mm Hg), development of infections, and endoscopic appearance (active bleeding, clot on varix, and shock).[16,24] Recurrent variceal bleeding is lower among patients who achieve a reduction in HVPG to less than 12 mm Hg or a 20% reduction in baseline HVPG values.[25] However, the role of HVPG-guided therapy remains unclear.[26] Predictors of mortality include the aforementioned factors in addition to hepatocellular carcinoma (HCC), worsening renal function, use of steroids, and advanced age.[20,22]

Child-Turcotte-Pugh Score

Traditionally the CTP score has been used to stratify patients at risk for death after AVB, with a higher CTP score associated with an increased mortality.[27] The CTP score is easy to use, but lack of standardized measurement of albumin and prothrombin time across laboratories and the use of subjective parameters limit its clinical use.

Model for End-Stage Liver Disease Score

MELD was shown to be superior to CTP score in predicting mortality after transjugular intrahepatic portosystemic shunt (TIPS) performed to prevent recurrent variceal bleeding.[28] However, in a retrospective study of 212 cirrhotic patients with AVB, CTP and MELD scores similarly predicted overall in-hospital mortality, but MELD was significantly better than CTP score for predicting in-hospital mortality directly related to variceal bleeding.[29]

Patients with a MELD score of 18 or higher were found to be at increased risk for death within the first 6 weeks, and for rebleeding within the first 5 days after the index bleed ($P<.001$ and $P<.04$, respectively). Furthermore, patients with a MELD score of at least 18, requiring 4 or more units of packed red blood cells (PRBC) within the first 24 hours of acute variceal hemorrhage (hazard ratio [HR] 11.3; $P<.001$) or having active bleeding at endoscopy (HR 9.9, $P<.001$) were at increased risk for death within 6 weeks.[16] In addition, MELD score was a significant predictor of mortality in patients with cirrhosis who were hospitalized with an AVB: every 1-point increase in the MELD score conferred an 8% and 11% increased risk of death at 5 days and 6 weeks, respectively.[16] A recent study of 128 patients also found MELD to be a powerful predictor of 6-week mortality in patients with early rebleeding after endoscopic band ligation for AVB. The mortality rate was 14.7% in patients with a MELD score of less than 21.5 and 71.7% in patients with MELD score of at least 21.5 at 6 weeks ($P<.001$).[30]

Reverter and colleagues[23] recently sought to improve the determination of risk for patients presenting with AVB using objective variables. The primary outcome was mortality within 6 weeks of incident bleed. Several previously proposed prognostic models were compared: these included the MELD score, CTP score, and predictive models proposed by D'Amico and colleagues[21] and Augustin and colleagues.[31] The MELD score was identified as the best model in terms of discrimination and overall performance. A MELD score of at least 19 predicted at least 20% mortality, and a MELD score of less than 11 predicted less than 5% mortality within 6 weeks of the AVB episode.

Hepatic Venous Pressure Gradient

Elevated HVPG is an independent predictor of mortality, with a purported 3% increase in mortality per 1-mm Hg increase in HVPG.[32] A single HVPG measurement greater than 20 mm Hg is associated with worse probability of survival (1-year mortality, 64% vs 20%; $P<.01$) and early rebleeding from varices.[15,33] Other factors that encapsulate advanced liver disease, such as serum sodium, are also important. A combination of hyponatremia (serum sodium <130 mmol/L) and HVPG greater than 20 mm Hg is associated with a significantly worse prognosis than either alone. However, it is unclear whether addition of HVPG to MELD of Child-Pugh stage based prediction significantly improves the predictive capabilities of a prognostic model.[33]

DIAGNOSIS

In patients with cirrhosis, 70% of upper gastrointestinal bleeds are due to AVB. Hence all patients with cirrhosis and upper gastrointestinal bleeds should be treated for varices unless evidence for other causes is available. A thorough history and physical examination are important in establishing a diagnosis. Patients usually present with hematemesis, but hematochezia and melena may also be present. On physical examination the presence of signs of chronic liver disease in patients with no known history of cirrhosis should be sought. Severity of blood loss should be estimated by hemodynamic and laboratory parameters. Resting tachycardia in the absence of other causes is the first sign of mild hypovolemic shock, and should not be ignored. In patients who are normotensive, orthostatics should be measured. Orthostatic hypotension suggests a loss of 15% of the blood volume. On the other hand, frank hypotension is associated with a 40% loss of blood volume.[34]

Endoscopy is the gold standard for the diagnosis of AVB. The diagnosis of variceal hemorrhage is made when diagnostic endoscopy shows 1 of the following: active bleeding from a varix, a white nipple overlying a varix, clots overlying a varix, or varices with blood in stomach and no other potential source of bleeding.[35]

Several other modalities have been proposed to predict the presence of varices in subjects who have not overtly bled.

Hepatic Venous Pressure Gradient

HVPG is a reliable method for indirectly evaluating the portal pressure gradient, establishing the effectiveness of treatment, and predicting the occurrence of complications in portal hypertension. Portal hypertension is present when the HVPG is greater than 5 mm Hg, but it is considered clinically significant when the HVPG is greater than 10 mm Hg. Esophageal varices do not bleed at an HVPG less than 12 mm Hg.[36,37] In patients without varices, an HVPG greater than 10 mm Hg has been shown to be the strongest predictor of the development of varices[6] and clinical decompensation of cirrhosis.[38] In patients with variceal hemorrhage, an HVPG of more than 20 mm Hg (measured within 24 hours after admission) is the best predictor of variceal rebleeding and mortality.[14] By contrast, a reduction in the HVPG to less than 12 mm Hg or a reduction of more than 20% from the baseline value is associated with a decreased risk of variceal hemorrhage and improved patient survival.[25,39] A meta-analysis that included 10 studies with 595 patients evaluated whether targeted HVPG reduction predicts variceal bleeding in patients with cirrhosis receiving nonselective β-blockers for primary prophylaxis. The relative risk (RR) of bleeding in patients achieving a reduction of HVPG to less than or equal to 12 mm Hg or at least 20% compared with baseline (overall responders) was RR = 0.27 (95% confidence interval [CI] 0.14–0.52), although significant heterogeneity between studies was reported.[40]

Liver and Spleen Stiffness

Measurement of liver and spleen stiffness, as a potential surrogate of elevated HVPG by either transient elastography or acoustic radiation force impulse elastography, has been shown to correlate with the presence of varices. Measurement of liver stiffness correlates reasonably well with the HVPG, particularly at HVPG values lower than 10 mm Hg.[41–45]

Platelet count and spleen size, when combined with spleen stiffness measurement, have been able to better predict the presence of varices. A platelet count of less than 88,000 has been found to be associated with the presence of esophagogastric varices.[46] In a meta-analysis of 20 studies (N = 3063), the ratio of platelet count to spleen diameter was found to have a high accuracy for diagnosing esophageal varices (EV).[47] A single score obtained by combining measurements of liver stiffness, spleen size, and platelet count has shown good accuracy for diagnosing and ruling out varices and portal hypertension in patients with cirrhosis. In a study of 90 patients with hepatitis B–related liver cirrhosis, a predictive model measuring liver stiffness × spleen diameter/platelet count was found to have a 94.7% negative predictive value and a 93.3% positive predictive value for diagnosing EV, and was able to calculate the risk of future bleeding from EV.[48–50]

Other Modalities

FibroTest (a panel of 5 biochemical markers of hepatic fibrosis), combined with age and gender, is a good predictor of liver fibrosis and EV.[51] In a prospective study of 130 patients, Fibrotest was found to have good correlation with HVPG, but only a moderate diagnostic value for the detection of severe portal hypertension in patients with cirrhosis.[52]

Endoscopic ultrasonography has also been used to study varices and identify increased risk for bleeding. The role of capsule endoscopy in diagnosing varices has been evolving and also shows promise. Two recent pilot studies demonstrated that capsule endoscopy is a safe and well-tolerated technique with which to diagnose EV.[53,54]

Multidetector-row computed tomography (MDCT) has shown promising results in the evaluation of EV. A recent study concluded that enhanced MDCT was able to localize the origin of bleeding in 96.4% cases preceding urgent endoscopy, and also led to significantly swifter detection of bleeding etiology at endoscopy.[55]

TREATMENT

Addressing issues related to stabilizing the airway, breathing, and circulation is paramount. The goals of management include hemodynamic resuscitation, control of bleeding, and prevention and treatment of complications (**Fig. 1**).

The initial focus of treatment is on delivery of adequate oxygen to the tissues by maintaining oxygen saturation, cardiac output, and hemoglobin concentration.

Patients with AVB are at risk of aspiration of gastric contents, including blood. This risk is especially high in patients with massive hematemesis and reduced consciousness during the endoscopic procedure. Patients with HE or delirium tremens may have difficulties maintaining their airway. Therefore, elective endotracheal intubation before upper endoscopy should be considered in this subset of patients. Intubation before endoscopy not only decreases the risk of aspiration but also makes endoscopic procedures easier to perform, especially when clearance of a large volume of retained blood is expected. Two large-bore intravenous accesses should be established for rapid administration of volume. However, many patients end up with a central venous catheter for aggressive resuscitation, central venous pressure monitoring, and administration of vasoactive medications. Assessment of blood loss should be made by history taking, physical examination, and laboratory tests. While waiting for blood, resuscitation should be initiated with plasma expanders. The choice of fluids for

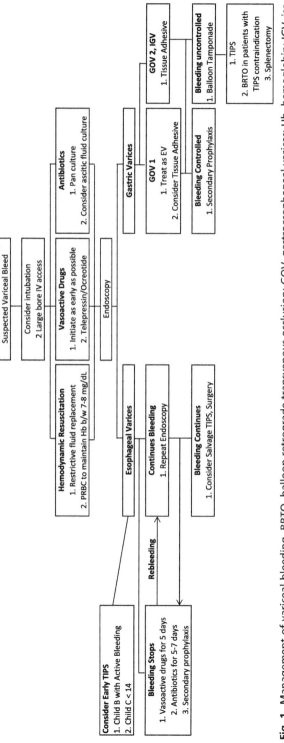

Fig. 1. Management of variceal bleeding. BRTO, balloon retrograde transvenous occlusion; GOV, gastroesophageal varices; Hb, hemoglobin; IGV, isolated gastric varices; IV, intravenous; PRBC, packed red blood cells; TIPS, transjugular intrahepatic portosystemic shunt. *Adapted from* Sarin SK, Kumar A, Angus PW, et al. Diagnosis and management of acute variceal bleeding: Asian Pacific Association for Study of the Liver recommendations. Hepatol Int 2011;5(2):607–24.

replacing the intravascular volume is a topic of debate.[20,32] Whatever the type of crystalloid used, the systolic blood pressure should be maintained around 90 to 100 mm Hg with a heart rate of less than 100 beats per minute.

Blood loss should be replaced with PRBC whenever possible to maintain hemoglobin between 7 and 8 mg/dL[20] except in patients with rapid ongoing bleeding or ischemic heart disease, in which case this threshold may be raised. A delicate balance should be maintained when administering blood or fluids, as on one hand hypervolemia has been shown to cause rebound increases in portal pressure and increase the risk of rebleeding and mortality, while on the other hypotension has been shown to increase the risk of infection, renal failure, rebleeding, and death.[56,57] Recently, the merits of a restrictive strategy of blood transfusion only when the hemoglobin drops below 7 g/dL in comparison with a liberal transfusion strategy (whenever hemoglobin drops below 9 g/dL) were shown, with higher survival seen among persons with Child-A and Child-B cirrhosis.[57] Patients with AVB usually have multiple derangements in clotting parameters secondary to their underlying chronic liver disease. However, these abnormalities do not correlate with the severity of bleeding. It is common practice to administer fresh frozen plasma and platelets to patients with elevated international normalized ratio and thrombocytopenia (platelets <50,000/μL), although the exact benefit of these measures is not established. A recent study suggested that patients with cirrhosis may at times instead be in a hypercoagulable state, owing to an imbalance between procoagulant and anticoagulant factors.[58] The use of fresh frozen plasma and platelets can also lead to expansion of the intravascular volume, leading to an increase in portal pressure.[59] The use of recombinant activated factor VII (the most common deficient clotting factor), which corrects prothrombin time in cirrhotics, is not routinely recommended.[60,61] Treatment with thrombopoietin[62] or desmopressin,[63] a drug that significantly decreases bleeding time in cirrhosis, has shown no clinical benefit in the setting of AVB.

Hepatic Encephalopathy

Patients having AVB may have HE at the time of presentation. In addition, AVB itself leads to worsening of HE, owing to the breakdown of blood to toxic proteins and portosystemic shunting. Sepsis, azotemia, and electrolyte disturbances that can occur in the context of AVB also tend to worsen HE. Sedation during endoscopy or intubation can also exacerbate HE. Change in mental status caused by HE should be differentiated from delirium resulting from alcohol withdrawal and Wernicke encephalopathy, as the treatment of these disorders is different. Lactulose should be used to treat HE. In a recent study, 70 patients with AVB were randomized to receive either lactulose or no lactulose. Only 5 patients (14%) who received lactulose developed HE, compared with 14 patients (40%) in the nonlactulose group ($P = .03$).[63]

Renal Failure

Renal failure develops in 11% of patients with AVB. Hypovolemia, sepsis, liver disease, and nephrotoxic medications contribute to renal failure. The risk of renal failure can be minimized by careful attention to volume status, maintenance of adequate urine output, aggressive treatment of sepsis, and avoidance of nephrotoxic drugs.[56]

Early Antibiotics

Approximately 20% patients of patients with AVB have infection at the time of admission, and an additional 50% acquire infections during their hospital stay.[64]

Infection in AVB is associated with increased mortality and early rebleeding.[65,66] The most frequent infections are spontaneous bacterial peritonitis (50%), urinary tract infections (25%), and pneumonia (25%), which are often caused by enteric aerobic gram-negative bacteremia.[67] A meta-analysis of 12 trials that compared antibiotic prophylaxis with placebo or no intervention found a significant benefit of prophylactic antibiotic use with regard to all-cause mortality (RR 0.79, 95% CI 0.63–0.98), mortality from bacterial infections (RR 0.43, 95% CI 0.19–0.97), bacterial infections (RR 0.35, 95% CI 0.26–0.47), rebleeding (RR 0.53, 95% CI 0.38–0.74), and days of hospitalization (mean difference −1.9 days, 95% CI −3.8 to 0.02).[68] In the last 2 decades infections caused by gram-positive cocci have markedly increased in the setting of extensive use of invasive procedures, frequent hospital admission, and use of antibiotic prophylaxis.[69]

The use of antibiotics in AVB is therefore recommended to help reduce infections and the risk of rebleeding and mortality.[69,70] Antibiotics should be started preferably before endoscopy and should be continued for 5 to 7 days. Quinolones have been the most used antibiotic, traditionally because of its ease of administration and low cost, but its use is now limited owing to increasing antibiotic resistance.[71]

A randomized controlled trial of 111 patients with advanced cirrhosis and AVB showed that the probability of developing possible or proven infection is higher with oral norfloxacin than with intravenous ceftriaxone (33% vs 11%, $P = .003$; 26% vs 11%, $P = .03$).[72] Therefore, professional societies have recommended that intravenous ceftriaxone should be considered over quinolones in patients with severely decompensated cirrhosis, high prevalence of quinolone resistance, or prior quinolone prophylaxis.[20] Newer antibiotics are being tested for their role in AVB. In a recent study, intravenous cefazolin was shown to be similar to ceftriaxone in preventing infections and reducing rebleeding among Child-A cirrhotic patients after endoscopic interventions for AVB, but inferior in Child-B and Child-C patients.[72] However, more rigorous studies are needed before cefazolin can be recommended. The final selection of antibiotics should be tailored to each individual, with due consideration to the local patterns of antibiotic resistance and patient allergies.

Vasoactive Drugs

The role of vasoactive medications in AVB is well established. This fact was reconfirmed in a recent meta-analysis of 30 randomized controlled trials including 3111 patients with AVB who were treated with vasopressin, somatostatin, or their analogues. The use of vasoactive agents was associated with a significantly lower risk of 7-day mortality (RR 0.74, 95% CI 0.57–0.95; $P = .02$), improved control of bleeding (RR 1.21, 95% CI 1.13–1.30; $P<.001$), shorter hospital stay, and lower transfusion requirements.[73] Vasoactive therapy should be started early and continued for 2 to 5 days. Studies comparing the various vasoactive medications have failed to demonstrate a significant difference in efficacy.[74] The choice of vasoactive drug should be made according to local resources and availability.

Timing of Endoscopy

The door to endoscopy time has been a topic of debate. Urgent endoscopy may have the advantages of earlier identification of bleeding, control of bleeding, risk stratification, and prevention of rebleeding,[74] but endoscopy-related complications may compromise these benefits.[75] Few studies concluded that delaying endoscopy in favor of pharmacologic treatment[76] may be as suitable an option, as endoscopic sclerotherapy and pharmacologic therapy were equally effective in controlling bleeding and survival, but the former was associated with more side effects.[76] However, in all these studies sclerotherapy instead of band ligation was performed, which is not the current standard of practice. Moreover, it has now been demonstrated that the combination of endoscopic intervention and pharmacologic treatment is superior to either therapy alone.[77]

Although there is a short delay in endoscopy on the weekends, a study of 36,734 patients presenting with esophageal variceal bleeding (EVB) showed that despite a short delay, there was no difference in mortality.[78] In a contrasting study including 311 cirrhotic patients with EVB, patients were divided into 2 groups of early and delayed endoscopy, taking 15 hours as the cutoff point. Patients in the delayed endoscopy group had a significantly increased risk of in-hospital mortality (odds ratio = 3.67; 95% CI 1.27–10.39; P = .016), independent of the severity of the underlying liver disease, comorbid conditions, hemodynamic status, and endoscopic treatment.[79] In a separate cohort study of 101 patients with AVB, patients presenting with hematemesis and active variceal bleeding observed during endoscopy had the poorest prognosis in terms of early rebleeding and mortality if they received delayed endoscopy. Their 6-week rebleeding and mortality rates were 38.9% and 52.8%, respectively, much higher than the rates of those who received early endoscopy. Contrary to these results, another study showed that the time to endoscopy had no effect on mortality in AVB. However, all patients who were included were hemodynamically stable.[80] Despite conflicting studies, all professional societies have recommended a door to endoscopy time of less than 12 hours in patients with suspected AVB.

Studies have shown that combined treatment with endoscopy and vasoactive drugs is more effective than either treatment alone. In a meta-analysis, combined pharmacologic and endoscopic treatment in comparison with endoscopic treatment alone was significantly more effective for initial control of bleeding (RR 1.12, 95% CI 1.02–1.23) and 5-day hemostasis (RR 1.28, 95% CI, 1.18–1.39).[20,77] In patients who rebleed, an attempt at repeat endoscopic control should be made. Otherwise, the patient should be considered for TIPS or surgery if liver transplantation is not an option. For patients who survive an episode of AVB, the most common approach for secondary prophylaxis is to combine daily nonselective β-blocker therapy with endoscopic variceal ligation every 3 to 4 weeks until obliteration of varices is achieved. Thereafter, endoscopic surveillance can be performed at varying intervals to determine if and when repeat band ligation is needed.[26]

Rescue Measures

In 10% to 20% of patients, AVB is unresponsive to initial endoscopic and/or pharmacologic treatment. Patients who are clinically stable and have mild bleeding can have a second attempt at endoscopy. If this fails, or if bleeding is severe or the patient is hemodynamically unstable, the patient should be offered rescue treatment.

Transjugular intrahepatic portosystemic shunt

TIPS serves as a side-to-side portosystemic anastomosis, and allows portal decompression without the need for major surgery. Traditionally TIPS has been used as a rescue therapy in patients with EVB who rebleed or do not respond to first-line endoscopic and pharmacologic therapy.[81] Factors associated with poor survival following TIPS include advanced age, emergency TIPS, alanine aminotransferase greater than 100 U/L, bilirubin greater than 3 mg/dL, pre-TIPS encephalopathy that is not related to bleeding, and MELD score. Because it is a procedure with high associated mortality, careful patient selection is needed. One study showed that early mortality is common in patients with a Child-Pugh score greater than 13 undergoing TIPS.[28]

The role of early TIPS in patients with advanced liver disease (Child-Pugh C disease, score 10–13) or HVPG 20 mm Hg or higher has been recently studied in 2 controlled trials.[82,83] In these selected patients, early TIPS (after the first index bleed) was associated with a significant reduction in failure of treatment and mortality if placed early (within 72 hours), before the patient deteriorates. In the first study, 52 patients with HVPG greater than 20 mm Hg were randomized to receive endoscopic sclerotherapy or uncovered TIPS within 24 hours of admission. Early TIPS placement significantly reduced treatment failure (12% vs 50%; $P =.0001$), in-hospital mortality (11% vs 38%), and 1-year mortality (35% vs 65%; $P<.05$).[83] However, the benefits of TIPS may have been overestimated, as the therapy used in the control group was not up to the current standards of endoscopic therapy for AVB. Patients in the control group did not receive combination therapy and the endoscopic treatment used was sclerotherapy, which is not the treatment of choice as per current recommendations. In the other recent study, early TIPS using a polytetrafluoroethylene-covered stent (placed within 72 hours) was compared with optimal medical therapy (endoscopic therapy plus vasoactive medications) in 63 high-risk (Child-Pugh class B with active bleeding or in Child-Pugh class C) patients with cirrhosis and AVB. Patients who were randomly assigned to receive TIPS had a significantly better chance of remaining free of bleeding at 1 year than those who received combined endoscopic and pharmacologic care (97% vs 50%). The rate of survival at 1 year was 86% in the TIPS group, compared with 61% in the medical therapy group. The rate of HE was similar in both groups.

Balloon tamponade
Balloon tamponade is used to temporarily control bleeding in cases of AVB where medical management and endoscopy have failed. Balloon tamponade has been shown to control bleeding in 90% of cases.[84] However, 50% of patients rebleed after removal of the tamponade tube. Complications such as aspiration, esophageal rupture, and necrosis develop in 30% of patients. The tube should be removed within 24 hours to reduce such complications. Balloon tamponade is a life-saving measure to temporarily control bleeding in patients with massive hemorrhage until a more definitive therapy can be undertaken.

Self-expandable metal stents
Self-expandable metal stents (SEMS) control bleeding by compression of the bleeding varices. Similar to balloon tamponade, they are used as a life-saving measure in refractory bleeding. SEMS are inserted over an endoscopically placed guide wire using a stent delivery device without the need for fluoroscopy.[85] Compared with balloon tamponade, these stents can be left in place for up to 2 weeks and can be easily removed by endoscopy. However, they are associated with a high risk of rebleeding after removal. Complications of SEMS include esophageal ulcerations, compression of the bronchi, and stent migration into the stomach. Recent data suggest that a self-expanding covered esophageal metal stent may be an alternative to the Sengstaken-Blakemore balloon in refractory EVB, with the advantage of less severe complications despite longer periods of treatment.[86] More studies are needed to establish the role of SEMS in refractory variceal bleeding.

Surgery
The role of surgery in EVB is limited to patients who fail medical measures and endoscopy. However, today surgical expertise for these procedures is greatly limited. Portal decompressive surgery and esophageal transection were highly effective in achieving hemostasis but were associated with a high mortality of 45% to 75%; such procedures are seldom carried out nowadays. In addition, in patients surviving the bleeding episode, portosystemic shunt surgery significantly increases the incidence of chronic

or recurrent HE. In a retrospective study of 82 patients who underwent salvage surgery for variceal bleeding, control of bleeding was achieved in 95% of patients. The in-hospital mortality rate was 15%, and was higher among patients undergoing emergency surgery and in those with cirrhotic portal hypertension.[87] Surgery should be performed in patients with Child-A cirrhosis only. The decision to perform surgery is based on local resources and expertise.

GASTRIC VARICES

The initial management of GV is similar to that of EVB, including the use of prophylactic antibiotics, careful replacement of intravascular volume with a restrictive transfusion policy, and the early administration of vasoactive drugs (terlipressin, somatostatin, or a somatostatin analogue).[20] Although no studies have been done, the combination of drug therapy plus endoscopic treatment seems to be rational for acute bleeding from GV.

In patients with acute bleeding from GV, endoscopic variceal obturation using tissue adhesives is the treatment of choice and controls bleeding in up to 90% of patients.[88] In patients with acute bleeding from gastroesophageal type 1 varices, treatment should be similar to that of esophageal varices or glue injection.[88] Randomized controlled trials comparing tissue adhesive with endoscopic scleroligation and endoscopic variceal ligation (EVL) for acute bleeding have shown that tissue adhesives are equally or more effective than EVL in the control of acute bleeding, and more effective than both in preventing rebleeding in a study that included patients with and without cirrhosis.[88,89]

A relatively large prospective, randomized trial compared gastric variceal obturation (GVO) using N-butyl-cyanoacrylate versus EVL in patients with acute gastric variceal hemorrhage. This study demonstrated that control of active bleeding was similar in both groups, but that rebleeding over a follow-up period of 1.6 to 1.8 years occurred significantly less in the GVO group (23% vs 47%).[90]

Transjugular Intrahepatic Portosystemic Shunt in Gastric Varices

TIPS plays a more significant role in bleeding GV than in bleeding EV. TIPS should be considered in patients with uncontrolled bleeding from GV or if bleeding recurs despite combined pharmacologic and endoscopic treatment. TIPS has been shown to control bleeding in 90% of cases, and reduces the rebleeding rate. A prospective study comparing salvage TIPS in patients with uncontrolled bleeding in gastric fundal varices (n = 28) versus uncontrolled EVB (n = 84) showed equal efficacy in control of hemorrhage in all but 1 patient in each group.[91] Recently, embolization of collaterals feeding GV along with TIPS has been done, but studies that support this practice are rare.[88] Studies comparing TIPS with glue injection have shown variable results. One prospective trial comparing TIPS and glue injection showed that TIPS is more effective in preventing rebleeding, with similar survival.[92] Another study suggested a worse cost-effectiveness ratio and a higher long-term morbidity rate when performing TIPS in a comparison with cyanoacrylate glue injection.[93]

Balloon Retrograde Transvenous Occlusion

Balloon retrograde transvenous occlusion (BRTO) is indicated in GV with gastrorenal shunt when endoscopic cyanoacrylate injection has failed and TIPS is contraindicated because of HE or old age.[88,94] BRTO is successful in controlling active gastric variceal bleeding in 95% of cases (91%–100%). The GV rebleed rate of successful BRTO is

3.2% to 8.7%. However, BRTO diverts blood into the portal circulation and increases the portal hypertension, thus aggravating EV (24%–37% at 1 year).[95]

Surgery

In selected cases, patients with GV and segmental/left-sided portal hypertension that is due to isolated splenic vein thrombosis may be candidates for splenectomy or splenic embolization as a means of definitive therapy.

REFERENCES

1. Garcia-Tsao G, Bosch J. Management of varices and variceal hemorrhage in cirrhosis. N Engl J Med 2010;362(9):823–32.
2. Cales P, Pascal JP. Natural history of esophageal varices in cirrhosis (from origin to rupture). Gastroenterol Clin Biol 1988;12(3):245–54 [in French].
3. D'Amico G, Pagliaro L, Bosch J. The treatment of portal hypertension: a meta-analytic review. Hepatology 1995;22(1):332–54.
4. D'Amico G. Esophageal varices: from appearance to rupture; natural history and prognostic indicators. In: Groszmann RJ, Bosch J, editors. Portal hypertension in the 21st century. Dordrecht: Springer; 2004. p. 147–54.
5. Sanyal AJ, Fontana RJ, Di Bisceglie AM, et al. The prevalence and risk factors associated with esophageal varices in subjects with hepatitis C and advanced fibrosis. Gastrointest Endosc 2006;64(6):855–64.
6. Navasa M, Pares A, Bruguera M, et al. Portal hypertension in primary biliary cirrhosis. Relationship with histological features. J Hepatol 1987;5(3):292–8.
7. Groszmann RJ, Garcia-Tsao G, Bosch J, et al. Beta-blockers to prevent gastroesophageal varices in patients with cirrhosis. N Engl J Med 2005;353(21): 2254–61.
8. Merli M, Nicolini G, Angeloni S, et al. Incidence and natural history of small esophageal varices in cirrhotic patients. J Hepatol 2003;38(3):266–72.
9. Grace ND. Prevention of initial variceal hemorrhage. Gastroenterol Clin North Am 1992;21(1):149–61.
10. North Italian Endoscopic Club for the Study, Treatment of Esophageal Varices. Prediction of the first variceal hemorrhage in patients with cirrhosis of the liver and esophageal varices. A prospective multicenter study. N Engl J Med 1988; 319(15):983–9.
11. McCormick PA, O'Keefe C. Improving prognosis following a first variceal haemorrhage over four decades. Gut 2001;49(5):682–5.
12. Chalasani N, Kahi C, Francois F, et al. Improved patient survival after acute variceal bleeding: a multicenter, cohort study. Am J Gastroenterol 2003;98(3):653–9.
13. Graham DY, Smith JL. The course of patients after variceal hemorrhage. Gastroenterology 1981;80(4):800–9.
14. Smith JL, Graham DY. Variceal hemorrhage: a critical evaluation of survival analysis. Gastroenterology 1982;82(5 Pt 1):968–73.
15. Moitinho E, Escorsell A, Bandi JC, et al. Prognostic value of early measurements of portal pressure in acute variceal bleeding. Gastroenterology 1999;117(3): 626–31.
16. Bambha K, Kim WR, Pedersen R, et al. Predictors of early re-bleeding and mortality after acute variceal haemorrhage in patients with cirrhosis. Gut 2008;57(6): 814–20.
17. Bosch J, Abraldes JG, Berzigotti A, et al. Portal hypertension and gastrointestinal bleeding. Semin Liver Dis 2008;28(1):3–25.

18. Kim T, Shijo H, Kokawa H, et al. Risk factors for hemorrhage from gastric fundal varices. Hepatology 1997;25(2):307–12.

19. Tripathi D, Therapondos G, Jackson E, et al. The role of the transjugular intrahepatic portosystemic stent shunt (TIPSS) in the management of bleeding gastric varices: clinical and haemodynamic correlations. Gut 2002;51(2):270–4.

20. Amitrano L, Guardascione MA, Manguso F, et al. The effectiveness of current acute variceal bleed treatments in unselected cirrhotic patients: refining short-term prognosis and risk factors. Am J Gastroenterol 2012;107(12):1872–8.

21. D'Amico G, De Franchis R, Cooperative Study Group. Upper digestive bleeding in cirrhosis. Post-therapeutic outcome and prognostic indicators. Hepatology 2003;38(3):599–612.

22. de Franchis R, Baveno VF. Revising consensus in portal hypertension: report of the Baveno V consensus workshop on methodology of diagnosis and therapy in portal hypertension. J Hepatol 2010;53(4):762–8.

23. Reverter E, Tandon P, Augustin S, et al. A MELD-based model to determine risk of mortality among patients with acute variceal bleeding. Gastroenterology 2014;146(2):412–9.e3.

24. Augustin S, Genescà J. Diagnostic and prognostic markers in liver cirrhosis. Dis Markers 2011;31(3):119–20.

25. D'Amico G, Garcia-Pagan JC, Luca A, et al. Hepatic vein pressure gradient reduction and prevention of variceal bleeding in cirrhosis: a systematic review. Gastroenterology 2006;131(5):1611–24.

26. Garcia-Tsao G, Sanyal AJ, Grace ND, et al. Practice Guidelines Committee of the American Association for the Study of Liver D, Practice Parameters Committee of the American College of G. Prevention and management of gastroesophageal varices and variceal hemorrhage in cirrhosis. Hepatology 2007;46(3):922–38.

27. Pugh RN, Murray-Lyon IM, Dawson JL, et al. Transection of the oesophagus for bleeding oesophageal varices. Br J Surg 1973;60(8):646–9.

28. Malinchoc M, Kamath PS, Gordon FD, et al. A model to predict poor survival in patients undergoing transjugular intrahepatic portosystemic shunts. Hepatology 2000;31(4):864–71.

29. Flores-Rendon AR, Gonzalez-Gonzalez JA, Garcia-Compean D, et al. Model for end stage of liver disease (MELD) is better than the Child-Pugh score for predicting in-hospital mortality related to esophageal variceal bleeding. Ann Hepatol 2008;7(3):230–4.

30. Chen WT, Lin CY, Sheen IS, et al. MELD score can predict early mortality in patients with rebleeding after band ligation for variceal bleeding. World J Gastroenterol 2011;17(16):2120–5.

31. Augustin S, Altamirano J, Gonzalez A, et al. Effectiveness of combined pharmacologic and ligation therapy in high-risk patients with acute esophageal variceal bleeding. Am J Gastroenterol 2011;106(10):1787–95.

32. Ripoll C, Banares R, Rincon D, et al. Influence of hepatic venous pressure gradient on the prediction of survival of patients with cirrhosis in the MELD era. Hepatology 2005;42(4):793–801.

33. Abraldes JG, Villanueva C, Banares R, et al. Hepatic venous pressure gradient and prognosis in patients with acute variceal bleeding treated with pharmacologic and endoscopic therapy. J Hepatol 2008;48(2):229–36.

34. Sarin SK, Kumar A, Angus PW, et al. Diagnosis and management of acute variceal bleeding: Asian Pacific Association for Study of the Liver recommendations. Hepatol Int 2011;5(2):607–24.

35. de Franchis R, Pascal JP, Ancona E, et al. Definitions, methodology and thera-peutic strategies in portal hypertension. A Consensus Development Workshop, Baveno, Lake Maggiore, Italy, April 5 and 6, 1990. J Hepatol 1992;15(1–2): 256–61.
36. Garcia-Tsao G, Groszmann RJ, Fisher RL, et al. Portal pressure, presence of gastroesophageal varices and variceal bleeding. Hepatology 1985;5(3): 419–24.
37. Groszmann RJ, Glickman M, Blei AT, et al. Wedged and free hepatic venous pressure measured with a balloon catheter. Gastroenterology 1979;76(2): 253–8.
38. Ripoll C, Groszmann R, Garcia-Tsao G, et al. Hepatic venous pressure gradient predicts clinical decompensation in patients with compensated cirrhosis. Gastroenterology 2007;133(2):481–8.
39. Abraldes JG, Tarantino I, Turnes J, et al. Hemodynamic response to pharmaco-logical treatment of portal hypertension and long-term prognosis of cirrhosis. Hepatology 2003;37(4):902–8.
40. Albillos A, Banares R, Gonzalez M, et al. Value of the hepatic venous pressure gradient to monitor drug therapy for portal hypertension: a meta-analysis. Am J Gastroenterol 2007;102(5):1116–26.
41. Vizzutti F, Arena U, Romanelli RG, et al. Liver stiffness measurement predicts se-vere portal hypertension in patients with HCV-related cirrhosis. Hepatology 2007;45(5):1290–7.
42. Shi KQ, Fan YC, Pan ZZ, et al. Transient elastography: a meta-analysis of diag-nostic accuracy in evaluation of portal hypertension in chronic liver disease. Liver Int 2013;33(1):62–71.
43. Sharma P, Kirnake V, Tyagi P, et al. Spleen stiffness in patients with cirrhosis in predicting esophageal varices. Am J Gastroenterol 2013;108(7):1101–7.
44. Bota S, Sporea I, Sirli R, et al. Can ARFI elastography predict the presence of significant esophageal varices in newly diagnosed cirrhotic patients? Ann Hep-atol 2012;11(4):519–25.
45. Takuma Y, Nouso K, Morimoto Y, et al. Measurement of spleen stiffness by acoustic radiation force impulse imaging identifies cirrhotic patients with esoph-ageal varices. Gastroenterology 2013;144(1):92–101.e2.
46. Zaman A, Hapke R, Flora K, et al. Factors predicting the presence of esopha-geal or gastric varices in patients with advanced liver disease. Am J Gastroen-terol 1999;94(11):3292–6.
47. Ying L, Lin X, Xie ZL, et al. Performance of platelet count/spleen diameter ratio for diagnosis of esophageal varices in cirrhosis: a meta-analysis. Dig Dis Sci 2012;57(6):1672–81.
48. Kim BK, Han KH, Park JY, et al. A liver stiffness measurement-based, noninva-sive prediction model for high-risk esophageal varices in B-viral liver cirrhosis. Am J Gastroenterol 2010;105(6):1382–90.
49. Kim BK, Kim do Y, Han KH, et al. Risk assessment of esophageal variceal bleeding in B-viral liver cirrhosis by a liver stiffness measurement-based model. Am J Gastroenterol 2011;106(9):1654–62, 1730.
50. Berzigotti A, Seijo S, Arena U, et al. Elastography, spleen size, and platelet count identify portal hypertension in patients with compensated cirrhosis. Gastroenterology 2013;144(1):102–11.e1.
51. Thabut D, Trabut JB, Massard J, et al. Non-invasive diagnosis of large oesopha-geal varices with FibroTest in patients with cirrhosis: a preliminary retrospective study. Liver Int 2006;26(3):271–8.

52. Thabut D, Imbert-Bismut F, Cazals-Hatem D, et al. Relationship between the Fibrotest and portal hypertension in patients with liver disease. Aliment Pharmacol Therapeut 2007;26(3):359–68.

53. Lapalus MG, Dumortier J, Fumex F, et al. Esophageal capsule endoscopy versus esophagogastroduodenoscopy for evaluating portal hypertension: a prospective comparative study of performance and tolerance. Endoscopy 2006; 38(1):36–41.

54. Eisen GM, Eliakim R, Zaman A, et al. The accuracy of PillCam ESO capsule endoscopy versus conventional upper endoscopy for the diagnosis of esophageal varices: a prospective three-center pilot study. Endoscopy 2006;38(1): 31–5.

55. Miyaoka Y, Amano Y, Ueno S, et al. The role of enhanced multi-detector-row computed tomography before urgent endoscopy in acute upper gastrointestinal bleeding. J Gastroenterol Hepatol 2014;29(4):716–22.

56. Cardenas A, Gines P, Uriz J, et al. Renal failure after upper gastrointestinal bleeding in cirrhosis: incidence, clinical course, predictive factors, and short-term prognosis. Hepatology 2001;34(4 Pt 1):671–6.

57. Villanueva C, Colomo A, Bosch A, et al. Transfusion strategies for acute upper gastrointestinal bleeding. N Engl J Med 2013;368(1):11–21.

58. Tripodi A, Primignani M, Chantarangkul V, et al. An imbalance of pro- vs anti-coagulation factors in plasma from patients with cirrhosis. Gastroenterology 2009;137(6):2105–11.

59. Youssef WI, Salazar F, Dasarathy S, et al. Role of fresh frozen plasma infusion in correction of coagulopathy of chronic liver disease: a dual phase study. Am J Gastroenterol 2003;98(6):1391–4.

60. Ejlersen E, Melsen T, Ingerslev J, et al. Recombinant activated factor VII (rFVIIa) acutely normalizes prothrombin time in patients with cirrhosis during bleeding from oesophageal varices. Scand J Gastroenterol 2001;36(10):1081–5.

61. Bosch J, Thabut D, Albillos A, et al. Recombinant factor VIIa for variceal bleeding in patients with advanced cirrhosis: a randomized, controlled trial. Hepatology 2008;47(5):1604–14.

62. Peck-Radosavljevic M, Wichlas M, Zacherl J, et al. Thrombopoietin induces rapid resolution of thrombocytopenia after orthotopic liver transplantation through increased platelet production. Blood 2000;95(3):795–801.

63. Sharma P, Agrawal A, Sharma BC, et al. Prophylaxis of hepatic encephalopathy in acute variceal bleed: a randomized controlled trial of lactulose versus no lactulose. J Gastroenterol Hepatol 2011;26(6):996–1003.

64. Chavez-Tapia NC, Barrientos-Gutierrez T, Tellez-Avila FI, et al. Antibiotic prophylaxis for cirrhotic patients with upper gastrointestinal bleeding. Cochrane Database Syst Rev 2010;(9):CD002907.

65. Goulis J, Armonis A, Patch D, et al. Bacterial infection is independently associated with failure to control bleeding in cirrhotic patients with gastrointestinal hemorrhage. Hepatology 1998;27(5):1207–12.

66. Augustin S, Muntaner L, Altamirano JT, et al. Predicting early mortality after acute variceal hemorrhage based on classification and regression tree analysis. Clin Gastroenterol Hepatol 2009;7(12):1347–54.

67. Sass DA, Chopra KB. Portal hypertension and variceal hemorrhage. Med Clin North Am 2009;93(4):837–53, vii–viii.

68. Chavez-Tapia NC, Barrientos-Gutierrez T, Tellez-Avila F, et al. Meta-analysis: antibiotic prophylaxis for cirrhotic patients with upper gastrointestinal bleeding - an updated Cochrane review. Aliment Pharmacol Ther 2011;34(5):509–18.

69. Fernandez J, Navasa M, Gomez J, et al. Bacterial infections in cirrhosis: epidemiological changes with invasive procedures and norfloxacin prophylaxis. Hepatology 2002;35(1):140–8.
70. Hou MC, Lin HC, Liu TT, et al. Antibiotic prophylaxis after endoscopic therapy prevents rebleeding in acute variceal hemorrhage: a randomized trial. Hepatology 2004;39(3):746–53.
71. Fernandez J, Ruiz del Arbol L, Gomez C, et al. Norfloxacin vs ceftriaxone in the prophylaxis of infections in patients with advanced cirrhosis and hemorrhage. Gastroenterology 2006;131(4):1049–56 [quiz: 1285].
72. Wu CK, Wang JH, Lee CH, et al. The outcome of prophylactic intravenous cefazolin and ceftriaxone in cirrhotic patients at different clinical stages of disease after endoscopic interventions for acute variceal hemorrhage. PLoS One 2013;8(4):e61666.
73. Wells M, Chande N, Adams P, et al. Meta-analysis: vasoactive medications for the management of acute variceal bleeds. Aliment Pharmacol Therapeut 2012;35(11):1267–78.
74. Thabut D, Bernard-Chabert B. Management of acute bleeding from portal hypertension. Best practice & research. Best Pract Res Clin Gastroenterol 2007; 21(1):19–29.
75. D'Amico G, Pietrosi G, Tarantino I, et al. Emergency sclerotherapy versus vasoactive drugs for variceal bleeding in cirrhosis: a Cochrane meta-analysis. Gastroenterology 2003;124(5):1277–91.
76. Escorsell A, Ruiz del Arbol L, Planas R, et al. Multicenter randomized controlled trial of terlipressin versus sclerotherapy in the treatment of acute variceal bleeding: the TEST study. Hepatology 2000;32(3):471–6.
77. Banares R, Albillos A, Rincon D, et al. Endoscopic treatment versus endoscopic plus pharmacologic treatment for acute variceal bleeding: a meta-analysis. Hepatology 2002;35(3):609–15.
78. Myers RP, Kaplan GG, Shaheen AM. The effect of weekend versus weekday admission on outcomes of esophageal variceal hemorrhage. Can J Gastroenterol 2009;23(7):495–501.
79. Hsu YC, Chung CS, Tseng CH, et al. Delayed endoscopy as a risk factor for in-hospital mortality in cirrhotic patients with acute variceal hemorrhage. J Gastroenterol Hepatol 2009;24(7):1294–9.
80. Cheung J, Soo I, Bastiampillai R, et al. Urgent vs. non-urgent endoscopy in stable acute variceal bleeding. Am J Gastroenterol 2009;104(5):1125–9.
81. Escorsell A, Banares R, Garcia-Pagan JC, et al. TIPS versus drug therapy in preventing variceal rebleeding in advanced cirrhosis: a randomized controlled trial. Hepatology 2002;35(2):385–92.
82. Garcia-Pagan JC, Caca K, Bureau C, et al. Early use of TIPS in patients with cirrhosis and variceal bleeding. N Engl J Med 2010;362(25):2370–9.
83. Monescillo A, Martinez-Lagares F, Ruiz del Arbol L, et al. Influence of portal hypertension and its early decompression by TIPS placement on the outcome of variceal bleeding. Hepatology 2004;40(4):793–801.
84. Avgerinos A, Armonis A. Balloon tamponade technique and efficacy in variceal haemorrhage. Scand J Gastroenterol Suppl 1994;207:11–6.
85. Escorsell A, Bosch J. Self-expandable metal stents in the treatment of acute esophageal variceal bleeding. Gastroenterol Res Pract 2011;2011:910986.
86. Hubmann R, Bodlaj G, Czompo M, et al. The use of self-expanding metal stents to treat acute esophageal variceal bleeding. Endoscopy 2006;38(9): 896–901.

87. Sharma A, Vijayaraghavan P, Lal R, et al. Salvage surgery in variceal bleeding due to portal hypertension. Indian J Gastroenterol 2007;26(1):14–7.
88. Garcia-Pagan JC, Barrufet M, Cardenas A, et al. Management of gastric varices. Clin Gastroenterol Hepatol 2014;12(6):919–28.e1.
89. Sarin SK, Jain AK, Jain M, et al. A randomized controlled trial of cyanoacrylate versus alcohol injection in patients with isolated fundic varices. Am J Gastroenterol 2002;97(4):1010–5.
90. Tan PC, Hou MC, Lin HC, et al. A randomized trial of endoscopic treatment of acute gastric variceal hemorrhage: N-butyl-2-cyanoacrylate injection versus band ligation. Hepatology 2006;43(4):690–7.
91. Chau TN, Patch D, Chan YW, et al. "Salvage" transjugular intrahepatic portosystemic shunts: gastric fundal compared with esophageal variceal bleeding. Gastroenterology 1998;114(5):981–7.
92. Lo GH, Liang HL, Chen WC, et al. A prospective, randomized controlled trial of transjugular intrahepatic portosystemic shunt versus cyanoacrylate injection in the prevention of gastric variceal rebleeding. Endoscopy 2007;39(8):679–85.
93. Procaccini NJ, Al-Osaimi AM, Northup P, et al. Endoscopic cyanoacrylate versus transjugular intrahepatic portosystemic shunt for gastric variceal bleeding: a single-center U.S. analysis. Gastrointest Endosc 2009;70(5):881–7.
94. Matsumoto A, Hamamoto N, Nomura T, et al. Balloon-occluded retrograde transvenous obliteration of high risk gastric fundal varices. Am J Gastroenterol 1999;94(3):643–9.
95. Saad WE, Sabri SS. Balloon-occluded retrograde transvenous obliteration (BRTO): technical results and outcomes. Semin Intervent Radiol 2011;28(3):333–8.

Primary Prophylaxis of Variceal Bleeding

Jawad A. Ilyas, MD, MS[a], Fasiha Kanwal, MD, MSHS[a,b],*

KEYWORDS

- Portal hypertension • Cirrhosis • Hemorrhage

KEY POINTS

- Both nonselective beta-blockers and endoscopic band ligation form the cornerstone of prophylactic therapy for varices.
- In the absence of accurate noninvasive markers of hepatic venous pressure gradient, variceal size, high-risk stigmata of variceal bleeding, and the stage of underlying liver disease dictate the choice of prophylactic therapy.
- The major challenge is to screen patients in a timely manner and institute a form of therapy that has the highest chance of success in terms of both compliance and effectiveness.
- Without systematic efforts targeted at reducing these gaps in health care delivery, recent advances in the efficacy of primary prophylaxis may not translate into effective varices care at the bedside.

BACKGROUND

Cirrhosis is a common and burdensome condition. It is responsible for approximately 1 million days of work lost and 32,000 annual deaths in the United States, and thus has a substantial effect on productivity and survival.[1] The high mortality in cirrhosis is attributable, in part, to the development of varices and subsequent hemorrhage. Despite substantial advances in medical management of variceal bleeding, each episode of active variceal bleeding is fatal in 30% of cases.[2,3]

Development of varices is a direct consequence of portal hypertension and reflects abnormal changes in both portal resistance and flow. Portal hypertension is commonly

Funding: This work is partly funded by the Houston Veterans Affairs Health Services Research and Development Center of Excellence HFP90-020.
Disclosures: No conflicts of interest exist.
Disclaimer: The views expressed in this article are those of the authors and do not necessarily represent the views of the Department of Veterans Affairs.
[a] Gastroenterology and Hepatology, Department of Medicine, Baylor College of Medicine, 6620 Main St., Houston, TX 77030, USA; [b] Center for Innovations in Quality, Effectiveness, and Safety (IQuESt), Michael E. DeBakey Veterans Affairs Medical Center, Houston, TX, USA
* Corresponding author. 2002 Holcombe Boulevard, Houston, TX 77030.
E-mail address: kanwal@bcm.edu

measured using the hepatic venous pressure gradient (HVPG), which is the difference between wedged and free hepatic venous pressure. Varices generally develop when the hepatic venous pressure gradient (HVPG) exceeds 5 to 10 mm Hg as a compensatory mechanism to decompress the portal system; variceal bleeding occurs when the HVPG exceeds 12 mm Hg.[4] Esophageal varices are present in approximately 40% of patients with cirrhosis and as many as 60% of patients with cirrhosis and ascites. In patients without varices, new varices develop at the rate of 5% to 8% per year.[4] In patients with small varices at the time of initial endoscopic screening, progression to large varices occurs at a rate of 10% to 15% per year.[4] One of the largest prospective studies that followed the natural history of variceal progression enrolled 206 patients with cirrhosis. Of these, 113 patients did not have varices at baseline and 93 patients had small varices. After an average follow-up of 37 months, 28% of patients (without varices) developed varices, whereas 31% of patients (with small varices) experienced progression in variceal size. The strongest predictors of progression were the Child-Pugh score at baseline, presence of stigmata of bleeding (red wale markings), baseline platelet count, and alcohol-related liver disease. The risk of variceal bleeding was significantly higher in the patients who had small varices at baseline compared with those who did not have varices (12% vs 2% at 2 years).[5] A more recent study using data from the HALT-C trial found a similar rate of de novo varices development and progression (26.2% and 35.3%, respectively) during a median follow-up of 48 months.[6] Hispanic race and lower baseline albumin level were both strongly associated with the risk of varices development.

Several clinical and physiologic factors are associated with the risk of first variceal hemorrhage. These include variceal location, size, appearance of the varices, underlying HVPG, and the degree of hepatic dysfunction.[1] Of these, HVPG is the most important and a potentially modifiable risk factor. HVPG serves as an accurate surrogate marker of variceal development, as well as the risk of variceal bleeding. In a systematic review of prospective studies, a reduction in the HVPG to 12 mm Hg or lower, or a reduction of 20% or more from baseline significantly reduced the risk of first variceal bleeding (pooled odds ratio 0.21, 95% confidence interval [CI] 0.05–0.80).[7] Therapies aimed at reducing the HVPG below this threshold can affect the progression of varices and reduce the risk of first variceal bleeding.

PRIMARY PROPHYLAXIS

Prophylaxis is derived from the Greek word *prophulaktikos*, meaning "prevention." Primary prophylaxis entails prevention of the first episode of variceal bleeding after diagnosis of varices. However, this concept can be expanded to (1) prevention of formation of varices (preprimary prophylaxis), (2) prevention of progression of variceal size (early-primary prophylaxis), and (3) prevention of the first episode of bleeding (primary prophylaxis).

SCREENING FOR VARICES

Although the point prevalence of varices in patients with cirrhosis is relatively high, most patients with cirrhosis may not have varices. As a result, guidelines recommend screening for the presence of varices in patients with cirrhosis[8–10] and initiating treatment targeted at primary prophylaxis for patients identified to have high-risk varices.

Esophagogastroduodenoscopy (EGD) is considered the gold standard for the diagnosis of varices. However, EGD is relatively expensive and requires specialized expertise to perform. Moreover, as mentioned previously, most patients undergoing EGD either do not have varices or have varices that do not require prophylactic treatment (see later in this article), thus substantially increasing the cost associated with screening with EGD. The alternative strategies to universal screening with EGD are empiric beta-blocker therapy (ie, without prior screening) or screening with less expensive and less invasive diagnostic tools.

A randomized controlled trial (RCT) showed that empiric, nonselective beta-blockers are ineffective in preventing varices in patients with cirrhosis and portal hypertension and are associated with an increased number of adverse events.[4] However, only a small proportion of patients included in this trial had Child class B cirrhosis (10%) and none had Child class C cirrhosis. Therefore, it is unclear if the strategy of empiric beta-blockers would be effective in patients with a high probability of underlying varices, such as those with decompensated cirrhosis. Nonetheless, in light of these data, beta-blockers cannot be recommended empirically in patients without documented varices.

Given its noninvasive nature and relative ease of administration, video capsule endoscopy (VCE) may play a role in screening for varices. However, a multicenter trial designed to assess the diagnostic performance of VCE in comparison with EGD found that EGD was superior to VCE in identifying patients with varices.[11] Overall, EGD identified esophageal varices in 180 (62.5%) of 292 patients. VCE identified esophageal varices in 152 of these patients (difference 15.6%; 95% CI 11.4–19.8 in favor of EGD). VCE had a sensitivity, specificity, positive predictive value (PPV), and negative predictive value (NPV) of 84%, 88%, 92%, and 77%, respectively, for identifying patients with esophageal varices compared with the gold standard of EGD. In differentiating between medium/large varices requiring treatment and absent/small varices requiring surveillance, the sensitivity, specificity, PPV, and NPV for VCE were 78%, 96%, 87%, and 92%, respectively. In another study, 120 patients with both cirrhotic and noncirrhotic portal hypertension underwent VCE followed by EGD at the time of screening.[12] The sensitivity, specificity, NPV, and PPV of VCE for diagnosis of varices was 77%, 86%, 69%, and 90%, respectively. The interobserver concordance was generally poor (diagnosis of varices 79.4%; grading of varices 66.4%; indication for prophylaxis 89.7%) in this study.

Several studies have evaluated the predictive accuracy of multidetector computerized tomography (CT) esophagography to detect and grade esophageal varices.[13,14] This procedure requires esophageal insufflation via a transnasal catheter and thus is minimally invasive. The study by Kim and colleagues[13] included 90 patients with cirrhosis (65 men, mean age 54.8 years); 30 patients had endoscopic evidence of large esophageal varices. There was close correlation and substantial agreement between endoscopic and CT esophagographic grades ($\kappa = 0.831$). CT esophagography performed well in differentiating between low- and high-risk varices with the area under the receiver operating characteristic curve (AUROC) of 0.93 to 0.95. Perri and colleagues[14] prospectively evaluated 102 patients who underwent both CT and endoscopic screening for gastroesophageal varices. The multidetector CT scan with intravenous contrast was highly sensitive in identifying large esophageal varices (sensitivity = 90% compared with EGD). However, the specificity was limited (specificity = 50%). Patients preferred CT scan over EGD in both studies.

The use of the platelet count/spleen diameter ratio has also been proposed as a noninvasive tool to predict the presence of varices. This ratio is calculated by dividing the platelet count (number/mm^3) by the maximum spleen diameter (in mm) as estimated by abdominal ultrasound. In using a cutoff value of 909, Giannini and colleagues[15] found that the PPV and NPV of platelet count/spleen diameter ratio for the presence of varices were 96% and 100%, respectively, the AUROC was 0.98.

However, restricting the analysis to patients with compensated cirrhosis (the population in which this index may have the highest clinical utility), the PPV dropped to 74%. In an independent multicenter cohort study, the PPV and NPV of the platelet count/spleen diameter ratio were 76.6% and 87.0%, respectively.[16] Neither study demonstrated this index to be a reliable predictor of varices.

In summary

- Several noninvasive and minimally invasive means of identifying patients with varices have been tested in the recent years. However, the predictive accuracy of these markers is still unsatisfactory.
- Until large prospective studies are conducted, EGD screening remains the principal means of assessing for the presence of varices.
- More studies are needed to ascertain whether the simplicity and improved patient tolerance of VCE or CT esophagography over EGD can increase the rate of adherence to screening programs. For the time being, these modalities may be used in selected patients who are unwilling or unable to undergo EGD.

PRE-PRIMARY PROPHYLAXIS

Currently, the most effective strategy in preventing development of varices is effective management of the underlying liver disease. For example, in a prospective study by Bruno and colleagues,[17] only one of the patients with chronic hepatitis C cirrhosis who achieved a sustained virological response (SVR) developed varices during a 12-year follow-up period. In contrast, 32% of untreated patients and 39% of patients who were treated but did not achieve SVR developed varices.

Thus, the most effective strategy in preventing development of varices in patients with cirrhosis is effective management of the underlying liver disease

PRIMARY PROPHYLAXIS IN PATIENTS WITH SMALL VARICES

There has been one meta-analysis evaluating the role of nonselective beta-blockers in the prevention of a first variceal bleed in patients with small varices.[18] Since the publication of this meta-analysis, 2 additional trials have evaluated this same question.[19,20] Combining these data, the incidence of first variceal bleeding was 2.5% in the treatment group compared with 7.4% in the control group over 2-year follow-up (a statistically nonsignificant difference).

Two of these studies investigated the efficacy of beta-blockers in preventing the enlargement of small varices with contradictory results. In the first study,[19] 2-year proportion of patients with large varices was higher in the propranolol group compared with the placebo group (31% vs 14%). However, more patients in the propranolol group had varices at baseline compared with the placebo group (52% vs 30%). Moreover, one-third of the patients in this study were lost to follow-up. In the second larger randomized trial,[20] patients with small varices treated with nadolol had a significantly slower progression to larger varices (11% at 3 years) than patients who received placebo (37% at 3 years). In this study, patients received beta-blockers within 3 ($\pm$2.5) months of varices diagnosis.

Collectively, these data suggest that the risk of variceal bleeding is low in patients with small varices, and that beta-blockers do not reduce this risk further, at least in the intermediate term. Beta-blockers may slow the progression of varices, but this effect needs to be confirmed in future studies. Patients with small varices and no high-risk features should undergo routine surveillance to monitor for development of variceal enlargement and high-risk features. Of note, none of these aforementioned studies presented data stratified on the basis of the severity of underlying liver disease or presence versus absence of high-risk endoscopic features to inform decisions based on these factors.

Given the available data, the American Association for Study of Liver Diseases (AASLD) and the Baveno V guidelines provide the following recommendations for patients who have small varices.

- In patients with cirrhosis and small varices that have not bled and have no criteria for increased risk of bleeding, beta-blockers can be used, although their long-term benefit has not been established
- In patients with cirrhosis and small varices that have not bled but have criteria for increased risk of bleeding (child class B or C or presence of red wale markings on varices), beta-blockers should be used for the prevention of first variceal hemorrhage.

PRIMARY PROPHYLAXIS IN PATIENTS WITH LARGE VARICES

The 2 most common treatment modalities used for primary prophylaxis of variceal bleeding in patients with large varices include the use of nonselective beta-blockers or endoscopic band ligation.

Nonselective Beta-Blockers

A meta-analysis of 11 randomized trials that included 1189 patients with medium to large varices evaluated the efficacy of beta-blockers (propranolol, nadolol) versus placebo in the prevention of first variceal bleed. The risk of first variceal bleed in patients with medium or large varices was significantly reduced by beta-blockers (30% vs 14%, number needed to treat = 10) during 2 years of follow-up.[18] The disadvantages of nonselective beta-blockers include relatively common contraindications and side effects (fatigue and shortness of breath) that preclude treatment or require discontinuation in 15% to 20% of patients.

These data support the use of beta-blockers for the primary prophylaxis of variceal bleeding in patients with large varices. Both the AASLD and Baveno V guidelines agree with using beta-blockers in this subgroup and provide the following recommendations.

- In patients with large varices that have not bled, nonselective beta-blockers may be recommended for the prevention of first variceal hemorrhage. This applies to patients with or without any high-risk features (Childs B or C and/or red wale markings on varices).

Choice of Nonselective Beta-Blocker

Both nadolol and propranolol have been recommended as agents of choice in primary prevention of variceal bleeding. Both drugs result in unopposed alpha adrenergic–mediated splanchnic vasoconstriction and reduction of portal inflow (as a result of reduction in cardiac output).[21] Dose titration can be achieved by monitoring patients' resting heart rate or their HVPG. When the heart rate is used, beta-blockers are up-titrated to achieve a 20% reduction from baseline or achieve a target heart rate of 55 to 60 beats per minute. In some European centers, HVPG is routinely measured to guide titration of therapy and is recommended in the Baveno V guidelines. A reduction of HVPG to 12 mm Hg or lower or to 20% or less of the baseline HVPG value reduces the risk of variceal bleeding.[7] However, HVPG monitoring is invasive and is not routinely practiced in the United States outside of clinical trials.

Carvedilol, a beta-blocker with alpha adrenergic activity also has been studied as a pharmacologic agent for primary prophylaxis.[10,22,23] Multiple studies examining the effects of carvedilol on portal hypertension have shown a dose-related decrease in HVPG (20% from baseline), which is higher than seen with propranolol.[24,25] A recent meta-analysis that included a total of 175 patients from 5 studies compared the hemodynamic effects of carvedilol with propranolol.[26] Carvedilol resulted in a greater reduction in HVPG both in the short term (mean weighted difference in HVPG −7.70 mm Hg [95% CI −12.40 to −3.00] at 60–90 minutes after drug administration) and the long term (mean weighted difference in HVPG −6.81 mm Hg [95% CI −11.35 to −2.26] after 7–90 days of therapy) (**Fig. 1**). The risk of failure to achieve a hemodynamic response with carvedilol was lower than that with propranolol (relative risk [RR] 0.66, 95% CI 0.44–1.00). Adverse events were more frequent and serious with carvedilol; however, this difference failed to reach statistical significance.

A recent trial examined 104 patients with esophageal varices (mean HVPG 20.4 mm Hg) who underwent HVPG monitoring before and during propranolol treatment (80–160 mg per day).[25] Patients without a hemodynamic response to propranolol (defined as lack of a reduction in HVPG ≥20% compared with baseline or an absolute value ≥12 mm Hg on repeat HVPG) or those who did not tolerate propranolol (n = 10) were treated with carvedilol (6.25–50 mg per day). Of the 67 patients who met these criteria for propranolol nonresponse, 56% achieved a hemodynamic response with carvedilol. The decrease in HVPG was significantly greater with carvedilol than with propranolol (−19% ± 10% vs −12% ± 11%, P<.001). During 2-year follow-up, variceal bleeding occurred in 5% of patients on carvedilol compared with 11% on propranolol (P = .04). This study demonstrated that carvedilol is a reasonable option for patients who do not respond to propranolol.

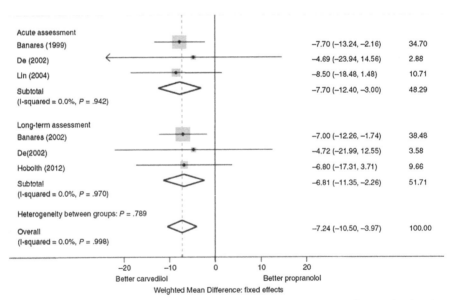

Fig. 1. Weighted mean difference in the hepatic venous pressure gradient reduction (expressed as percentage decrease) between carvedilol and propranolol in RCTs assessing both acute and long-term effect. (*From* Sinagra E, Perricone G, D'Amico M, et al. Systematic review with meta-analysis: the haemodynamic effects of carvedilol compared with propranolol for portal hypertension in cirrhosis. Aliment Pharmacol Ther 2014;39(6):565; with permission.)

Endoscopic Variceal Ligation

Endoscopic variceal ligation (EVL) has been compared with no therapy and beta-blockers in several randomized trials (with 5 meta-analyses[27–31]) in patients with medium to large varices. A meta-analysis that included a total of 601 patients from 5 trials comparing prophylactic EVL with untreated controls found that EVL decreased the risk of first variceal hemorrhage (RR 0.36), hemorrhage-related mortality (RR 0.20), and all-cause mortality (RR 0.55) compared with no treatment.[27]

A recent Cochrane review included 19 randomized trials that compared the efficacy of EVL versus beta-blockers in preventing first variceal bleeding.[31] Most trials only included patients with large or high-risk esophageal varices, defined as either having red signs (such as red wale markings, cherry red spots, or hematocystic spots) or as large varices (tortuous varices protruding into at least one-third of the esophageal lumen, or pseudotumorous varices, or at least 5 mm or at least 2 mm plus at least one red color sign). EVL was performed with conventional or multiband ligators and was repeated at 3-week to 4-week intervals until the varices were eradicated. On average, 2 to 3 sessions were necessary to achieve variceal eradication. Subsequently, patients were followed at 3-month to 6-month intervals and EVL was repeated in the case of variceal recurrence. Most of the trials used propranolol, one trial assessed nadolol, and one assessed carvedilol. The beta-blocker dose was adjusted to achieve a 20% to 25% reduction in heart rate or a resting heart rate of 55 beats per minute or less.

Upper gastrointestinal bleeding was diagnosed in 14% of patients randomized to EVL compared with 20% in the beta-blocker group. EVL reduced variceal bleeding compared with nonselective beta-blockers (RR 0.67; 95% CI 0.46–0.98); however, the beneficial effect of EVL on bleeding was not confirmed in subgroup analyses of trials with adequate randomization. Reporting of side effects was inconsistent and difficult to summarize in the analysis. A total of 9 of 190 patients (n = 4 trials) developed bleeding and 49 of the 221 patients (n = 5 trials) developed transient dysphagia or retrosternal pain after band ligation. Among patients randomized to beta-blockers, the most frequently noted adverse event was hypotension in 57 of 329 patients (n = 6 trials). There was no difference in the rates of overall mortality between the 2 treatment groups, and these results have been consistent across all published meta-analyses (**Fig. 2**).

These data demonstrate that both EVL and beta-blockers may be used as primary prophylaxis in high-risk esophageal varices, although EVL may have a greater beneficial effect in terms of rates of variceal bleeding. However, all trials in the systematic review included patients with high risk of variceal bleeding (large varices, or medium varices with red signs) and most patients had Child class B or C cirrhosis. Therefore, these data cannot be generalized to patients with medium to large varices who do not have other endoscopic high-risk stigmata (red signs) or to patients with Child class A cirrhosis.

Two RCTs examined the efficacy of EVL versus carvedilol for primary prophylaxis of esophageal variceal bleeding. One of these studies was included in the Cochrane systematic review discussed previously (Tripathi and colleagues[22]); the second trial was published after the completion of the Cochrane review (Shah and colleagues[23]). Both trials included patients without prior history of variceal bleeding who were identified to have medium to large varices on endoscopy. In the study by Tripathi and colleagues,[22] only 10% of patients randomized to carvedilol developed variceal bleeding compared with 23% of those randomized to EVL, and this difference was likely related to noncompliance with the EVL protocol. The rates of variceal

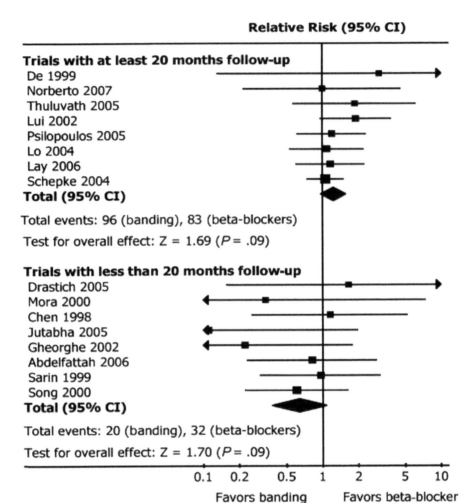

Fig. 2. Meta-analysis of mortality in randomized trials comparing endoscopic band ligation versus nonselective beta-blockers in primary prophylaxis of esophageal variceal bleeding, stratified by duration of follow-up. (*From* Gluud LL, Klingenberg S, Nikolova D, et al. Banding ligation vs beta-blockers as primary prophylaxis in esophageal varices: systematic review of randomized trials. Am J Gastroenterol 2007;102:2845; with permission.)

bleeding were similar between the 2 interventions in the study by Shah and colleagues[23] (8.5% vs 6.9%, respectively). There were no significant differences in overall mortality in both studies. Both studies showed that carvedilol was safe and the rate of serious adverse events leading to drug discontinuation was relatively small (0.02% and 0.12%, respectively).[22,23] Collectively, these data suggest that carvedilol is as (if not more) efficacious than EVL in preventing a first episode of variceal bleeding.

Use of EVL versus beta-blockers also has been examined in a cost-effectiveness study.[32] When considering only cost per life year (LY) as the outcome, the incremental cost-effectiveness ratio (ICER) of the strategy using initial EVL compared with beta-blocker use exceeded the benchmark of $50,000 per LY, with an ICER of $98,407 per LY saved. However, when quality of life was considered, EVL was cost-effective compared with beta-blockers (incremental cost utility ratio of $25,548 per quality-adjusted LY). The choice of treatment ultimately should be based on local resources and expertise, patient preferences, and characteristics.

The AASLD and Baveno V guidelines provide the following recommendations regarding patients with medium to large varices:

- In patients with medium/large varices that have not bled and have a high risk of hemorrhage (Child class B/C or variceal red wale markings on endoscopy), EVL may be recommended for the prevention of first variceal hemorrhage
- In patients with medium/large varices that have not bled and are not at the highest risk of hemorrhage, EVL should be considered in patients with contraindications or intolerance or noncompliance to beta-blockers
- The choice of treatment should be based on local resources and expertise, patient preference and characteristics, side effects, and contraindications

UNAPPROVED MODALITIES FOR PRIMARY PROPHYLAXIS

Endoscopic sclerotherapy, surgical shunts, and transjugular intrahepatic portosystemic shunts (TIPS) have been proposed as potential options for primary prophylaxis of variceal bleeding. Endoscopic sclerotherapy has failed to show a benefit when compared with either sham therapy or nonselective beta-blockers in controlled trials.[33] Both surgical shunts and TIPS have not been studied in the context of primary prophylaxis and therefore cannot be recommended at this time.

SURVEILLANCE ENDOSCOPY

Given the natural history of varices, expert consensus panels have determined that surveillance endoscopies should be performed every 2 years in patients with compensated cirrhosis who have small varices. Surveillance endoscopies should be performed annually in those with decompensated cirrhosis.[8] However, there are no direct data evaluating the effectiveness of these recommendations. The AASLD guidelines provide the following recommendations:

- In patients with small varices that have not bled and who are not receiving beta-blockers, EGD should be repeated in 2 years
- If there is evidence of hepatic decompensation, EGD should be done at that time and repeated annually
- In patients with small varices, who receive beta-blockers, a follow-up EGD is not necessary
- If a patient is placed on a nonselective beta-blocker and it is adjusted to the maximal tolerated dose, then follow-up surveillance EGD is unnecessary
- If a patient is treated with EVL, it should be repeated every 1 to 2 weeks until obliteration, with the first surveillance EGD performed 1 to 3 months after obliteration and then every 6 to 12 months to check for variceal recurrence

PRIMARY PROPHYLAXIS OF GASTRIC VARICES

Gastric varices are found in approximately 20% of patients with portal hypertension. Gastric variceal hemorrhage is more severe and has a higher mortality than esophageal variceal bleeding.[34] There are limited data on primary prophylaxis of gastric variceal bleeding. An RCT examined 89 patients with cirrhosis and gastric varices (gastroesophageal varices type 2 and isolated gastric varices type 1) and compared the efficacy of cyanoacrylate injections, beta-blockers and placebo in primary pro-phylaxis of variceal bleeding.[35] After a mean follow-up of 26 months, the bleeding rates in the cyanoacrylate, beta-blocker, and placebo groups were 13%, 28%, and 45%, respectively ($P = .003$). In addition, the actuarial probability of survival was higher in the cyanoacrylate group compared with the placebo group (90% vs 72%, respectively). Given the relative paucity of data and risks associated with injec-tion therapy, neither the AASLD nor Baveno V guidelines recommend cyanoacrylate injection therapy for primary prophylaxis of gastric variceal bleeding. More studies are needed to determine the optimal method of preventing bleeding in these high-risk patients.

GAPS AND FUTURE DIRECTIONS

There is a need for better understanding the fundamental and basic mechanisms behind development and progression of portal hypertension. A better foundation can potentially lead to more targeted and effective prophylactic measures. EGD is the current gold standard for diagnosis of varices; however, it remains an inva-sive test with potential risks. The adherence rates to screening could potentially be increased by developing more accurate noninvasive methods for varices detection. Future research also needs to focus on identifying noninvasive measures of HVPG monitoring and tailoring prophylactic therapy based on HVPG (6–10 mm Hg vs >10 mm Hg).

SUMMARY

In summary, both nonselective beta-blockers and endoscopic band ligation form the cornerstone of prophylactic therapy for varices. In the absence of accurate noninva-sive markers of HVPG, variceal size, high-risk stigmata of variceal bleeding, and the stage of underlying liver disease dictate the choice of prophylactic therapy. The major challenge is to screen patients in a timely manner and institute a form of therapy that has the highest chance of success in terms of both compliance and effectiveness. Specifically, in a retrospective cohort study of 550 patients with cirrhosis who sought care at 3 Department of Veterans Affairs facilities between 2000 and 2007, we found that only 24.3% (95% CI 20.2%–28.3%) of patients had an upper endoscopy during the first year after their cirrhosis diagnosis and 60% (95% CI 50.2%–70.7%) of pa-tients with varices received any form of primary prophylaxis of variceal bleeding.[36] Without systematic efforts targeted at reducing these gaps in health care delivery, recent advances in the efficacy of primary prophylaxis may not translate into effective varices care at the bedside.

REFERENCES

1. Garcia-Tsao G, Bosch J. Management of varices and variceal hemorrhage in cirrhosis. N Engl J Med 2010;362:823–32.
2. Smith JL, Graham DY. Variceal hemorrhage: a critical evaluation of survival anal-ysis. Gastroenterology 1982;82:968–73.
3. Graham DY, Smith JL. The course of patients after variceal hemorrhage. Gastro-enterology 1981;80:800–9.
4. Groszmann RJ, Garcia-Tsao G, Bosch J, et al. Beta-blockers to prevent gastroesophageal varices in patients with cirrhosis. N Engl J Med 2005;353:2254–61.

5. Merli M, Nicolini G, Angeloni S, et al. Incidence and natural history of small esophageal varices in cirrhotic patients. J Hepatol 2003;38:266–72.
6. Fontana RJ, Sanyal AJ, Ghany MG, et al. Factors that determine the development and progression of gastroesophageal varices in patients with chronic hepatitis C. Gastroenterology 2010;138:2321–31, 2331.
7. D'Amico G, Garcia-Pagan JC, Luca A, et al. Hepatic vein pressure gradient reduction and prevention of variceal bleeding in cirrhosis: a systematic review. Gastroenterology 2006;131:1611–24.
8. Garcia-Tsao G, Sanyal AJ, Grace ND, et al. Prevention and management of gastroesophageal varices and variceal hemorrhage in cirrhosis. Hepatology 2007;46:922–38.
9. Sarin SK, Kumar A, Angus PW, et al. Primary prophylaxis of gastroesophageal variceal bleeding: consensus recommendations of the Asian Pacific Association for the Study of the Liver. Hepatol Int 2008;2:429–39.
10. de FR. Revising consensus in portal hypertension: report of the Baveno V consensus workshop on methodology of diagnosis and therapy in portal hypertension. J Hepatol 2010;53:762–8.
11. de FR, Eisen GM, Laine L, et al. Esophageal capsule endoscopy for screening and surveillance of esophageal varices in patients with portal hypertension. Hepatology 2008;47:1595–603.
12. Lapalus MG, Ben SE, Gaudric M, et al. Esophageal capsule endoscopy vs. EGD for the evaluation of portal hypertension: a French prospective multicenter comparative study. Am J Gastroenterol 2009;104:1112–8.
13. Kim SH, Kim YJ, Lee JM, et al. Esophageal varices in patients with cirrhosis: multidetector CT esophagography—comparison with endoscopy. Radiology 2007; 242:759–68.
14. Perri RE, Chiorean MV, Fidler JL, et al. A prospective evaluation of computerized tomographic (CT) scanning as a screening modality for esophageal varices. Hepatology 2008;47:1587–94.
15. Giannini E, Botta F, Borro P, et al. Platelet count/spleen diameter ratio: proposal and validation of a non-invasive parameter to predict the presence of oesophageal varices in patients with liver cirrhosis. Gut 2003;52:1200–5.
16. Giannini EG, Zaman A, Kreil A, et al. Platelet count/spleen diameter ratio for the noninvasive diagnosis of esophageal varices: results of a multicenter, prospective, validation study. Am J Gastroenterol 2006;101:2511–9.
17. Bruno S, Crosignani A, Facciotto C, et al. Sustained virologic response prevents the development of esophageal varices in compensated, Child-Pugh class A hepatitis C virus-induced cirrhosis. A 12-year prospective follow-up study. Hepatology 2010;51:2069–76.
18. D'Amico G, Pagliaro L, Bosch J. Pharmacological treatment of portal hypertension: an evidence-based approach. Semin Liver Dis 1999;19:475–505.
19. Cales P, Oberti F, Payen JL, et al. Lack of effect of propranolol in the prevention of large oesophageal varices in patients with cirrhosis: a randomized trial. French-Speaking Club for the Study of Portal Hypertension. Eur J Gastroenterol Hepatol 1999;11:741–5.
20. Merkel C, Marin R, Angeli P, et al. A placebo-controlled clinical trial of nadolol in the prophylaxis of growth of small esophageal varices in cirrhosis. Gastroenterology 2004;127:476–84.
21. Villanueva C, Aracil C, Colomo A, et al. Acute hemodynamic response to beta-blockers and prediction of long-term outcome in primary prophylaxis of variceal bleeding. Gastroenterology 2009;137:119–28.

22. Tripathi D, Ferguson JW, Kochar N, et al. Randomized controlled trial of carvedilol versus variceal band ligation for the prevention of the first variceal bleed. Hepatology 2009;50:825–33.

23. Shah HA, Azam Z, Rauf J, et al. Carvedilol vs. esophageal variceal band ligation in the primary prophylaxis of variceal hemorrhage: a multicentre randomized controlled trial. J Hepatol 2014;60(4):757–64.

24. Banares R, Moitinho E, Piqueras B, et al. Carvedilol, a new nonselective beta-blocker with intrinsic anti-Alpha1-adrenergic activity, has a greater portal hypotensive effect than propranolol in patients with cirrhosis. Hepatology 1999; 30:79–83.

25. Reiberger T, Ulbrich G, Ferlitsch A, et al. Carvedilol for primary prophylaxis of variceal bleeding in cirrhotic patients with haemodynamic non-response to propranolol. Gut 2013;62:1634–41.

26. Sinagra E, Perricone G, D'Amico M, et al. Systematic review with meta-analysis: the haemodynamic effects of carvedilol compared with propranolol for portal hypertension in cirrhosis. Aliment Pharmacol Ther 2014;39(6):557–68.

27. Imperiale TF, Chalasani N. A meta-analysis of endoscopic variceal ligation for primary prophylaxis of esophageal variceal bleeding. Hepatology 2001;33:802–7.

28. Khuroo MS, Khuroo NS, Farahat KL, et al. Meta-analysis: endoscopic variceal ligation for primary prophylaxis of oesophageal variceal bleeding. Aliment Pharmacol Ther 2005;21:347–61.

29. Gluud LL, Klingenberg S, Nikolova D, et al. Banding ligation versus beta-blockers as primary prophylaxis in esophageal varices: systematic review of randomized trials. Am J Gastroenterol 2007;102:2842–8.

30. Li L, Yu C, Li Y. Endoscopic band ligation versus pharmacological therapy for variceal bleeding in cirrhosis: a meta-analysis. Can J Gastroenterol 2011;25:147–55.

31. Gluud LL, Krag A. Banding ligation versus beta-blockers for primary prevention in oesophageal varices in adults. Cochrane Database Syst Rev 2012;(8):CD004544.

32. Imperiale TF, Klein RW, Chalasani N. Cost-effectiveness analysis of variceal ligation vs. beta-blockers for primary prevention of variceal bleeding. Hepatology 2007;45:870–8.

33. Avgerinos A, Armonis A, Manolakopoulos S, et al. Endoscopic sclerotherapy plus propranolol versus propranolol alone in the primary prevention of bleeding in high risk cirrhotic patients with esophageal varices: a prospective multicenter randomized trial. Gastrointest Endosc 2000;51:652–8.

34. Sarin SK, Lahoti D, Saxena SP, et al. Prevalence, classification and natural history of gastric varices: a long-term follow-up study in 568 portal hypertension patients. Hepatology 1992;16:1343–9.

35. Mishra SR, Sharma BC, Kumar A, et al. Primary prophylaxis of gastric variceal bleeding comparing cyanoacrylate injection and beta-blockers: a randomized controlled trial. J Hepatol 2011;54:1161–7.

36. Buchanan P, Kramer J, El-Serag H, et al. The quality of care provided to patients with varices. Am J Gastroenterol 2014;109(7):934–40.

Endoscopic Hemostasis in Acute Esophageal Variceal Bleeding

Andrés Cárdenas, MD, MMSc, AGAF[a], Anna Baiges, MD[b],
Virginia Hernandez-Gea, MD, PhD[b],
Juan Carlos Garcia-Pagan, MD, PhD[b,*]

KEYWORDS

- Endoscopy • Hemostasis • Acute variceal bleeding • Portal hypertension

KEY POINTS

- Acute variceal bleeding (AVB) is a serious complication of patients with portal hypertension.
- Initial management includes appropriate volume replacement, transfusion of blood to keep hemoglobin levels around 7 to 8 g/dL, antibiotic prophylaxis, and endotracheal intubation in selected cases.
- Standard of care mandates early administration of vasoactive drug therapy followed by endoscopic band ligation (EBL) or injection endoscopic sclerotherapy (if EBL cannot be performed) within the first 12 hours of patient presentation.
- Patients who fail endoscopic hemostasis therapy may require the temporary placement of balloon tamponade or an esophageal stent; however, experience with esophageal stents is limited and use of balloon tamponade is associated with potentially lethal complications such as aspiration and perforation of the esophagus.
- Both modalities should be available for potential use and all patients surviving an episode of AVB should undergo secondary prophylaxis in order to prevent variceal rebleeding.

The development of portal hypertension in cirrhosis changes the natural course of patients with chronic liver disease because it has several consequences, including the development of gastroesophageal varices, variceal bleeding, ascites, hepatorenal syndrome, and hepatic encephalopathy. The initial appearance of varices in patients

[a] GI/Endoscopy Unit, Hospital Clinic, Institut d'Investigacions Biomèdiques August Pi-Sunyer (IDIBAPS), Ciber de Enfermedades Hepáticas y Digestivas (CIBEREHD), Barcelona, Spain; [b] Barcelona Hepatic Hemodynamic Laboratory, Liver Unit, Hospital Clinic, Institut d'Investigacions Biomèdiques August Pi-Sunyer (IDIBAPS), Ciber de Enfermedades Hepáticas y Digestivas (CIBEREHD), Barcelona, Spain
* Corresponding author. Hepatic Hemodynamic Laboratory, Liver Unit, Hospital Clinic, Villarroel 170, Barcelona 08036, Spain.
E-mail address: jcgarcia@clinic.ub.es

Gastroenterol Clin N Am 43 (2014) 795–806
http://dx.doi.org/10.1016/j.gtc.2014.08.009
0889-8553/14/$ – see front matter © 2014 Elsevier Inc. All rights reserved.

with compensated cirrhosis indicates a progression of the disease from a low-risk state to an intermediate state, but once bleeding occurs this indicates decompensation and an increased risk of death.[1] Although mortalities caused by acute variceal bleeding (AVB) have declined from nearly 60% to 15% to 20% at 6 weeks in the past 3 to 4 decades, there is still a significant risk of recurrence and of morbidity and mortality.[2–4] All patients surviving an AVB should therefore receive secondary prophylaxis.[5] This article reviews the current management approach of patients with AVB with particular emphasis on endoscopic hemostatic techniques for bleeding varices.

NATURAL HISTORY AND DIAGNOSIS OF ACUTE VARICEAL BLEEDING

Patients with esophageal varices have an incidence of AVB that ranges from 4% to 15% per year depending on the severity of liver disease, variceal size, presence of red wale markings, and a hepatic venous pressure gradient (HVPG) value greater than 12 mm Hg.[6–8] In most cases (80%), patients with cirrhosis and gastrointestinal bleeding have gastroesophageal varices as the cause of hemorrhage. Thus upper gastrointestinal bleeding in patients with cirrhosis must be presumed to be variceal in origin until proved otherwise. Although the clinical history is highly reliable in assuming the diagnosis of AVB, the gold standard for the diagnosis is upper endoscopy. Endoscopy can show active blood spurting or oozing from a varix (this can be present in 15% of patients) (**Fig. 1**), a white nipple or clot adherent to a varix, or the presence of varices without other potential sources of bleeding in the upper gastrointestinal tract. Although acute bleeding from varices may cease spontaneously in nearly half of patients, rebleeding rates are significantly high (30%–40%) if patients are not treated appropriately.[9,10] The highest risk occurs within the 48 hours following the index bleed and most of the rebleeding episodes occur with the first 14 days. Initial endoscopic failure to control bleeding occurs most commonly in patients with Child class C cirrhosis, concomitant bacterial infection, portal vein thrombosis, active spurting of a varix, and an HVPG greater than 20 mm Hg.[11–15]

Survival from an episode of AVB has improved greatly: from 42% in the 1980s[10] to the current rates of 80% to 85%.[3,4,16–19] This improvement has been caused by overall improvements in intensive care, volume repletion, pharmacologic and endoscopic therapy, implementation of transjugular intrahepatic portosystemic shunts

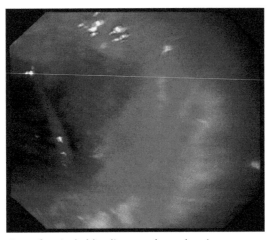

Fig. 1. Endoscopic view of actively bleeding esophageal varix.

(TIPS), and prophylaxis for bacterial infections. Current estimates of mortality from uncontrolled bleeding are 4% to 8%.[11] Approximately one-third of the deaths are a direct consequence of bleeding and the remainder are caused by liver failure, infections, and renal failure.[20]

Recent studies stress the importance of identifying good prognostic markers in patients with episodes of acute bleeding. Although it is well known that HVPG greater than 20 mm Hg is associated with a high risk of 5-day treatment failure to control bleeding, obtaining this measurement is invasive and not available in all centers.[14,15] However, easily obtainable clinical variables (Child-Pugh class C, systolic blood pressure <100 mm Hg at admission, and nonalcoholic causes of cirrhosis) are also associated with 5-day treatment failure to control bleeding,[14] which means that the presence of any of these variables on admission helps clinicians to plan aggressive management and further therapies that may be needed if there is no good response to initial standard-of-care treatment.

INITIAL MANAGEMENT

The most important initial step in providing adequate care for patients with AVB consists of (1) providing optimal hemodynamic management with cautious correction of hypovolemia, (2) preventing complications, and (3) stopping the hemorrhage. An established protocol that takes into account adequate volume resuscitation, airway management, prophylactic antibiotics, administration of vasoconstrictors, and therapeutic endoscopy should be followed in all cases of AVB.

A decision to secure the airway before endoscopy should be considered in patients with hepatic encephalopathy and those actively vomiting blood because of the high risk of pulmonary aspiration. Although there are scarce data on this practice and some investigators claim intubation is not safe, others have shown benefits in improving patient outcome.[21,22] Volume resuscitation with plasma expanders should be instituted in order to keep systolic blood pressure at 100 mm Hg. This measure ensures adequate tissue perfusion with avoidance of hemodynamic shock; hemodynamic shock can cause renal failure, which is associated with an increased risk of death.[20,23] In contrast, overtransfusion should be avoided because it may induce rebound increases in portal pressure and variceal rebleeding.[24,25] Blood transfusions should aim for a hemoglobin (Hb) level of 7 g/dL, except in patients with active ongoing bleeding or with ischemic heart disease.[23] A recent study that compared a restrictive transfusion policy that administered blood products if Hb levels decreased to less than 7 g/dL with a liberal policy (transfusion if Hb <9 g/dL) showed that the probability of survival was significantly higher in patients with cirrhosis and Child-Pugh class A or B disease who were assigned to the restrictive policy group. Moreover, within the first 5 days, the portal-pressure gradient increased significantly in patients in the liberal strategy group but not in patients assigned to the restrictive strategy group.[25]

There are no evidence-based data to support the routine use of platelet transfusion or fresh frozen plasma administration. Current consensus and expert opinion suggest that, in patients with platelet counts less than 50,000 per μL and/or with an International Normalized Ratio greater than 1.5, it is prudent, weighing the risks and benefits, to consider transfusion of platelets and/or fresh frozen plasma before the procedure.[26] Bacterial infections are a poor prognostic indicator in AVB.[12] The most common infections are spontaneous bacterial peritonitis, urinary tract infections, and pneumonia. Prophylactic antibiotics in patients with AVB reduce the risk of rebleeding and mortality,[27–29] thus all patients on admission should receive them. Norfloxacin 400 mg by mouth twice daily for 7 days may be given; however, patients with hypovolemic shock, ascites, malnutrition, encephalopathy, or bilirubin greater than 3 mg/dL should receive intravenous ceftriaxone (1 g/d) because it is more effective than oral norfloxacin in the prophylaxis of bacterial infections in patients with cirrhosis and AVB.[29]

Prompt initiation of vasoactive drugs and timing of endoscopy should be planned from the time the patient arrives at the hospital. This promptness facilitates establishing a diagnosis and performing therapy. Emergency endoscopy should be performed within the first 12 hours after admission.[23,30] If patients are actively vomiting blood, it should be performed once the patient has been hemodynamically stabilized in a monitored unit. Recent data indicate that the early placement of TIPS (within 72 hours) for patients with AVB with Child B actively bleeding or Child C cirrhosis (<13 points) is associated with a significant reduction in rebleeding and mortality and thus should be considered in such cases.[31]

SPECIFIC TREATMENT
Vasoconstrictors

In suspected variceal bleeding, vasoactive drugs (which reduce portal pressure and decrease variceal blood flow) need to be given as soon as possible and before upper endoscopy. This advice is supported by randomized controlled trials (RCTs) and meta-analyses showing that the use of vasoactive drugs achieves hemostasis and reduces the rate of active bleeding, making endoscopy easier to perform for diagnostic and therapeutic purposes.[32–36] In addition, these drugs reduce rebleeding and all-cause mortality among patients with cirrhosis and AVB.[36] Two types of drugs are used: vasopressin and its analogues (terlipressin) and somatostatin and its analogues (octreotide/vapreotide) (**Table 1**).

Endoscopy

Endoscopy is one of the cornerstones of AVB management because it confirms the diagnosis and allows therapy during the same session. Endoscopic therapies for varices are designed to reduce variceal wall tension by obliteration of the varix. The 2 endoscopic methods available for AVB are endoscopic sclerotherapy (EST) and endoscopic band ligation (EBL) (**Fig. 2**). Endoscopic therapy should be used in conjunction with vasoconstrictors. This strategy is strongly supported by several trials and guidelines showing that the efficacy of both emergency EST and EBL is significantly improved when they are associated with pharmacologic treatment.[23,37–40]

Endoscopic sclerotherapy
For AVB, this technique consists of the injection of a sclerosing agent into the variceal lumen (intravariceal injection); this causes thrombosis of the varix and inflammation of the surrounding mucosa that with time creates a scar over the esophageal wall. EST is performed with an injection catheter (needle tip, 23 or 25 gauge) and the sclerosant

Table 1
Vasoconstrictors used in AVB. All drugs are administered for a minimum of 2 days and may be administered for up to 5 days

Drug	Dose
Terlipressin	IV bolus 2 mg every 4 h for 24–48 h then 1 mg every 4 h
Somatostatin	IV bolus 250 μg followed by infusion of 250–500 μg/h
Octreotide	IV bolus of 50–100 μg followed by infusion of 50 μg/h
Vapreotide	IV bolus of 50 μg followed by infusion of 50 μg/h

Abbreviation: IV, intravenous.

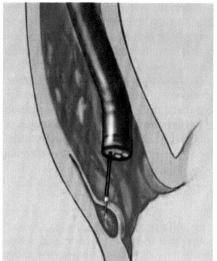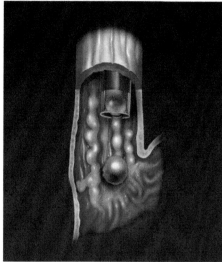

Fig. 2. Endoscopic techniques for esophageal varices. EST (*right*) and EBL (*left*). (*From* AGA Institute Gastroslides. Cirrhosis and Portal Hypertension. Available at: https://www. gastroslides.org.)

solution. The most common sclerosants are ethanolamine oleate (5%), polidocanol (1%–2%), or sodium morrhuate (5%).[41,42] The first injection of 1 to 2 mL of the sclerosant should be placed immediately below (distal to) the bleeding site. Afterward, the remaining varices are injected with 1 to 2 mL adjacent to the bleeding varix. The main objective is to target the lower esophagus near the gastroesophageal (GE) junction. In most cases, up to 15 mL of a sclerosant solution are required. The advantages of using EST for AVB are mainly related to the technique being user friendly because the injection catheter fits through the working channel of a diagnostic gastroscope and does not require a second oral intubation. In addition, there is rapid formation of a thrombus. Drawbacks include a variety of local and systemic side effects, including substernal chest pain, fever, dysphagia, and pleural effusion.[43–45] Esophageal ulcers are common and in 20% of patients they may cause bleeding.[43–45] Bacteremia may occur in up to 35% of patients and lead to other complications such as spontaneous bacterial peritonitis or distal abscesses.[45,46] Other complications include esophageal strictures, perforations, mediastinitis, pericarditis, chylothorax, esophageal motility disorders, and acute respiratory distress syndrome.[43,44]

Endoscopic band ligation
This technique consists of placing elastic bands on the varices in order to occlude the varix and cause thrombosis and the subsequent necrosis of the mucosa. The bands fall off in 5 to 8 days leaving a superficial mucosal ulceration that heals and eventually scars.[47] Clinical trials and a meta-analysis have shown that EBL is better than EST for all major outcomes, including initial control of bleeding (primary hemostasis), recurrent bleeding, side effects, time to variceal obliteration, and survival.[48–50]

There are several multiband devices available for EBL; the most common are the Saeed Multiple Ligator (Wilson-Cook Medical, Inc) and the Speedband (Boston Scientific Corporation). They have between 4 and 10 preloaded bands, but in most cases the ligators with 6 or 7 bands are used. All work on the same principle, which is placement of elastic bands on the varix after it is sucked into a clear plastic cylinder attached to the tip of the endoscope. After the diagnostic endoscopy is performed and the variceal bleeding site is identified, the endoscope is withdrawn and the ligation device is loaded. After reintubation with the ligation device placed on the endoscope, the varix (usually in the distal third of the esophagus) is identified and the tip is pointed toward it and continuous suction applied so that it fills the cap. Once inside the cap has a red-out sign, the band can be deployed (**Fig. 3**). After the varix is ligated, the endoscope should not be advanced, to avoid dislodgement of the bands, which is why banding should always commence in the most distal portion of the esophagus near the GE junction. Bands are applied in a spiral pattern progressing the esophagus up (proximally) until all major columns of varices of the lower third of the esophagus (usually no more than 10 cm above the GE junction) are banded. If there is active bleeding and there is a limited view, the bands should be placed at the GE junction. This method reduces ongoing bleeding and further bands can be fired afterward until active bleeding ceases.

Complications of EBL include transient dysphagia and chest pain, which are common and respond well to analgesics as well as an oral suspension of antacids. Patients should commence liquids for the first 12 hours and then progress to soft foods. Shallow ulcers at the site of bands are common but rarely bleed. The use of a proton pump inhibitor per os decreases the size of ulcers but does not prevent them from bleeding.[51] Severe but rare complications, such as massive bleeding from ulcers or rarely from variceal rupture, esophageal perforation, esophageal strictures, and altered esophageal motility, may occur with EBL.[52]

Both EST and EBL have been shown to be highly effective in the control of AVB, with an immediate efficacy of between 80% and 90%.[53] Two well-performed RCTs specifically comparing EBL and EST in AVB[49,50] have clearly shown that treatment with EBL along with vasoconstrictors is associated with greater efficacy and safety, and improved mortality, compared with EST and vasoconstrictors. In addition, in another 8 trials these 2 modalities were also compared in AVB and in the prevention of rebleeding. A meta-analysis of the 10 trials shows that EBL is better than EST in the initial control of bleeding, and is associated with fewer adverse events and improved mortality.[54] In addition, EST, but not EBL, may induce a sustained increase in portal pressure after the procedure.[55] Therefore, EBL should be the endoscopic therapy of choice in AVB. Although we prefer EBL to EST for an episode of AVB, in the setting of active hemorrhage or torrential bleeding EBL is sometimes difficult to perform because of a lack of visibility. Therefore, both techniques are reasonable options in the setting of AVB.

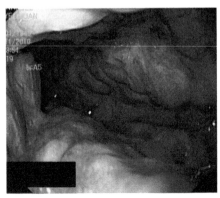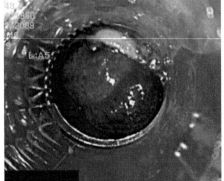

Fig. 3. Endoscopic view of large varices with red spots (*left*) and endoscopic view of a successfully placed band on a varix (*right*).

Other Methods

Sengstaken-Blakemore tubes and esophageal stents

Balloon tamponade of the esophagus may be required in patients with uncontrolled bleeding or in patients with such massive and profuse bleeding in whom an upper endoscopy cannot safely be performed. Pneumatic compression of the fundus and the distal esophagus stops bleeding in approximately 85% of cases. The problem is that recurrence after balloon deflation, which must occur within 48 hours of placement, is high (50%) and major complications, including aspiration pneumonia and esophageal perforation, may occur in up to 30% of patients.[56] Given the high success rates of current endoscopic and pharmacologic therapies, balloon tamponade is uncommonly performed. A recently introduced, fully covered, self-expandable metallic stent (Ella-Danis, Czech Republic) for AVB may be useful in cases for which balloon tamponade is considered (**Fig. 4**).[57–59] The stent may be placed blindly or over a guidewire previously passed to the stomach. The stent has a distal balloon that is inflated with a syringe to ensure proper location in the gastric cardia and distal esophagus so no fluoroscopy is needed. The stent can be left in place for up to 7 to 10 days and can be retrieved by endoscopy with a hook system. Although there are limited data for its use, a multicenter RCT (published in abstract form) comparing esophageal stenting with balloon tamponade in 28 patients with AVB refractory to medical and endoscopic treatment and/or with massive bleeding precluding endoscopy has shown esophageal stents to be more effective and safer than balloon tamponade for the temporary control of AVB.[60]

Cyanoacrylate glue and Hemospray

Although endoscopic injection of cyanoacrylate glue is mainly used for patients who bleed from gastric varices, its use has also been proposed for patients with AVB. There are 2 small studies that indicate that injection of cyanoacrylate glue (1 mL per injection) is safe and effective for patients with AVB.[61,62] However rebleeding rates are higher compared with EBL.[61] In one study, there were no technical difficulties in performing secondary prophylaxis with EBL.[62] Other hemostasis methods seem promising as hemostatic techniques for patients with variceal bleeding. Three small

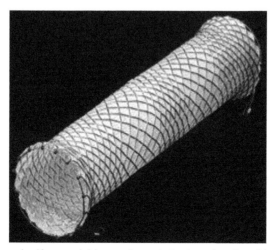

Fig. 4. A fully covered self-expandable esophageal stent can be placed in the esophagus as rescue therapy in patients in whom variceal bleeding cannot be controlled with EBL or EST.

case series indicate that Hemospray (hemostatic powder), which is used for nonvariceal gastrointestinal bleeding, is effective in controlling bleeding from portal gastropathy and gastric varices, but there are no data in patients with acute esophageal variceal hemorrhage.[63–65] These emerging hemostasis modalities therefore may be useful for those patients in whom EBL or EST fails to achieve primary hemostasis at index endoscopy, but additional comparative data are needed.

Failures

Approximately 10% to 15% of patients do not respond to the current first-line therapies.[23] In such cases, if the patient is stable, a second therapeutic endoscopy may be performed. However, if this is unsuccessful or there is massive bleeding, the patient should be considered for TIPS because it is considered the rescue therapy of choice.[23,38] This topic is beyond the scope of this article and is discussed elsewhere.[66]

SUMMARY

AVB is a serious complication of patients with portal hypertension. Initial management includes appropriate volume replacement, transfusion of blood to keep Hb levels around 7 to 8 g/dL, antibiotic prophylaxis, and endotracheal intubation in selected cases. Standard of care mandates starting vasoactive drug therapy early followed by EBL or injection EST (if EBL cannot be performed) within the first 12 hours of patient presentation. Pharmacologic agents may be administered for up to 5 days. Patients who fail endoscopic hemostasis therapy may require the temporary placement of balloon tamponade or an esophageal stent. However, experience with esophageal stents is limited and the use of balloon tamponade is associated with potentially lethal complications such as aspiration and perforation of the esophagus. Therefore, both modalities should be available for potential use. All patients surviving an episode of AVB should undergo secondary prophylaxis in order to prevent variceal rebleeding. An algorithm foe the management of AVB is shown in **Fig 5**.

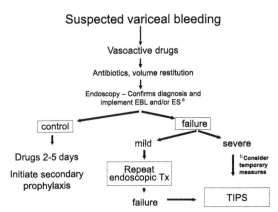

Fig. 5. Recommended treatment algorithm for a patient with an episode of acute esophageal variceal bleeding. [a] Placement of TIPS (within 72 hours) for patients with AVB with Child B actively bleeding or Child C cirrhosis (<13 points) is associated with a significant reduction in rebleeding and mortality and can be considered in such cases. [b] Temporizing measures include placement of an esophageal stent or balloon tamponade. Experience with esophageal stents is limited and use of balloon tamponade can be associated with potentially lethal complications such as pulmonary aspiration and perforation of the esophagus. EBL, endoscopic band ligation; ES, endoscopic sclerotherapy; Tx, treatment.

REFERENCES

1. D'Amico G, Garcia-Tsao G, Pagliaro L. Natural history and prognostic indicators of survival in cirrhosis: a systematic review of 118 studies. J Hepatol 2006;44:217–31.
2. O'Brien J, Triantos C, Burroughs AK. Management of varices in patients with cirrhosis. Nat Rev Gastroenterol Hepatol 2013;10:402–12.
3. Chalasani N, Kahi C, Francois F, et al. Improved patient survival after acute variceal bleeding: a multicenter, cohort study. Am J Gastroenterol 2003;98:653–9.
4. Carbonell N, Pauwels A, Serfaty L, et al. Improved survival after variceal bleeding in patients with cirrhosis over the past two decades. Hepatology 2004;40:652–9.
5. Bosch J, Garcia-Pagan JC. Prevention of variceal rebleeding. Lancet 2003;361:952–4.
6. de Franchis R, Primignani M. Natural history of portal hypertension in patients with cirrhosis. Clin Liver Dis 2001;5:645–63.
7. The North Italian Endoscopic Club for the Study and Treatment of Esophageal Varices. Prediction of the first variceal hemorrhage in patients with cirrhosis of the liver and esophageal varices. A prospective multicenter study. N Engl J Med 1988;319:983–9.
8. Groszmann RJ, Bosch J, Grace ND, et al. Hemodynamic events in a prospective randomized trial of propranolol versus placebo in the prevention of a first variceal hemorrhage. Gastroenterology 1990;99:1401–7.
9. D'Amico G, Pagliaro L, Bosch J. Pharmacological treatment of portal hypertension: an evidence-based approach. Semin Liver Dis 1999;19:475–505.
10. Graham D, Smith J. The course of patients after variceal hemorrhage. Gastroenterology 1981;80:800–6.
11. D'Amico G, de Franchis R. Upper digestive bleeding in cirrhosis. Post-therapeutic outcome and prognostic indicators. Hepatology 2003;38:599–612.
12. Goulis J, Armonis A, Patch D, et al. Bacterial infection is independently associated with failure to control bleeding in cirrhotic patients with gastrointestinal hemorrhage. Hepatology 1998;27:1207–12.
13. Ben Ari Z, Cardin F, McCormick AP, et al. A predictive model for failure to control bleeding during acute variceal haemorrhage. J Hepatol 1999;31:443–50.
14. Abraldes JG, Villanueva C, Banares R, et al. Hepatic venous pressure gradient and prognosis in patients with acute variceal bleeding treated with pharmacologic and endoscopic therapy. J Hepatol 2008;48:229–36.
15. Monescillo A, Martinez-Lagares F, Ruiz-del-Arbol L. Influence of portal hypertension and its early decompression by TIPS placement on the outcome of variceal bleeding. Hepatology 2004;40:793–801.
16. Bambha K, Kim WR, Pedersen R, et al. Predictors of early re-bleeding and mortality after acute variceal haemorrhage in patients with cirrhosis. Gut 2008;57:814–20.
17. Hsu SC, Chen CY, Weng YM, et al. Comparison of 3 scoring systems to predict mortality from unstable upper gastrointestinal bleeding in cirrhotic patients. Am J Emerg Med 2014;32. pii:S0735-6757(14) 00015–1.
18. Reverter E, Tandon P, Augustin S, et al. A MELD-based model to determine risk of mortality among patients with acute variceal bleeding. Gastroenterology 2014;146:412–9.
19. Jairath V, Rehal S, Logan R, et al. Acute variceal haemorrhage in the United Kingdom: patient characteristics, management and outcomes in a nationwide audit. Dig Liver Dis 2014;46. pii:S1590-658(13) 00698–1.

20. Cardenas A, Gines P, Uriz J, et al. Renal failure after upper gastrointestinal bleeding in cirrhosis: incidence, clinical course, predictive factors, and short-term prognosis. Hepatology 2001;34:671–6.

21. Koch DG, Arguedas MR, Fallon MB. Risk of aspiration pneumonia in suspected variceal hemorrhage: the value of prophylactic endotracheal intubation prior to endoscopy. Dig Dis Sci 2007;52:2225–8.

22. Rudolph SJ, Landsverk BK, Freeman ML. Endotracheal intubation for airway protection during endoscopy for severe upper GI hemorrhage. Gastrointest Endosc 2003;57:58–61.

23. de Franchis R, Faculty BV. Revising consensus in portal hypertension: report of the Baveno V consensus workshop on methodology of diagnosis and therapy in portal hypertension. J Hepatol 2010;53:762–8.

24. Castaneda B, Debernardi-Venon W, Bandi JC. The role of portal pressure in the severity of bleeding in portal hypertensive rats. Hepatology 2000;31:581–6.

25. Villanueva C, Colomo A, Bosch A, et al. Transfusion strategies for acute upper gastrointestinal bleeding. N Engl J Med 2013;368:11–21.

26. Caldwell SH, Hoffman M, Lisman T, et al, Coagulation in Liver Disease Group. Coagulation disorders and hemostasis in liver disease: pathophysiology and critical assessment of current management. Hepatology 2006;44:1039–46.

27. Hou MC, Lin HC, Liu TT. Antibiotic prophylaxis after endoscopic therapy prevents rebleeding in acute variceal hemorrhage: a randomized trial. Hepatology 2004;39:746–53.

28. Chavez-Tapia NC, Barrientos-Gutierrez T, Tellez-Avila F, et al. Meta-analysis: antibiotic prophylaxis for cirrhotic patients with upper gastrointestinal bleeding - an updated Cochrane Review. Aliment Pharmacol Ther 2011;34:509–18.

29. Fernandez J, Ruiz-del-Arbol L, Gomez C, et al. Norfloxacin vs ceftriaxone in the prophylaxis of infections in patients with advanced cirrhosis and hemorrhage. Gastroenterology 2006;131:1049–56.

30. Chen PH, Chen WC, Hou MC, et al. Delayed endoscopy increases re-bleeding and mortality in patients with hematemesis and active esophageal variceal bleeding: a cohort study. J Hepatol 2012;57:1207–13.

31. Garcia-Pagan JC, Caca K, Bureau C, et al. Early use of TIPS in patients with cirrhosis and variceal bleeding. N Engl J Med 2010;362:2370–9.

32. Ioannou G, Doust J, Rockey DC. Terlipressin for acute variceal hemorrhage. Cochrane Database Syst Rev 2003;(1):CD002147.

33. Gotzsche PC, Hrobjartsson A. Somatostatin analogues for acute bleeding oeso-phageal varices. Cochrane Database Syst Rev 2008;(3):CD000193.

34. Escorsell A, Ruiz-del-Arbol L, Planas R, et al. Multicenter randomized controlled trial of terlipressin versus sclerotherapy in the treatment of acute variceal bleeding: the TEST study. Hepatology 2000;32:471–6.

35. Corley DA, Cello JP, Adkisson W, et al. Octreotide for acute esophageal variceal bleeding: a meta-analysis. Gastroenterology 2001;120:946–54.

36. Wells M, Chande N, Adams P, et al. Meta-analysis: vasoactive medications for the management of acute variceal bleeds. Aliment Pharmacol Ther 2012;35:1267–78.

37. D'Amico G, Pietrosi G, Tarantino I, et al. Emergency sclerotherapy versus vaso-active drugs for variceal bleeding in cirrhosis: a Cochrane meta-analysis. Gastroenterology 2003;124:1277–91.

38. Garcia-Tsao G, Sanyal AJ, Grace ND, et al. Prevention and management of gastroesophageal varices and variceal hemorrhage in cirrhosis. Hepatology 2007;46(3):922–38.

39. Villanueva C, Ortiz J, Sabat M, et al. Somatostatin alone or combined with emergency sclerotherapy in the treatment of acute esophageal variceal bleeding: a prospective randomized trial. Hepatology 1999;30:384–9.
40. Banares R, Albillos A, Rincon D, et al. Endoscopic treatment versus endoscopic plus pharmacologic treatment for acute variceal bleeding: a meta-analysis. Hepatology 2002;35:609–15.
41. Villanueva C, Colomo A, Aracil C, et al. Current endoscopic therapy for variceal bleeding. Best Pract Res Clin Gastroenterol 2008;22:261–78.
42. Park WG, Yeh RW, Triadafilopoulos G. Injection therapies for variceal bleeding disorders of the GI tract. Gastrointest Endosc 2008;67:313–23.
43. Baillie J, Yudelman P. Complications of endoscopic sclerotherapy of esophageal varices. Endoscopy 1992;24:284–91.
44. Lee JG, Lieberman DA. Complications related to endoscopic hemostasis techniques. Gastrointest Endosc Clin N Am 1996;6:305–21.
45. Rolando N, Gimson A, Philpott-Howard J, et al. Infectious sequelae after endoscopic sclerotherapy of oesophageal varices: role of antibiotic prophylaxis. J Hepatol 1993;18:290–4.
46. Selby WS, Norton ID, Pokorny CS, et al. Bacteremia and bacterascites after endoscopic sclerotherapy for bleeding esophageal varices and prevention by intravenous cefotaxime: a randomized trial. Gastrointest Endosc 1994;40:680–4.
47. Baron TH, Wong Kee Song LM. Endoscopic variceal band ligation. Am J Gastroenterol 2009;104:1083–5.
48. Laine L, El-Newhi HM, Migikovsky B, et al. Endoscopic ligation compared with sclerotherapy for the treatment of bleeding esophageal varices. Ann Intern Med 1993;119:1–7.
49. Villanueva C, Piqueras M, Aracil C, et al. A randomized controlled trial comparing ligation and sclerotherapy as emergency endoscopic treatment added to somatostatin in acute variceal bleeding. J Hepatol 2006;45:560–7.
50. Lo GH, Lai KH, Cheng JS, et al. Emergency banding ligation versus sclerotherapy for the control of active bleeding from esophageal varices. Hepatology 1997;25:1101–4.
51. Shaheen NJ, Stuart E, Schmitz SM, et al. Pantoprazole reduces the size of postbanding ulcers after variceal band ligation: a randomized, controlled trial. Hepatology 2005;41:588–94.
52. Garcia-pagan JC, Bosch J. Endoscopic band ligation in the treatment of portal hypertension. Nat Clin Pract Gastroenterol Hepatol 2005;2:526–35.
53. Qureshi W, Adler DG, Davila R, et al. ASGE guideline: the role of endoscopy in the management of variceal hemorrhage, updated 2005. Gastrointest Endosc 2005;62:651–5.
54. Abraldes JG, Bosch J. The treatment of acute variceal bleeding. J Clin Gastroenterol 2007;41(Suppl 3):S312–7.
55. Avgerinos A, Armonis A, Stefanidis G, et al. Sustained rise of portal pressure after sclerotherapy, but not band ligation, in acute variceal bleeding in cirrhosis. Hepatology 2004;39:1623–30.
56. Avgerinos A, Klonis C, Rekoumis G, et al. A prospective randomized trial comparing somatostatin, balloon tamponade and the combination of both methods in the management of acute variceal haemorrhage. J Hepatol 1991;13:78–83.
57. Hubmann R, Bodlaj G, Czompo M, et al. The use of self-expanding metal stents to treat acute variceal bleeding. Endoscopy 2006;38:896–901.

58. Holster IL, Kuipers EJ, van Buuren HR, et al. Self-expandable metal stents as definitive treatment for esophageal variceal bleeding. Endoscopy 2013;45: 485–8.

59. Dechêne A, El Fouly AH, Bechmann LP, et al. Acute management of refractory variceal bleeding in liver cirrhosis by self-expanding metal stents. Digestion 2012;85:185–91.

60. Escorcell CA, Pavel O, Morillas R, et al. Self-expandable esophageal metal stent vs balloon tamponade in esophageal variceal bleeding refractory to medical and endoscopic treatment: a multicenter randomized controlled trial. Hepatology 2013;58(S1):LB16.

61. Ljubicić N, Bisćanin A, Nikolić M, et al. A randomized-controlled trial of endoscopic treatment of acute esophageal variceal hemorrhage: N-butyl-2-cyanoacrylate injection vs. variceal ligation. Hepatogastroenterology 2011;58: 438–43.

62. Cipolletta L, Zambelli A, Bianco MA, et al. Acrylate glue injection for acutely bleeding oesophageal varices: a prospective cohort study. Dig Liver Dis 2009;41:729–34.

63. Smith LA, Morris AJ, Stanley AJ. The use of Hemospray in portal hypertensive bleeding; a case series. J Hepatol 2014;60:457–60.

64. Stanley AJ, Smith LA, Morris AJ. Use of hemostatic powder (Hemospray) in the management of refractory gastric variceal hemorrhage. Endoscopy 2013; 45(Suppl 2):E86–7.

65. Holster IL, Poley JW, Kuipers EJ, et al. Controlling gastric variceal bleeding with endoscopically applied hemostatic powder (Hemospray™). J Hepatol 2012;57: 1397–8.

66. D'Amico M, Berzigotti A, Garcia-Pagan JC. Refractory acute variceal bleeding: what to do next? Clin Liver Dis 2010;14:297–305.

Endoscopic Management of Gastric Variceal Bleeding

Frank Weilert, MD[a], Kenneth F. Binmoeller, MD[b],*

KEYWORDS

- Gastric varices • Endoscopic ultrasound • Cyanoacrylate • Coil embolization

KEY POINTS

- Gastric varices occur in 20% of patients with portal hypertension, but have a 65% risk of bleeding with high mortality due to high intravariceal pressure.
- Endoscopic treatment with cyanoacrylate injection is recommended as first-line therapy (Baveno IV, American Association for the Study of Liver Disease guidelines).
- Systemic embolization of cyanoacrylate injection is a major, potentially fatal complication.
- Endoscopic ultrasound (EUS) guidance enables direct intravascular delivery of therapy and selective targeting of feeder vessels.
- EUS-guided delivery of a coil followed by glue is a novel approach that may reduce the risk of glue embolization and improve treatment outcomes.

INTRODUCTION

Gastric varices (GVs) are less common than esophageal varices, but may be present in up to 20% of patients with portal hypertension. As many as 65% of GVs will bleed over 2 years.[1] The cumulative risk of bleeding of incidentally detected GVs at 1, 3, and 5 years has been reported to be 16%, 36%, and 44%, respectively.[2] The estimated incidence of bleeding from GVs in the United States is approximately 7000 cases per year.[3] The mortality from the first variceal bleed has remained high, at 20% within 6 weeks of the index bleed.[4] There is also a high risk of rebleeding, ranging from 3% to 89%, following initial intervention.[5,6] More effective primary and secondary treatment modalities are needed. This article discusses the evolving role of endoscopic treatment of GVs.

[a] Department of Gastroenterology, Waikato Hospital, Pembroke Street, Hamilton 2001, New Zealand; [b] Interventional Endoscopy Services, California Pacific Medical Center, 2351 Clay Street, 6th Floor, San Francisco, CA 94115, USA
* Corresponding author.
E-mail address: BinmoeK@sutterhealth.org

Gastroenterol Clin N Am 43 (2014) 807–818
http://dx.doi.org/10.1016/j.gtc.2014.08.010
0889-8553/14/$ – see front matter © 2014 Elsevier Inc. All rights reserved.

Endoscopic Classification of Gastric Varices

GVs differ in morphology, pathophysiology, natural history, and response to endoscopic treatment. The vascular anatomy of GVs is classified into 2 types: type 1 (localized type) consists of a single varicose vessel with almost the same diameter as the inflow/outflow vein, and type 2 (diffuse type) consists of multiple varicose vessels with complex vascular connections.[1] Gastric varices may exist as extensions of esophageal varices as 2 types: gastroesophageal varices type 1 (GOV1) are found along the lesser curvature, and gastroesophageal varices type 2 (GOV2) are found at the cardia. Isolated GVs (IGVs) exist as 2 types: IGV1s are located in the fundus, and IGV2s are sporadic. These distinctions are important in predicting the frequency of bleeding and the response to treatment.[7] IGVs have the highest flow rates, are larger in size, and have deeper feeding vessels, resulting in more severe bleeding episodes.[8,9]

Endoscopic Treatment of Gastric Varices

Endoscopic therapy of variceal bleeding has become established as first-line therapy as recommended by the Baveno IV consensus[10] and American Association for the Study of Liver Disease guidelines.[11] Variceal ligation has performed well in the treatment of esophageal varices; however, results with GVs have not been favorable.[5] Sclerosants have had less success in the treatment of GVs, because they are associated with a high incidence of complications, including gastric ulcerations and perforation, and recurrent bleeding rates of 37% to 89%.[5,6,8]

Direct endoscopic cyanoacrylate (CYA) injection of bleeding GVs (**Fig. 1**), first described by Soehendra and colleagues[12] in 1986, is widely considered first-line endoscopic therapy.[10] N-butyl-2-cyanoacrylate (Histoacryl) has been used in a number of sizable case series with hemostasis rates of greater than 90%, variceal obliteration rates of 70% to 90%, and rebleeding rates less than 30%.[7,13] As secondary prophylaxis, cyanoacrylate injection has been shown to reduce rebleeding rates as

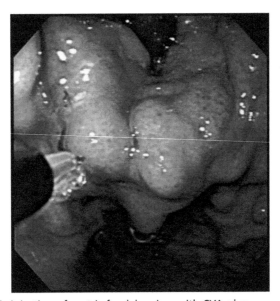

Fig. 1. Endoscopic injection of gastric fundal varices with CYA glue.

compared with band ligation[2] and propranolol.[14] As primary prophylaxis, cyanoacrylate has been shown to reduce the risk of bleeding and mortality from GOV2 or IGV1 greater than 10 mm diameter as compared with propranolol alone.[15]

Cyanoacrylate Glues and Injection Technique

A variety of cyanoacrylate glue monomers are commercially available, differing in the length of their alkyl group. N-butyl-2-cyanoacrylate (NB2-CYA), with a 4-carbon alkyl group, has been most widely used for the treatment of GVs. The polymerization time of NB2-CYA is rapid and can result in premature solidification of the glue in the needle or entrapment of the needle within the varix. NB2-CYA is therefore diluted with Lipiodol (ratios from 1:1 to 1:1.6). The injection catheter needs to be primed with distilled water, and then 1 mL of the glue-lipiodol mixture is injected, followed by flushing with water (to clear a catheter dead space of approximately 1 mL) to deliver the entire glue contents from the catheter into the varix. The 2-octyl-cyanoacrylate (2O-CYA) has a longer polymerization time due to a longer carbon alkyl group (8) and therefore can be injected without dilution and more slowly.[16] The injection catheter is primed (and flushed) with saline because there is no risk of premature solidification within the catheter. Rengstorff and Binmoeller[16] reported on the use of 2O-CYA in 25 patients with GVs with similar hemostasis rates and a 4% rebleeding rate over 11 months.

In preparation for endoscopic injection of cyanoacrylate, the endoscope tip is coated with silicone oil, as well as flushed oil through the instrument channel to minimize the risk of glue adherence that can lead to endoscope damage. The injection needle catheter is primed with either sterile water for NB2-CYA injection or saline for 2O-CYA injection. Saline should not be used for NB2-CYA injection because it accelerates the polymerization time, which may lead to premature clogging of the needle. An initial injection with water or saline should be free flowing into the varix and not forming a submucosal injection. Glue is injected into the varix in aliquots of 0.5 to 1.0 mL. The injection time will vary depending on the choice of cyanoacrylate and amount of dilution; undiluted NB2-CYA must be rapidly injected over seconds, whereas undiluted 2O-CYA can be more slowly injected over a minute. After the glue has been injected, the glue in the catheter dead space is flushed out with sterile water or saline. Continuously flushing will keep the needle patent for a possible repeat injection. The varix is palpated with a blunt-tipped instrument to confirm "hardness" from glue obliteration; if the varix is still soft, then additional injections are performed.

Noncyanoacrylate Glues

Noncyanoacrylate sealants, including fibrin glue and thrombin, have been used to arrest variceal bleeding in small uncontrolled case series.[17,18] Thrombin plus ethanolamine was found to be equivalent to ethanolamine alone in 1 randomized controlled trial.[19] In 2 retrospective studies, thrombin reportedly achieved hemostasis in bleeding GVs in 75% to 94%.[20,21] There have been no reported adverse events, specifically, no reports of distant embolization of thrombin. Bovine thrombin (with its putative risk of Creutzfeld-Jacob disease) has been replaced by human formulation, but still does not negate the potential risk of unknown infections (pooled from 4000–5000 plasma donors). Rebleeding rates of 12% to 30%, usually within 3 months, are still of concern,[17,20,21] and obliteration of the feeding varix is achieved in only 6%.[21]

Cyanoacrylate Glue Embolization

The most serious adverse events of CYA glue injection therapy is systemic embolization.[22] A recent study by Romero-Castro and colleagues[23] documented a high frequency of pulmonary embolization in 58% of patients treated with NB2-CYA diluted

1:1 with lipiodol. Fortunately, most of these patients were asymptomatic. Sepsis has been reported secondary to embolized glue acting as a septic focus.[24–34] Emboliza-tion into the arterial circulation (via a patent foramen ovale or arteriovenous pulmonary shunt) can result in stroke and multiorgan infarction.[33,35] Factors that may increase the embolization risk before the glue has hardened include overdilution of NB2-CYA with lipiodol, excessively rapid injection, injection of too large a volume of glue in a single injection, and IGV1 that has high blood-flow rates. Other adverse events described were visceral fistulization,[36] which may occur after accidental paravariceal injection.[14] Entrapment of the needle in the varix by glue[37,38] and damage to the scope also have been reported.

Endoscopic Ultrasound–Guided Cyanoacrylate Injection

Delivery of CYA under endoscopic ultrasound (EUS) guidance has the advantage of enabling precise delivery of glue into the varix lumen. EUS also enables assessment with Doppler to confirm vessel obliteration after treatment. This may have prognostic significance, as rebleeding risk after CYA injection has been linked to residual patency of treated varices.[39,40] Furthermore, treatment can be performed without dependency on direct varix visualization; even in the presence of retained food or blood that may obstruct the endoscopic view, the varix lumen can be accurately targeted for glue injection.

EUS can identify the main feeding vein system, which derives from the left gastric vein trunk, the posterior gastric vein, short gastric vein, or outflowing venous sys-tem[40,41] with gastrorenal shunts.[42] Romero-Castro and colleagues[43] described a small case series targeting the perforating "feeder vessel," rather than the varix lumen proper, under EUS guidance. Targeting the perforating vessel conceptually may mini-mize the amount of CYA needed to achieve obliteration of GV and thereby reduce the risk of embolization. The glue-lipiodol mixture enabled fluoroscopic visualization of the injected vessel and confirmation that the feeder vessel had been accurately targeted. No rebleeding or complications were observed. The limitation of this approach is that identification of the perforating vessel with EUS can be difficult and time consuming. Importantly, as the perforating vessel may be afferent or efferent, contrast medium must be injected before treatment to determine directional flow relative to the varix.

Endoscopic Ultrasound-Guided Coiling

Two small cases series have described deployment of commercially available stain-less steel coils. Levy and colleagues[44] used a 22-gauge needle loaded with a "micro-coil." The stylet was used to advance the constrained coil to the tip of the needle. Once the needle was inserted into the largest (1.4 cm) varix, the stylet was further advanced to deliver the coil. Two additional coils were placed into separate varices. Although rebleeding occurred and repeat EUS therapy performed, the previously treated vari-ces were shown to be thrombosed. Two additional coils were placed into untreated varices. Romero-Castro and colleagues[45] used a 19-gauge needle to deliver 0.035-inch coils of 50 to 150-mm length (coil diameter of 8–15 mm after deployment). In one patient with a large gastrorenal shunt, the investigators failed to achieve oblitera-tion of GVs despite deployment of 13 coils. A further 9 coils were deployed at a sub-sequent treatment session. The investigators did not comment on cost, but this becomes a consideration when large numbers of coils are required to achieve obliter-ation. Romero-Castro and colleagues[23] recently reported on a retrospective 4-year cohort study, comparing EUS-guided therapy using CYA to coil embolization in 30 pa-tients (23% never bled), with IGV1 in 15, GOV2 in 14, and GOV1 in 1 patient, respec-tively. Two-thirds had CYA injection, and one-third received coil insertion targeting perforating veins in 29 of 30 patients. The overall obliteration rate was 97%. A higher number of treatment sessions was required to achieve complete obliteration in the CYA versus coil group (P = NS), but a single session achieved complete obliteration in 82% of the coiled group. Adverse events were significantly higher in the CYA (58%) versus the coil (9%) group (P<.01), predominantly related to radiological documentation of 9 asymptomatic pulmonary emboli and 2 symptomatic patients with chest pain and fever, respectively.

Endoscopic Ultrasound-Guided Coiling and Cyanoacrylate Injection

In an ex vivo study, we deployed a coil in a container of heparinized blood, followed by injection of 1 mL CYA glue. The glue immediately adhered to the synthetic fibers on the coil and both coil and adherent glue were removed in one piece from the container (**Fig. 2**). Outside the container, the glue firmly adhered to the coil and no residual glue was identified in the container. The deployment of a coil before CYA injection may serve several functions: (1) the coil itself may contribute to varix obliteration and hemostasis, (2) the coil concentrates the glue at the site of coil deployment, and (3) the coil may prevent glue embolization.

We reported our first use of combined coil and CYA injection as "rescue" treatment after standard endoscopy-guided CYA treatment failed in a patient with massive gastric fundal variceal (GFV) bleeding.[46] We injected 2O-CYA after deployment of a single coil in a series of 30 patients with large gastric fundal varices.[47] The procedure (**Box 1**) was successful in all patients, with immediate hemostasis achieved for active bleeding (**Fig. 3**). The average volume of CYA injected was 1.4 mL per patient after coil deployment. Of note, this was 1 mL less than the average amount injected per patient in our previous study using the same CYA injected alone. There was no damage to the echoendoscope related to glue injections and no procedure-related complications. Of 24 patients who underwent follow-up endoscopy, 23 (96%) had complete GFV obliteration after a single treatment session, with no intravariceal flow on EUS color Doppler imaging. Recurrent bleeding from GFV developed in 1 patient at 21 days.

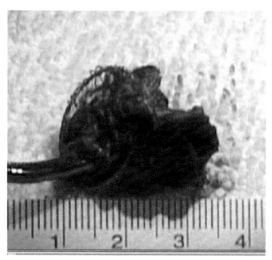

Fig. 2. Ex vivo demonstration of CYA glue adherence to the synthetic fibers of a coil, removed in one piece after coil and glue were deposited in a container filled with heparinized blood.

Box 1
Endoscopic ultrasound (EUS)-guided coil-and-glue injection (California Pacific Medical Center protocol)

1. Prophylactic intravenous broad-spectrum antibiotics are mandatory before the procedure.

2. Standard upper endoscopy allows for classification of the varices and assesses for active bleeding (direct visualization not required during active bleeding).

3. EUS with a curvilinear array echoendoscope and intraluminal water filling of the gastric fundus for improved sonographic visualization.

4. EUS-guided varix puncture:

    Standard 19 or 22-G fine needle aspiration (FNA) needle (depending on coil size selected) is used.

    FNA needle is primed with sterile saline.

    Preferred needle trajectory is a transesophageal-transcrural path from the distal esophagus.

    Varix puncture is confirmed by blood aspiration or saline injection (bubbles visualized endosonographically).

5. EUS-guided coil deployment:

    Advancement of the coil using the needle stylet as a pusher.

    The coil is sonographically visualized during deployment as a curved echogenicity.

    Careful advancement of the coil required to maintain the needle within the varix lumen.

6. EUS-guided glue injection:

    After coil deployment, blood is again aspirated to confirm intravariceal position before delivery of cyanoacrylate injection. One milliliter of 2-octyl-cyanoacrylate is injected over 30 to 45 seconds.

    Normal saline is then flushed to expel the glue in the dead space of the catheter.

    The EUS scope is carefully withdrawn with the FNA needle sheath advanced within the working channel to prevent glue damage.

7. Post coil and glue assessment:

    The varix is re-interrogated with EUS and color Doppler to confirm absence of flow.

    Additional injections of 1 mL glue or repeat combination of coil and glue are used as needed to achieve complete obliteration.

    The varix can be endoscopically probed with a closed forceps to assess for induration from glue solidification.

This patient underwent a second successful treatment with EUS-guided coil and CYA. No patient required surgical or percutaneous shunt procedures.

Transesophageal Injection

The gastric fundus is well visualized on EUS with the transducer positioned in the distal esophagus (**Fig. 4**). We therefore elected to treat GFV from the esophagus with the echoendoscope in an orthograde position. Apart from enabling EUS-guided access to GFV, this transesophageal approach is not hindered by gastric contents, such as blood and food, which tend to accumulate in the fundus. There is also no disruption of the gastric mucosa overlying the varix, which is usually thinned and at high risk of "back-bleeding" after varix puncture. The transesophageal approach also allows

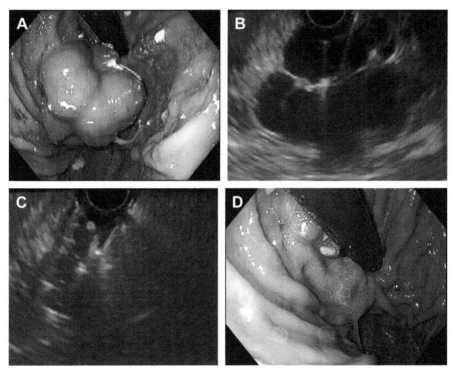

Fig. 3. Obliteration of gastric fundal varices by using coils and 2O-CYA. (*A*) Large, type 1 isolated gastric varices conglomerate. (*B*) EUS showing deployment of coil into varix. (*C*) EUS showing echogenic glue-filling varix. (*D*) Appearance at 3 months.

visualization of the diaphragmatic crus muscle, which is typically "sandwiched" between the esophageal and gastric fundic walls (see **Fig. 4**). When visualized, we intentionally included the crus muscle in our path of access to GFV ("transcrural" puncture), hypothesizing that the crus muscle, a thick fibromuscular bundle approximately 1 cm in thickness, acts as a stabilizing "backboard" to GFV.

Radiologic Therapy of Gastric Varices

Radiological intervention is used as a rescue strategy when endoscopic treatment fails or as primary intervention when endoscopic expertise is not available.

Transjugular intrahepatic portosystemic shunt

Decompression of the portal system by placement of a transjugular intrahepatic portosystemic shunt (TIPS) is frequently used for the treatment of portal hypertension and its complications.[48] The effectiveness of TIPS has been well documented in the treatment of acute variceal bleeding,[10,49] the prevention of recurrent variceal bleeding,[50] and the management of refractory ascites.[51] Patients with GV have a lower porto-caval pressure gradient due to extensive, spontaneous portosystemic shunts, explaining reduced efficacy in patients with GV.[52]

Balloon-occluded retrograde transvenous obliteration

Balloon-occluded retrograde transvenous obliteration (B-RTO) is a method of treating GVs that are associated with a gastrorenal shunt by angiographic injection of a

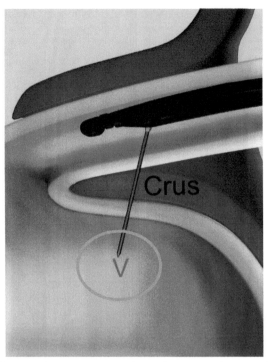

Fig. 4. Anatomic diagram showing transesophageal-transcrural approach to gastric fundal varices.

sclerosant. A balloon is inflated to occlude the gastrorenal shunt to stagnate blood flow. Drawbacks include worsening of esophageal varices, hepatic and renal toxicity related to a high volume of injected sclerosant, and embolism (pulmonary and cerebral). Combination of B-RTO with endoscopic treatment may improve clinical outcomes. Akahoshi and colleagues[53] compared endoscopic CYA injection with CYA plus B-RTO as a secondary prevention strategy, and showed the addition of B-RTO significantly reduced cumulative rebleeding rates at 5 years and the number of treatment sessions. Balloon occluded endoscopic injection sclerotherapy (BO-EIS) is a variation of B-RTO where a sclerosant is injected endoscopically after selective angiographic balloon occlusion. A randomized trial comparing BO-EIS to B-RTO showed the 2 techniques to achieve an 89% to 90% obliteration of GV, but with a significant reduction in the volume of sclerosant using BO-EIS with no worsening of esophageal varices.[54] Modified percutaneous transhepatic variceal embolization with or without B-RTO[55] was found to be superior to endoscopic CYA obliteration with reduced 3-year rebleeding rates (49% vs 84%).

Forward-View Echoendoscope

A limitation of the conventional curved linear array (CLA) echoendoscope is the oblique-viewing optics, which can make it difficult to endoscopically visualize gastric fundal varices. Maneuvering the echoendoscope into retroflexion to visualize the fundus is challenging. The recent availability of the forward-view (FV) CLA echoendoscope addresses this limitation. In addition, the FV-CLA echoendoscope has several conceptual advantages for EUS-guided treatment: (1) more perpendicular needle orientation to the target lesion, (2) uniaxis instrumentation imparting an increased forward transfer of force to the tip of the needle, and (3) accessory water jet channel for water filling and irrigation. The tip of FV-CLA can be angled to provide nearly perpendicular needle access to the fundus from the distal esophagus. These advantages have been previously described in other clinical applications of the FV-CLA echoendoscope.[56,57]

SUMMARY

Endoscopic therapy of GVs related to portal hypertension needs to be part of the basic skill set of the interventional endoscopist. This entails a thorough knowledge of the range of interventional options available, including CYA injection technique. The integration of EUS guidance is a logical evolution due to the unique ability to sonographically visualize GVs before, during, and after treatment. The role of EUS-guided intravascular delivery of coils, CYA glue, or their combination remains to be defined. Deployment of a coil before glue injection may reduce the risk of glue embolization, which can be fatal. The recent availability of the FV-CLA echoendoscope with front-view optics similar to a standard gastroscope contributes to the conceptual integration of sonographic and endoscopic guidance in delivery of therapy in GV.

REFERENCES

1. Arakawa M, Masuzaki T, Okuda K. Pathomorphology of esophageal and gastric varices. Semin Liver Dis 2002;22:73–82.
2. Tan P, Hou M, Lin H, et al. A randomized trial of endoscopic treatment of acute gastric variceal hemorrhage: N-butyl-2-cyanoacrylate injection versus band ligation. Hepatology 2006;43(4):690–7.
3. Caldwell S. Gastric varices: is there a role for endoscopic cyanoacrylate, or are we entering the BRTO era? Am J Gastroenterol 2012;107(12):1784–90.
4. D'Amico G, de Franchis R. End-of-the-century reappraisal of 6-week outcome of upper gastrointestinal bleeding in cirrhosis. A prospective study. Gastroenterology 1999;117:A1199.
5. Trudeau W, Prindiville T. Endoscopic injection sclerosis in bleeding gastric varices. Gastrointest Endosc 1986;32:264–8.
6. Sarin S. Long-term follow-up of gastric variceal sclerotherapy: an eleven-year experience. Gastrointest Endosc 1997;46:8–14.
7. Petersen B, Barkun A, Carpenter S, et al. Tissue adhesives and fibrin glue. Gastrointest Endosc 2004;60(3):327–33.
8. Sarin S, Lahoti D, Saxena S. Prevalence, classification and natural history of gastric varices: a long-term follow-up study in 568 portal hypertension patients. Hepatology 1992;16:1343–9.
9. de Franchis R, Primignani M. Natural history of portal hypertension in patients with cirrhosis. Clin Liver Dis 2001;5:645–63.
10. de Franchis R. Evolving consensus in portal hypertension. Report of the Baveno IV consensus workshop on methodology of diagnosis and therapy in portal hypertension. J Hepatol 2005;43(1):167–76.
11. Garcia-Tsao G, Sanyal A, Grace N, et al. Prevention and management of gastroesophageal varices and variceal hemorrhage in cirrhosis. Hepatology 2007;46(3):922–38.
12. Soehendra N, Grimm H, Nam V. N-butyl-2-cyanoacrylate: a supplement to endoscopic sclerotherapy. Endoscopy 1986;19:221–4.

13. Rengstorff D, Binmoeller K. A pilot study of 2-octyl cyanoacrylate injection for treatment of gastric fundal varices in humans. Gastrointest Endosc 2004;59:553–8.
14. Binmoeller K. Glue for gastric varices: some sticky issues. Gastrointest Endosc 2000;52(2):298–301.
15. Mishra S, Chander Sharma B, Kumar A, et al. Endoscopic cyanoacrylate injection versus beta-blocker for secondary prophylaxis of gastric variceal bleed: a randomised controlled trial. Gut 2010;59(6):729–35.
16. Mishra S, Sharma B, Kumar A, et al. Primary prophylaxis of gastric variceal bleeding comparing cyanoacrylate injection and beta-blockers: a randomized controlled trial. J Hepatol 2011;54(6):1161–7.
17. Datta D, Vlavianos P, Alisa A, et al. Use of fibrin glue (beriplast) in the management of bleeding gastric varices. Endoscopy 2003;35(8):675–8.
18. Heneghan M, Byrne A, Harrison P. An open pilot study of the effects of a human fibrin glue for endoscopic treatment of patients with acute bleeding from gastric varices. Gastrointest Endosc 2002;56(3):422–6.
19. Kitano S, Hashizume M, Yamaga H, et al. Human thrombin plus 5 per cent ethanolamine oleate injected to sclerose oesophageal varices: a prospective randomized trial. Br J Surg 1989;76(7):715–8.
20. Przemioslo R, McNair A, Williams R. Thrombin is effective in arresting bleeding from gastric variceal hemorrhage. Dig Dis Sci 1999;44(4):778–81.
21. Yang W, Tripathi D, Therapondos G, et al. Endoscopic use of human thrombin in bleeding gastric varices. Am J Gastroenterol 2002;97(6):1381–5.
22. Seewald S, Leong T, Imazu H, et al. A standardized injection technique and regimen ensures success and safety of N-butyl-2-cyanoacrylate injection for the treatment of gastric fundal varices. Gastrointest Endosc 2008;68:447–54.
23. Romero-Castro R, Ellrichmann M, Ortiz-Moyano C, et al. EUS-guided coil versus cyanoacrylate therapy for the treatment of gastric varices: a multicenter study. Gastrointest Endosc 2013;78(5):711–21.
24. Berry P, Cross T, Orr D. Clinical challenges and images in GI. Pulmonary embolization of Histoacryl "glue" causing hypoxia and cardiovascular instability. Gastroenterology 2007;133(5):1413.
25. Chang C, Shiau Y, Chen T, et al. Pyogenic portal vein thrombosis as a reservoir of persistent septicaemia after cyanoacrylate injection for bleeding gastric varices. Digestion 2008;78:139–43.
26. Saracco G, Giordanino C, Roberto N, et al. Fatal multiple systemic embolisms after injection of cyanoacrylate in bleeding gastric varices of a patient who was noncirrhotic but with idiopathic portal hypertension. Gastrointest Endosc 2007;65(2):345–7.
27. Shim C, Cho Y, Kim J, et al. A case of portal and splenic vein thrombosis after Histoacryl injection therapy in gastric varices. Endoscopy 1996;28(5):461.
28. Liu C, Tsai F, Liang P, et al. Splenic vein thrombosis and Klebsiella pneumoniae septicaemia after endoscopic gastric variceal obturation therapy with N-butyl-2-cyanoacrylate. Gastrointest Endosc 2006;63(2):336–8.
29. Wright G, Matuli W, Zambreanu L, et al. Recurrent bacteremia due to retained embolized glue following variceal obliteration. Endoscopy 2009;41(Suppl 2): E56–7.
30. Cheng P, Sheu B, Chen C, et al. Splenic infarction after histoacryl injection for bleeding gastric varices. Gastrointest Endosc 1998;48(4):426–7.
31. Yu L, Hsu C, Tseng J, et al. Splenic infarction complicated by splenic artery occlusion after N-butyl-2-cyanoacrylate injection for gastric varices: a case report. Gastrointest Endosc 2005;61(2):343–5.

32. Turler A, Wolff M, Dorlars D, et al. Embolic and septic complications after sclero-therapy of fundic varices with cyanoacrylate. Gastrointest Endosc 2001;53(2): 228–30.

33. Tan Y, Goh K, Kamarulzaman A, et al. Multiple systemic embolisms with septi-cemia after gastric variceal obliteration with cyanoacrylate. Gastrointest Endosc 2002;55(2):276–8.

34. Wahl P, Lammer F, Conen D, et al. Septic complications after injection of N-butyl-2-cyanoacrylate: a report of two cases and review. Gastrointest Endosc 2004; 59(7):911–6.

35. Abdullah A, Sachithanandan S, Tan O, et al. Cerebral embolism following N-butyl-2-cyanoacrylate injection for oesophageal postbanding ulcer bleed: a case report. Hepatol Int 2009;3(3):504–8.

36. Battaglia G, Morbin T, Paternello E, et al. Visceral fistula as a complication of endoscopic treatment of esophageal and gastric varices using isobutyl-2-cyanoacrylate: a report of two cases. Gastrointest Endosc 2000;52(2):267–70.

37. Dhiman R, Chawla Y, Taneja S. Endoscopic sclerotherapy of gastric variceal bleeding with N-butyl-2-cyanoacrylate. J Clin Gastroenterol 2002;35:222–7.

38. Bhasin D, Sharma B, Prasad H. Endoscopic removal of sclerotherapy needle from gastric varix after N-butyl-2-cyanoacrylate injection. Gastrointest Endosc 2000;51:497–8.

39. Lee Y, Chan F, Ng E, et al. EUS-guided injection of cyanoacrylate for bleeding gastric varices. Gastrointest Endosc 2000;52:168–74.

40. Iwase H, Suga S, Morise K. Color Doppler endoscopic ultrasonography for the evaluation of gastric varices and endoscopic obliteration with cyanoacrylate glue. Gastrointest Endosc 1995;41:150–4.

41. Hino S, Kakutani H, Ikeda H. Hemodynamic analysis of esophageal varices using color Doppler endoscopic ultrasonography to predict recurrence after endoscopic treatment. Endoscopy 2001;33:869–72.

42. Kakutani H, Hino S, Ikeda K. Use of the curved linear-array echo endoscope to identify gastrorenal shunts in patients with gastric fundal varices. Endoscopy 2004;36:710–4.

43. Romero-Castro R, Pellicer-Bautista F, Jimenez-Saenz M. EUS-guided injection of cyanoacrylate in perforating feeding veins in gastric varices: results in 5 cases. Gastrointest Endosc 2007;66:402–7.

44. Levy M, Wong Kee Song L, Kendrick M. EUS-guided coil embolization for re-fractory ectopic variceal bleeding. Gastrointest Endosc 2008;67:572.

45. Romero-Castro R, Pellicer-Bautista F, Giovannini M. Endoscopic ultrasound (EUS)-guided coil embolization therapy in gastric varices. Endoscopy 2010; 42(Suppl 2):E35–6.

46. Sanchez-Yague A, Shah J, Nguyen-Tang T. EUS-guided coil embolization of gastric varices after unsuccessful endoscopic glue injection. Gastrointest En-dosc 2009;69:AB6.

47. Binmoeller K, Weilert F, Shah J, et al. EUS-guided transesophageal treatment of gastric fundal varices with combined coiling and cyanoacrylate glue injection. Gastrointest Endosc 2011;74(5):1019–25.

48. Colombato L. The role of transjugular intrahepatic portosystemic shunt (TIPS) in the management of portal hypertension. J Clin Gastroenterol 2007;41: S344–51.

49. Boyer T, Haskal Z. AASLD practice guideline. The role of transjugular intra-hepatic portosystemic shunt in the management of portal hypertension. Hepa-tology 2005;41:1–15.

50. D'Amico G, Pagliaro L, Bosch J. The treatment of portal hypertension: a meta-analytic view. Hepatology 1995;22:332–53.

51. Gines P, Uriz J, Calahorra B. Transjugular intrahepatic portosystemic shunt versus repeated paracentesis plus intravenous albumin for refractory ascites in cirrhosis. A multicenter randomized comparative study. Gastroenterology 2002;123:1839–47.

52. Sanyal A, Freedman A, Luketic V, et al. The natural history of portal hypertension after transjugular intrahepatic portosystemic shunts. Gastroenterology 1997; 112(3):889–98.

53. Akahoshi T, Tomikawa M, Kamori M, et al. Impact of balloon-occluded retrograde transvenous obliteration on the management of isolated fundal gastric variceal bleeding. Hepatol Res 2012;424:385–93.

54. Shiba M, Higuchi K, Nakamura K, et al. Efficacy and safety of balloon-occluded endoscopic injection sclerotherapy as a prophylactic treatment for high risk gastric fundal varices: a prospective, randomized, comparative trial. Gastrointest Endosc 2002;56(4):522–8.

55. Wang J, Tian XG, Li Y, et al. Comparison of modified percutaneous transhepatic variceal embolization and endoscopic cyanoacrylate injection for gastric variceal bleeding. World J Gastroenterol 2013;19(5):706–14.

56. Nguyen-Tang T, Shah J, Sanchez-Yague A. Use of the front-view forward-array echoendoscope to evaluate right colonic subepithelial lesions. Gastrointest Endosc 2010;72:606–10.

57. Binmoeller K. Optimizing interventional EUS: the echoendoscope in evolution. Gastrointest Endosc 2007;66:917–9.

Nonendoscopic Management Strategies for Acute Esophagogastric Variceal Bleeding

 CrossMark

Sanjaya K. Satapathy, MBBS, MD, DM[a], Arun J. Sanyal, MBBS, MD[b],*

KEYWORDS

- Portal hypertension • Variceal hemorrhage • Variceal bleeding • Varices • TIPS
- Portosytemic shunt • BRTO

KEY POINTS

- Initial stabilization and resuscitation is imperative in the management of acute variceal bleeding along with attention at prevention of associated complications such as hepatic encephalopathy, acute renal injury, spontaneous bacterial peritonitis, and sepsis.
- Urgent attention at achieving hemostasis through endoscopic means remains the key and should be supported by pharmacotherapy aiming at reducing portal venous pressure.
- Patients failing initial treatment should be rescued with transjugular intrahepatic portosystemic shunt, balloon-occluded retrograde transvenous obliteration, or rarely surgical shunts.

Acute variceal bleeding is a potentially life-threatening complication of portal hypertension defined as elevation of hepatic venous pressure gradient (HVPG) to greater than 5 mm Hg. Portal hypertension is classified as prehepatic, intrahepatic, or posthepatic, intrahepatic being the form most often caused by cirrhosis, irrespective of the cause.[1] Portal hypertension results in redistribution and increased blood flow through the coronary veins and the short gastric veins, resulting in esophageal and gastric varices. Gastroesophageal varices begin to form at a pressure gradient of 8 to 10 mm Hg, with bleeding risk increased at a gradient of 12 mm Hg.[1] In patients without varices, esophageal varices develop and grow in size at a rate of about 7%

Author Disclosures: Authors disclose no direct financial interest in the subject matter discussed in the article. No grants received in preparation of this article.

[a] Division of Surgery, Methodist University Hospital Transplant Institute, University of Tennessee Health Sciences Center, Memphis, TN 38104, USA; [b] Division of Gastroenterology, Department of Internal Medicine, Virginia Commonwealth University School of Medicine, MCV Box 980341, Richmond, VA 23298-0341, USA
* Corresponding author.
E-mail address: asanyal@mcvh-vcu.edu

per year as a result of ongoing portal hypertension.[2,3] Variceal rupture could potentially occur in about one-third of patients, with the highest rates observed in patients with HVPG greater than 20 mm Hg[4] and/or Child C patients with large varices with red wale markings.[5,6] Acute variceal bleeding occurs in 25% to 40% of cirrhotic patients and carries a mortality of 25% to 30%, making it one of the most dreaded complications of portal hypertension.[7] Bleeding usually occurs at the gastroesophageal junction because varices are most superficial and have the thinnest wall at this anatomic location. Approximately 50% of the acute variceal bleeding ceases spontaneously.[8] After an index bleeding episode, most of the episodes of rebleeding occurs in the first 6 weeks[9,10] and more than 50% of such rebleeding episodes occur within 3 to 4 days from the time of the initial bleeding episode.[9,11–14] The risk factors for early rebleeding are severe initial bleeding as defined by a hemoglobin less than 8 g/dL, gastric variceal bleeding, thrombocytopenia, encephalopathy, alcohol-related cirrhosis, large varices, active bleeding during endoscopy, and a high HVPG.[11–16] In the long term, approximately 70% of subjects experience further variceal bleeding and have a similar risk of mortality within the first year.[17,18] Age greater than 60 years, large esophageal varices, severity of liver disease, continued alcoholism, renal failure, and presence of a hepatoma increase the risk of rebleeding.[12,19]

Before the advent of pharmacotherapy, endoscopic therapy, and shunt procedures for control of variceal bleeding, almost 40% of patients with acute variceal hemorrhage died within 6 weeks, one-third rebled at 6 weeks, and only about one-third survived beyond 1 year.[9]

Significant advances have been observed in the last 2 decades in the management of acute variceal bleeding by both endoscopic and nonendoscopic means and have resulted in significant reductions in both morbidity and mortality from this potentially life-threatening condition. Endoscopic treatment is important and remains the cornerstone in the management of acute variceal bleeding, and newer techniques are continuing to evolve. The current article, however, intends to highlight only the current nonendoscopic treatment approaches for control of acute variceal bleeding and recent developments.

MANAGEMENT OF ACUTE VARICEAL BLEEDING
General Management

Acute variceal bleeding is a potentially life-threatening event. Most patients vomit blood but hematochezia and melena might be the only initial symptoms. Hemodynamic stability depends on the amount of blood lost; presentation could include symptoms of orthostatic hypotension to hemorrhagic shock. Despite advances in therapy, up to 40% of patients still die from exsanguinating bleeding. Of note, most deaths are unrelated to bleeding per se and are rather caused by complications of bleeding such as liver failure, infections, and hepatorenal syndrome.[20,21] The degree of liver dysfunction, creatinine level, hypovolemic shock, active bleeding on endoscopy, and presence of hepatocellular carcinoma are important determinants of adverse outcome.[20–24] Thus, the management of patients with acute variceal bleeding includes not only treatment and control of active bleeding but also the prevention of rebleeding, hepatic encephalopathy, infections, and renal failure.[25] Available therapeutic options to control bleeding include medical and endoscopic treatment, balloon tamponade, placement of fully covered self-expandable metallic stents, transjugular intrahepatic portosystemic shunt (TIPS), and surgical shunts. Nowadays, the initial approach is a combination of vasoactive drugs, antibiotics, and endoscopic therapy,[26] followed by a more aggressive approach in patients failing first-line treatment.

ASSESSMENT OF SEVERITY OF BLEEDING

Assessment of the severity of variceal bleeding is of paramount importance to risk stratify the level of resuscitation. The Baveno II Consensus Conference[27] defined an episode of acute variceal bleeding as clinically significant when there is blood transfusion requirement of at least 2 units and a systolic pressure less than 100 mm Hg, or a postural drop of 20 mm Hg and/or pulse rate greater than 100 beats per minute at time of patient presentation (ie, time zero). Management of acute variceal hemorrhage includes hemodynamic resuscitation, prevention and treatment of complications, and control of bleeding.

Resuscitation

Correction of hypovolemia

The foremost step is the assessment of intravascular volume loss and replacement with crystalloids and packed red blood cells to keep systolic blood pressure at least at 90 to 100 mm Hg and the heart rate less than 100 beats/min, with a hemoglobin level around 7 to 8 g/dL (hematocrit of 21–24). Care must be taken to avoid overtransfusion because this can cause a rebound increase in portal pressure and precipitate early rebleeding.[28,29] Fresh frozen plasma and platelets (particularly for a platelet count <50,000/mL) have often been used to correct coagulopathy. These measures do not adequately correct the coagulopathy and could potentially induce volume overload and rebound portal hypertension.[30] The use of recombinant factor VII has been shown to improve hemostasis rates, but it does not improve survival.[31]

Aspiration precaution

Patients with acute variceal hemorrhage are at very high risk for aspiration pneumonia, which often progresses to multiorgan failure and has been associated with a very high mortality. It is therefore imperative to pay attention to the airway and protect the airway by prophylactic intubation when mental status is impaired, delirium tremens is imminent, or bleeding is too severe for the patient to maintain the integrity of their airway.

Prevention and Treatment of Associated Complications

Antibiotic prophylaxis

Bacterial infection is documented in 30% to 40% of cirrhotic patients on admission or within the first week after variceal bleeding, associated with an increased in-hospital mortality.[23,32] The most common infections in these patients are spontaneous bacterial peritonitis and bacteremia, followed by urinary tract infections and pneumonia. Most infections are due to enterobacteria.[23,33] Antibiotic prophylaxis significantly increases both the proportion of patients free from infection and the mean survival rate at 14 days.[33]

Currently, it is recommended that short-term antibiotic prophylaxis, a measure that reduces bacterial infections,[34] variceal rebleeding,[35] and death,[34] be used in every patient with cirrhosis admitted with gastrointestinal hemorrhage.[36,37] The choice of antibiotics, however, is not standardized as different antibiotics have been used in different trials, and given different local antibiotic susceptibility patterns and different availability, it is unlikely that a definitive trial in this area will be performed. Quinolones in uncomplicated patients[38] and ceftriaxone in high-risk patients with advanced liver disease (ascites, encephalopathy, jaundice, and malnutrition) or previous therapy with quinolones is a reasonable choice.[39]

Hepatic encephalopathy

Hepatic encephalopathy is frequently precipitated after acute variceal hemorrhage. Digested blood in the gastrointestinal tract provides a source of extra protein, which is a source of excess ammonia and other toxic amines. Because of portosystemic shunting, the normal first-pass extraction by the liver is decreased and the circulating levels of these toxins increase, thereby contributing to the development of hepatic encephalopathy. Hepatic encephalopathy is also worsened by sepsis, azotemia, and electrolyte disturbances that can occur in the context of a variceal bleed. Of note, sedation used during endoscopy or for airway intubation may also contribute to altered mental status in such patients. Management of hepatic encephalopathy in the setting of acute variceal bleeding includes aggressive therapy with lactulose, either orally or by means of a nasogastric tube, in patient with altered mental status once bleeding is controlled and the gut is known to be functional. Although the role of rifaximin and other antibiotics for the treatment of encephalopathy in the setting of acute variceal bleeding is unclear, recent studies have shown a combination therapy of lactulose with rifaximin may be more useful than lactulose alone.[40] For patients with persistent hepatic encephalopathy, especially those with Grade IV hepatic encephalopathy without improvement despite withdrawal of sedation and aggressive use of lactulose, an imaging study of the head (computed tomography scan or magnetic resonance imaging) and electroencephalogram should be considered.

Acute renal failure

Acute renal failure in a patient with cirrhosis is a severe complication and often a harbinger of death,[24] whereas serum creatinine is a key component of the model for end-stage liver disease score, a well-established predictor of mortality.[41] Renal failure in a patient with acute variceal bleeding is also a predictor of increased mortality, hence physicians should not just focus on the bleeding alone, but measures should be taken to prevent the occurrence of renal failure.[42] The risk of renal failure can be minimized by careful attention to volume status, avoidance and aggressive treatment of sepsis, and avoidance of nephrotoxic drugs. An indwelling catheter should be used to monitor urine output, and the fluids administered should be tailored to maintain an output of at least 50 cc/h.

Achievement of Hemostasis

In the context of active bleeding, it is imperative to begin therapy quickly and control bleeding. Several modalities are available as first-line treatment of the achievement of hemostasis. These include pharmacologic treatment, endoscopic sclerotherapy, and variceal ligation. Several other modalities of treatment are available in patients failing standard measures as a rescue therapy such as balloon tamponade, placement of esophageal covered metal stent, TIPS, balloon-occluded retrograde transvenous obliteration (BRTO), and so on; a detailed discussion of these is beyond the scope of this article. Nonendoscopic measures to achieve hemostasis are discussed later in this article.

Balloon tamponade

Balloon tamponade is aimed at obtaining temporary hemostasis by direct compression of bleeding varices. The use of balloon tamponade for the treatment of acute esophageal variceal bleeding was introduced by Sengstaken and Blakemore.[43] The Minnesota tube is a modified version with an aspiration channel above the esophageal balloon. For uncontrolled bleeding from gastric varices, the Linton-Nicholas tube is preferred.[44] Balloon tamponade is highly successful in stopping bleeding in experienced hands,[45-51] but recurrence is observed in about 50% of the patients within 24 hours following deflation of the balloon. Major complications, the most lethal of which is esophageal rupture, have been observed in 6% to 20% of patients,[52] occurring more frequently in series in which tubes were inserted by inexperienced staff.[47] It should be noted that balloon tamponade is only a bridging procedure for a more definitive procedure later on.

Pharmacotherapy

Based on the principle of hydromechanics, portal pressure is determined by intravascular resistance and blood flow. In portal hypertension, the intrahepatic vascular resistance (IHVR) and splanchnic blood flow are the 2 main contributors to portal pressure.[53] IHVR is under dynamic regulation; postprandial increases in splanchnic blood flow is always associated with an autonomic down-regulation, leading to no alteration in portal pressure. However, in patients with cirrhosis, this delicate balance is lost, and the IHVR is significantly upregulated by mechanical and hemodynamic factors, which is further aggravated by splanchnic vasodilation.[54] The resultant increase in portal pressure is the antecedent to variceal bleeding with its associated morbidity and high mortality.[55,56] Most drugs currently used to treat varices and/or variceal hemorrhage cause splanchnic vasoconstriction, leading to a reduction in portal venous inflow and consequently to a decrease in portal pressure.

Vasopressin Vasopressin (antidiuretic hormone) is a powerful vasoconstrictor that acts at the level of V1 receptors located in the smooth muscle of the arteries inducing contraction by activating phospholipase C and increasing cytosolic calcium $[Ca^{++}]$ level through the inositol triphosphate pathway.[57] The ability of vasopressin to control variceal bleeding is caused by powerful splanchnic arteriolar vasoconstriction, which decreases the portal inflow and thus the portal pressure.[58] Unfortunately, vasopressin also causes profound systemic vasoconstriction with increased peripheral resistance and reduced cardiac output, heart rate, and coronary blood flow, leading to myocardial ischemia and/or infarction, cardiac arrhythmias, mesenteric ischemia, extremity ischemia, and cerebrovascular accidents in a sizable proportion of patients. In clinical trials, 32% to 64% of the patients treated with vasopressin experienced adverse effects and almost 25% had to be taken off the drug. Fatal complications caused by vasopressin also have been reported.[59,60] The systemic vasoconstrictive adverse effects of vasopressin may be minimized by the concomitant use of nitrates.[61–63] Vasopressin is administered as a continuous infusion at a rate of 0.2 to 0.4 U/min that may be increased to 0.6 U/min if required. Therapy is maintained for 24 hours after the control of bleeding. Vasopressin rarely is used today in the management of variceal bleeding because of its adverse effect profile.

Terlipressin (Glypressin) Triglycyl-lysl-vasopressin (terlipressin), a synthetic analogue of vasopressin, is in itself inactive but is activated after the glycyl residue is cleaved releasing vasopressin slowly and continuously causing splanchnic vasoconstriction.[64–66] Terlipressin has a longer biological half-life and is administered every 4 hours, and thus continuous infusion is not needed. Terlipressin does not increase the plasminogen activator activity, as is seen with vasopressin, but has similar effects on the coronary vasculature.

Somatostatin and analogues Somatostatin is a naturally occurring peptide originally named for its growth hormone–inhibiting properties.[67,68] Somatostatin causes an increase in splanchnic vascular resistance by causing vasoconstriction resulting in decrease in the portal blood inflow. The vasoconstriction is mediated by inhibiting the release of splanchnic vasodilator hormones like glucagon and vasoactive intestinal peptide.[69,70] In addition, somatostatin also acts by preventing post-prandial hyperemia and also causes a modest decrease in the hepatic blood flow and the wedged hepatic venous pressure (WHVP).[71–75] Somatostatin has a short half-life and is rapidly cleared from the blood. Somatostatin is given as an intravenous bolus of 250 μg, followed by a continuous infusion of 250 μg/h; the therapy is continued for 2 to 5 days if successful. A bolus of somatostatin markedly decreases the HVPG by 52% at 1 minute, 19% at 3 minutes, and 13% at 5 minutes.[76]

In current clinical practice and clinical trials, the synthetic analogues of somatostatin, namely octreotide and vapreotide, have been most widely used in the management of acute variceal bleeding and have a longer duration of action. Octreotide produces a modest decline in the WHVP[77] and a variable effect on intravariceal pressure.[78] Additionally, it significantly decreases azygos blood flow and has an excellent safety profile in the absence of the systemic circulatory adverse effects as seen with vasopressin. Octreotide is a synthetic analogue of somatostatin with longer half-life. It is administered as an initial bolus of 50 μg, followed by an infusion of 50 μg/h.[79] The complication rates with somatostatin and octreotide are few but can include mild hyperglycemia and abdominal cramping.

Radiological intervention
Transjugular intrahepatic portosystemic shunt for acute variceal bleeding TIPS is an artificial channel within the liver that establishes communication between the inflow portal vein and the outflow hepatic vein. The procedure is usually performed by an interventional radiologist, who creates the shunt using a fluoroscopy-guided endovascular approach, with the jugular vein as the usual entry site, from which a catheter is advanced to gain access to the patient's hepatic vein by traveling from the superior vena cava into the inferior vena cava and finally the hepatic vein. Once the catheter is in the hepatic vein, a branch of the portal vein within the liver is then catheterized with placement of an expandable stent from the hepatic vein into the branch of the portal vein. The success rate with TIPS for decompression of the portal vein is high—more than 90% of cases in most case series.[80–86] Guidelines have been established by the Society of Interventional Radiology for creation of a TIPS, and the consensus was that a technically successful outcome is creation of the shunt with a decrease in portal pressure to less than 12 mm Hg that should be achieved in 95% of patients, and resolution of the complication of portal hypertension should be achieved in 90% of cases.[87,88]

In general, pharmacologic therapy and endoscopic banding achieve control of variceal bleeding in most of the cases; failures to standard therapy occur in about 10% to 20% of patients, and in these subgroups TIPS could potentially be lifesaving. As discussed earlier, the success rate of TIPS to achieve decompression of the portal vein is more than 90%,[80–86] nevertheless, mortality at 6 weeks among patients treated with rescue TIPS for uncontrolled index bleeding and rebleeding is very high (35%), reflecting the severity of their underlying liver disease as well as additional organ dysfunction that may have occurred owing to hypotension, infection, and aspiration.[89]

It is thus important to identify patients at high risk of failing standard therapy, because these patients could potentially be offered TIPS early on. The most important predictor of failure to standard therapy is HVPG greater than 20 mm Hg measured within 24 hours of admission.[4,90] Unfortunately, such measurements are not feasible in most centers, and Child's status is used as a surrogate marker, because Child's C status correlates with the likelihood of having an HVPG above 20 mm Hg in more than 85% of patients.[90] To verify the utility of preemptive TIPS, 2 trials in patients with acute variceal hemorrhage at high risk of failing standard therapy were conducted. In the first, a single-center trial, 52 patients with an HVPG greater than 20 mm Hg were randomized to (uncoated) TIPS within 24 hours of admission versus continuing standard therapy.[91] In the second trial, a multicenter European study, 63 Child class C patients (excluding those with the highest scores of 14 and 15) or Child class B patients with active bleeding were randomized to (polytetrafluoroethylene-coated) TIPS within 24 to 72 hours of admission versus continued standard therapy.[92] Both trials showed a significant advantage of TIPS with a reduction in composite outcomes (failure to control bleeding or early rebleeding) and, importantly, a significantly higher survival. Usefulness of early TIPS in acute variceal hemorrhage and high risk of treatment failure has been further confirmed in a recent retrospective trial with a lower incidence of failure to control bleeding or rebleeding as well as reduced mortality.[93] These studies recommended that early (preemptive) TIPS (<72 hours) should be considered for patients with variceal bleeding who are Child class C (14 points) or are Child class B with active bleeding (**Fig. 1**).[94] A recent economic modeling study has further confirmed early TIPS insertion is to be a cost-effective intervention in selected high-risk patients.[95] Importantly, the subpopulation of patients with variceal bleeding who would be candidates for early TIPS represent less than 20% of the patients admitted with this complication. In the rest of the patients, the majority, TIPS is considered second-line therapy and is reserved for patients who fail standard therapy.

Balloon-occluded retrograde transvenous obliteration The BRTO procedure is an endovascular technique that causes occlusion of outflow portosystemic shunt, such as a gastrorenal shunt, using an occlusion balloon followed by the endovascular injection of a sclerosing agent directly into the gastrovariceal system/complex.[96–100] For the conventional BRTO procedure, a large infradiaphragmatic "left-sided" portosystemic collateral is required.[101–103] The most common shunt to be occluded during a conventional BRTO procedure is a gastrorenal shunt, which provides venous outflow in 90% of gastric varices cases. The remaining 10% of gastric varices drain through a gastrocaval shunt (infradiaphragmatically) or other less common transdiaphragmatic veins. Preprocedural imaging is important in assessing the sites, types, and morphology of these portosystemic shunts.[104]

Bleeding esophageal varices that cannot be controlled medically and endoscopically would warrant a TIPS procedure and not a BRTO.[92,105] Bleeding from gastric varices that are small and exhibit slow flow by endoscopic Doppler ultrasound can be sclerosed (or "glued") endoscopically and may not necessarily require a BRTO procedure. However, if there are large fundal and/or cardia gastric varices exhibiting high flow, some endoscopists would defer to a BRTO procedure due to concerns about causing intravascular (usually systemic venous) nontarget embolization of the

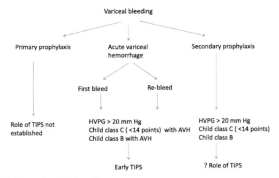

Fig. 1. Role of TIPS in variceal bleeding.

sclerosant. Obviously, if bleeding is from combined gastric and esophageal varices, then the esophageal varices can be managed by endoscopy and large high-flow gastric varices could be managed by BRTO. In the presence of large high-flow gastric varices and prominent but not bleeding esophageal varices, preemptive esophageal variceal banding may be warranted because BRTO exacerbates portal hypertension and may aggravate esophageal varices.[106–108]

Portal vein thrombosis creates a special situation; risks and benefits of BRTO should be carefully considered in the presence of portal vein thrombosis. Gastrorenal shunts and splenorenal shunts, if present, are portosystemic collaterals that naturally occur and promote hepatofugal flow. In the presence of a thrombosed main portal vein, occlusion of the gastrorenal shunt, a by-product of the BRTO procedure, would potentially cause mesenteric venous hypertension, mesenteric ischemia, and possibly thrombosis of the entire splanchnic portal venous circulation. Chronic occlusion of the main portal vein with cavernous transformation may provide sufficient outflow for the portal venous system after occluding the portosystemic shunts, and therefore it may be acceptable to proceed with the BRTO.[104]

BRTO has shown considerable effectiveness in controlling gastric variceal bleeding with low rebleed rates. It has many advantages versus TIPS in that it is less invasive and can be performed on patients with poor hepatic reserve and encephalopathy (and may even improve both). However, its by-product is occlusion of a spontaneous hepatofugal (TIPS equivalent) shunt and could potentially increase in portal hypertension with aggravation of esophageal varices and ascites. With the increasing experience with the management of gastric varices, a tailored approach based on the anatomy of the patient, clinical features of portal hypertension, and hepatic reserve management can be better selected for either endoscopy, TIPS, or BRTO.

SURGICAL PROCEDURES

Surgical procedures in patients with acute or recurrent variceal bleeding are limited to a very small portion of patients in whom medical and/or endoscopic control of bleeding was not achievable and in situations when TIPS is not an option because of technical or anatomic problems such as complete thrombosis of the portal vein. Surgical procedures are primarily based on creation of a shunt to decompress the portal vasculature or nonshunt operations such as esophageal transection or devascularization of the gastroesophageal junction. Shunt operations have been further categorized as nonselective if they derive all portal blood flow to the inferior vena cava bypassing the liver, such as portacaval shunt, and selective if they are intended to at least partly preserve the portal blood flow to the liver, such as the distal splenorenal shunt or the calibrated small-diameter portacaval H-graft shunt. It is to be noted that despite such categorization, the selectivity of these shunts is never completely achieved or is mostly lost during follow-up.[109] It is probably for these reasons, no major differences in clinical outcomes among these 2 types of shunt are found at medium- or long-term follow-up.[2]

Portal decompressive surgery and esophageal transection are highly effective in achieving hemostasis.[52,110] However, despite the success in controlling bleeding, the mortality of these patients is still high (approximately 45%–75%).[52,110] Not uncommonly, patients surviving these episodes are fraught with chronic or recurrent portal systemic encephalopathy.[52] The calibrated small-diameter portacaval H-graft shunt has reduced encephalopathy in comparison with total portacaval shunt in the only randomized controlled trial reported.[111] In addition, portacaval shunts alter vascular anatomy, which further complicates future liver transplant surgery.

SUMMARY

Variceal bleeding is a potentially life-threatening complication of portal hypertension. Patients presenting with acute bleeding not only needs attention for treatment directed at emergent hemostasis but also needs therapy directed at hemodynamic resuscitation, protection of the airway, prevention, and treatment of complications including prophylactic use of antibiotics. Currently available first-line treatment of acute esophageal variceal bleeding includes a combination of nonendoscopic treatment aimed at reducing portal pressure as well as endoscopic treatment with band ligation, sclerotherapy. Patients failing first-line therapy are triaged for TIPS or surgically created shunts as rescue procedures. Balloon tamponade and use of self-expandable metal stents are used as a bridge to more definitive treatment. Management of gastric varices is particularly challenging; treatment includes early institution of pharmacotherapy, in combination with endoscopic therapy with cyanoacrylate, TIPS, and BRTO. This choice depends on the size of the varices, portal vein patency, presence or absence of gastrorenal shunt, hepatic reserve, and local expertise. Advances in pharmacologic agents, improved endoscopic techniques, and advances in the use of coated stents for TIPS will hopefully pave the way for improved control of hemostasis, ultimately further reducing the morbidity and mortality in patients with acute variceal bleeding. Ultimately, liver transplantation remains the only definitive treatment and provides long-term survival in those who have advanced liver failure and variceal bleeding.

REFERENCES

1. Garcia-Tsao G, Groszmann RJ, Fisher RL, et al. Portal pressure, presence of gastroesophageal varices and variceal bleeding. Hepatology 1985;5: 419–24.
2. Groszmann RJ, Garcia-Tsao G, Bosch J, et al. Beta-blockers to prevent gastroesophageal varices in patients with cirrhosis. N Engl J Med 2005; 353:2254–61.
3. Merli M, Nicolini G, Angeloni S, et al. Incidence and natural history of small esophageal varices in cirrhotic patients. J Hepatol 2003;38:266–72.
4. Moitinho E, Escorsell A, Bandi JC, et al. Prognostic value of early measurements of portal pressure in acute variceal bleeding. Gastroenterology 1999;117: 626–31.
5. Beppu K, Inokuchi K, Koyanagi N, et al. Prediction of variceal hemorrhage by esophageal endoscopy. Gastrointest Endosc 1981;27:213–8.
6. North Italian Endoscopic Club for the Study and Treatment of Esophageal Varices. Prediction of the first variceal hemorrhage in patients with cirrhosis of the liver and esophageal varices. A prospective multicenter study. N Engl J Med 1988;319:983–9.
7. Wright AS, Rikkers LF. Current management of portal hypertension. J Gastrointest Surg 2008;9:992–1005.
8. Prandi D, Rueff B, Roche-Sicot J, et al. Life-threatening hemorrhage of the digestive tract in cirrhotic patients. An assessment of the postoperative mortality after emergency portacaval shunt. Am J Surg 1976;131:204–9.
9. Graham DY, Smith JL. The course of patients after variceal hemorrhage. Gastroenterology 1981;80:800–9.
10. Smith JL, Graham DY. Variceal hemorrhage: a critical evaluation of survival analysis. Gastroenterology 1982;82:968–73.

11. McCormick PA, Jenkins SA, McIntyre N, et al. Why portal hypertensive varices bleed and bleed: a hypothesis. Gut 1995;36:100–3.
12. de Franchis R, Primignani M. Why do varices bleed? Gastroenterol Clin North Am 1992;21:85–101.
13. Pagliaro L, D'Amico G, Luca A, et al. Portal hypertension: diagnosis and treatment. J Hepatol 1995;23:36–44.
14. Boyer TD. Natural history of portal hypertension. Clin Liver Dis 1997;1:31–44.
15. Sarin SK, Lahoti D, Saxena SP, et al. Prevalence, classification, and natural history of gastric varices: a long-term follow-up study in 568 portal hypertension patients. Hepatology 1992;16:1343–9.
16. Ready JB, Robertson AD, Goff JS, et al. Assessment of the risk of bleeding from esophageal varices by continuous monitoring of portal pressure. Gastroenterology 1991;100:1403–10.
17. Burroughs AK, Jenkins WJ, Sherlock S, et al. Controlled trial of propranolol for the prevention of recurrent variceal hemorrhage in patients with cirrhosis. N Engl J Med 1983;309:1539–42.
18. Burroughs AK, McCormick PA. Prevention of variceal rebleeding. Gastroenterol Clin North Am 1992;21:119–47.
19. de Dombal FT, Clarke JR, Clamp SE, et al. Prognostic factors in upper GI bleeding. Endoscopy 1986;18:6–10.
20. Augustin S, Muntaner L, Altamirano JT, et al. Predicting early mortality after acute variceal hemorrhage based on classification and regression tree analysis. Clin Gastroenterol Hepatol 2009;7:1347–54.
21. D'Amico G, De Franchis R. Upper digestive bleeding in cirrhosis. Post-therapeutic outcome and prognostic indicators. Hepatology 2003;38:599–612.
22. Augustin S, Altamirano J, González A, et al. Effectiveness of combined pharmacologic and ligation therapy in high-risk patients with acute esophageal variceal bleeding. Am J Gastroenterol 2011;106:1787–95.
23. Bernard B, Cadranel JF, Valla D, et al. Prognostic significance of bacterial infection in bleeding cirrhotic patients: a prospective study. Gastroenterology 1995; 108:1828–34.
24. Cárdenas A, Ginès P, Uriz J, et al. Renal failure after upper gastrointestinal bleeding in cirrhosis: incidence, clinical course, predictive factors, and short-term prognosis. Hepatology 2001;34(Pt 1):671–6.
25. García-Pagán JC, Reverter E, Abraldes JG, et al. Acute variceal bleeding. Semin Respir Crit Care Med 2012;33:46–54.
26. Bañares R, Albillos A, Rincón D, et al. Endoscopic treatment versus endoscopic plus pharmacologic treatment for acute variceal bleeding: a meta-analysis. Hepatology 2002;35:609–15.
27. de Franchis R. Developing consensus in portal hypertension. J Hepatol 1996; 25(3):390–4.
28. Kravetz D, Bosch J, Arderiu M, et al. Hemodynamic effects of blood volume restitution following a hemorrhage in rats with portal hypertension due to cirrhosis of the liver: influence of the extent of portal-systemic shunting. Hepatology 1989;9:808–14.
29. Kravetz D, Sikuler E, Groszmann RJ. Splanchnic and systemic hemodynamics in portal hypertensive rats during hemorrhage and blood volume restitution. Gastroenterology 1986;90:1232–40.
30. Youssef WI, Salazar F, Dasarathy S, et al. Role of fresh frozen plasma infusion in correction of coagulopathy of chronic liver disease: a dual phase study. Am J Gastroenterol 2003;98:1391–4.

31. Bosch J, Thabut D, Bendtsen F, et al. Recombinant factor VIIa for upper gastro-intestinal bleeding in patients with cirrhosis: a randomized, double-blind trial. Gastroenterology 2004;127:1123–30.
32. Deschenes M, Villeneuve JP. Risk factors for the development of bacterial infections in hospitalized patients with cirrhosis. Am J Gastroenterol 1999;94: 2193–7.
33. Soares-Weiser K, Brezis M, Tur-Kaspa R, et al. Antibiotic prophylaxis of bacterial infections in cirrhotic inpatients: a meta-analysis of randomized controlled trials. Scand J Gastroenterol 2003;38:193–200.
34. Bernard B, Grange JD, Khac EN, et al. Antibiotic prophylaxis for the prevention of bacterial infections in cirrhotic patients with gastrointestinal bleeding: a meta-analysis. Hepatology 1999;29:1655–61.
35. Hou MC, Lin HC, Liu TT, et al. Antibiotic prophylaxis after endoscopic therapy prevents rebleeding in acute variceal hemorrhage: a randomized trial. Hepatology 2004;39:746–53.
36. de Franchis R. Evolving consensus in portal hypertension report of the Baveno IV consensus workshop on methodology of diagnosis and therapy in portal hypertension. J Hepatol 2005;43:167–76.
37. Garcia-Tsao G, Sanyal AJ, Grace ND, et al, Practice Guidelines Committee of the American Association for the Study of Liver Diseases, Practice Parameters Committee of the American College of Gastroenterology. Prevention and management of gastroesophageal varices and variceal hemorrhage in cirrhosis. Hepatology 2007;46:922–38.
38. Rimola A, García-Tsao G, Navasa M, et al. Diagnosis, treatment and prophylaxis of spontaneous bacterial peritonitis: a consensus document. International Ascites Club. J Hepatol 2000;32:142–53.
39. Fernández J, Ruiz del Arbol L, Gómez C, et al. Norfloxacin vs ceftriaxone in the prophylaxis of infections in patients with advanced cirrhosis and hemorrhage. Gastroenterology 2006;131:1049–56 [quiz: 1285].
40. Sharma BC, Sharma P, Lunia MK, et al. A randomized, double-blind, controlled trial comparing rifaximin plus lactulose with lactulose alone in treatment of overt hepatic encephalopathy. Am J Gastroenterol 2013;108(9):1458–63.
41. Kremers WK, van IJperen M, Kim WR, et al. MELD score as a predictor of pre-transplant and post-transplant survival in OPTN/UNOS status 1 patients. Hepatology 2004;39:764–9.
42. Fallatah HI, Al Nahdi H, Al Khatabi M, et al. Variceal hemorrhage: Saudi tertiary center experience of clinical presentations, complications and mortality. World J Hepatol 2012;4:268–73.
43. Sengstaken RW, Blakemore AH. Balloon tamponage for the control of hemorrhage from esophageal varices. Ann Surg 1950;131:781–9.
44. Terés J, Cecilia A, Bordas JM, et al. Esophageal tamponade for bleeding varices. Controlled trial between the Sengstaken-Blakemore tube and the Linton-Nachlas tube. Gastroenterology 1978;75:566–9.
45. Panés J, Terés J, Bosch J, et al. Efficacy of balloon tamponade in treatment of bleeding gastric and esophageal varices. Results in 151 consecutive episodes. Dig Dis Sci 1988;33:454–9.
46. Cook D, Laine L. Indications, technique, and complications of balloon tamponade for variceal gastrointestinal bleeding. J Intensive Care Med 1992;7: 212–8.
47. Chojkier M, Conn HO. Esophageal tamponade in the treatment of bleeding varices. A decadel progress report. Dig Dis Sci 1980;25:267–72.

48. Hunt PS, Korman MG, Hansky J, et al. An 8-year prospective experience with balloon tamponade in emergency control of bleeding esophageal varices. Dig Dis Sci 1982;27:413–6.

49. Fort E, Sautereau D, Silvain C, et al. A randomized trial of terlipressin plus nitroglycerin vs. balloon tamponade in the control of acute variceal hemorrhage. Hepatology 1990;11:678–81.

50. Paquet KJ, Feussner H. Endoscopic sclerosis and esophageal balloon tamponade in acute hemorrhage from esophagogastric varices: a prospective controlled randomized trial. Hepatology 1985;5:580–3.

51. Pitcher JL. Safety and effectiveness of the modified Sengstaken-Blakemore tube: a prospective study. Gastroenterology 1971;61:291–8.

52. D'Amico G, Pagliaro L, Bosch J, et al. The treatment of portal hypertension: a meta-analytic review. Hepatology 1995;22:332–54.

53. Cichoz-Lach H, Celiński K, Słomka M, et al. Pathophysiology of portal hypertension. J Physiol Pharmacol 2008;59(Suppl 2):231–8.

54. Moneta GL, Taylor DC, Helton WS, et al. Duplex ultrasound measurement of postprandial intestinal blood flow: effect of meal composition. Gastroenterology 1988;95:1294–301.

55. Albillos A, Bañares R, González M, et al. The extent of the collateral circulation influences the postprandial increase in portal pressure in patients with cirrhosis. Gut 2007;56:259–64.

56. Bellis L, Berzigotti A, Abraldes JG, et al. Low doses of isosorbide mononitrate attenuate the postprandial increase in portal pressure in patients with cirrhosis. Hepatology 2003;37:378–84.

57. Schmid PG, Sharabi FM, Guo GB, et al. Vasopressin and oxytocin in the neural control of the circulation. Fed Proc 1984;43:97–102.

58. Reichen J. Liver function and pharmacological considerations in pathogenesis and treatment of portal hypertension. Hepatology 1990;11:1066–78.

59. Kravetz D, Bosch J, Teres J, et al. Comparison of intravenous somatostatin and vasopressin infusions in treatment of acute variceal hemorrhage. Hepatology 1984;4:442–6.

60. Conn HO, Ramsby GR, Storer EH, et al. Intra-arterial vasopressin in the treatment of upper gastrointestinal hemorrhage: a prospective, controlled clinical trial. Gastroenterology 1975;68:211–21.

61. Tsai YT, Lay CS, Lai KH, et al. Controlled trial of vasopressin plus nitroglycerin vs. vasopressin alone in the treatment of bleeding esophageal varices. Hepatology 1986;6:406–9.

62. Gimson AE, Westaby D, Hegarty J, et al. A randomized trial of vasopressin and vasopressin plus nitroglycerin in the control of acute variceal hemorrhage. Hepatology 1986;6:410–3.

63. Bosch J, Groszmann RJ, Garcia-Pagan JC, et al. Association of transdermal nitroglycerin to vasopressin infusion in the treatment of variceal hemorrhage: a placebo-controlled clinical trial. Hepatology 1989;10:962–8.

64. Burroughs AK, Panagou E. Pharmacological therapy for portal hypertension: rationale and results. Semin Gastrointest Dis 1995;6:148–64.

65. Berzigotti A, Bosch J. Pharmacologic management of portal hypertension. Clin Liver Dis 2014;18:303–17.

66. Blei AT. Vasopressin analogs in portal hypertension: different molecules but similar questions. Hepatology 1986;6:146–7.

67. Bloom SR, Polak JM. Somatostatin. Br Med J (Clin Res Ed) 1987;295:288–90.

68. Brazeau P, Vale W, Burgus R, et al. Hypothalamic polypeptide that inhibits the secretion of immunoreactive pituitary growth hormone. Science 1973;179:77–9.
69. Reichlin S. Somatostatin. N Engl J Med 1983;309:1495–501.
70. Reichlin S. Somatostatin (second of two parts). N Engl J Med 1983;309: 1556–63.
71. Baxter JN, Jenkins SA. Somatostatin: an alternative to sclerotherapy? Scand J Gastroenterol Suppl 1994;207:17–22.
72. Merkel C, Gatta A, Zuin R, et al. Effect of somatostatin on splanchnic hemodynamics in patients with liver cirrhosis and portal hypertension. Digestion 1985; 32:92–8.
73. Consolo F, Pustorino S. Theoretical and physiopharmacological bases of the somatostatin treatment in digestive diseases. Minerva Chir 1992;47:723–9 [in Italian].
74. Hanisch E, Doertenbach J, Usadel KH, et al. Somatostatin in acute bleeding oesophageal varices. Pharmacology and rationale for use. Drugs 1992;44: 24–35.
75. Sieber CC, Stalder GA. Pathophysiological and pharmacotherapeutic aspects of portal hypertension. Schweiz Med Wochenschr 1993;123:3–13 [in German].
76. Cirera I, Feu F, Luca A, et al. Effects of bolus injections and continuous infusions of somatostatin and placebo in patients with cirrhosis: a double-blind hemodynamic investigation. Hepatology 1995;22:106–11.
77. McKee R. A study of octreotide in oesophageal varices. Digestion 1990;45: 60–4.
78. Jenkins SA, Baxter JN, Corbett WA, et al. Effects of a somatostatin analogue SMS 201–995 on hepatic haemodynamics in the pig and on intravariceal pressure in man. Br J Surg 1985;72:1009–12.
79. Abraldes JG, Bosch J. Somatostatin and analogues in portal hypertension. Hepatology 2002;35:1305–12.
80. Boyer TD. Transjugular intrahepatic portosystemic shunt: current status. Gastroenterology 2003;124:1700–10.
81. Rössle M, Haag K, Ochs A, et al. The transjugular intrahepatic portosystemic stent-shunt procedure for variceal bleeding. N Engl J Med 1994;330:165–71.
82. Luketic VA, Sanyal AJ. Esophageal varices. II. TIPS (transjugular intrahepatic portosystemic shunt) and surgical therapy. Gastroenterol Clin North Am 2000; 29:387–421.
83. Cello JP, Ring EJ, Olcott EW, et al. Endoscopic sclerotherapy compared with percutaneous transjugular intrahepatic portosystemic shunt after initial sclerotherapy in patients with acute variceal hemorrhage. A randomized, controlled trial. Ann Intern Med 1997;126:858–65.
84. Sanyal AJ, Freedman AM, Luketic VA, et al. Transjugular intrahepatic portosystemic shunts compared with endoscopic sclerotherapy for the prevention of recurrent variceal hemorrhage. A randomized, controlled trial. Ann Intern Med 1997;126:849–57.
85. Cabrera J, Maynar M, Granados R, et al. Transjugular intrahepatic portosystemic shunt versus sclerotherapy in the elective treatment of variceal hemorrhage. Gastroenterology 1996;110:832–9.
86. Barton RE, Rosch J, Saxon RR, et al. TIPS: short- and long-term results: a survey of 1750 patients. Semin Intervent Radiol 1995;12:364–7.
87. Haskal ZJ, Martin L, Cardella JF, et al. Quality improvement guidelines for transjugular intrahepatic portosystemic shunts. J Vasc Interv Radiol 2001;12:131–6.

88. Haskal ZJ, Martin L, Cardella JF, et al. Quality improvement guidelines for transjugular intrahepatic portosystemic shunts. J Vasc Interv Radiol 2003;14: S265–70.

89. Boyer TD, Haskal ZJ, American Association for the Study of Liver Diseases. The role of Transjugular Intrahepatic Portosystemic Shunt (TIPS) in the management of portal hypertension: update 2009. Hepatology 2010;51(1):306.

90. Abraldes JG, Villanueva C, Banares R, et al. Hepatic venous pressure gradient and prognosis in patients with acute variceal bleeding treated with pharmacologic and endoscopic therapy. J Hepatol 2008;48:229–36.

91. Monescillo A, Martinez-Lagares F, Ruiz-del-Arbol L, et al. Influence of portal hypertension and its early decompression by TIPS placement on the outcome of variceal bleeding. Hepatology 2004;40:793–801.

92. Garcia-Pagan JC, Caca K, Bureau C, et al. Early use of TIPS in patients with cirrhosis and variceal bleeding. N Engl J Med 2010;362:2370–9.

93. Garcia-Pagán JC, Di Pascoli M, Caca K, et al. Use of early-TIPS for high-risk variceal bleeding: results of a post-RCT surveillance study. J Hepatol 2013;58(1): 45–50.

94. de Franchis R. Revising consensus in portal hypertension: report of the Baveno V consensus workshop on methodology of diagnosis and therapy in portal hypertension. J Hepatol 2010;53:762–8.

95. Harman DJ, McCorry RB, Jacob RP, et al. Economic modelling of early transjugular intrahepatic portosystemic shunt insertion for acute variceal haemorrhage. Eur J Gastroenterol Hepatol 2013;25(2):201–7.

96. Kanagawa H, Mima S, Kouyama H, et al. Treatment of gastric fundal varices by balloon-occluded retrograde transvenous obliteration. J Gastroenterol Hepatol 1996;11(1):51–8.

97. Kiyosue H, Mori H, Matsumoto S, et al. Transcatheter obliteration of gastric varices. Part 1. Anatomic classification. Radiographics 2003;23(4):911–20.

98. Kiyosue H, Mori H, Matsumoto S, et al. Transcatheter obliteration of gastric varices: part 2. Strategy and techniques based on hemodynamic features. Radiographics 2003;23(4):921–37 [discussion: 937].

99. Chikamori F, Kuniyoshi N, Shibuya S, et al. Transjugular retrograde obliteration for chronic portosystemic encephalopathy. Abdom Imaging 2000;25: 567–71.

100. Hiraga N, Aikata H, Takaki S, et al. The long-term outcome of patients with bleeding gastric varices after balloon-occluded retrograde transvenous obliteration. J Gastroenterol 2007;42(8):663–72.

101. Saad WE, Darcy MD. Transjugular intrahepatic portosystemic shunt (TIPS) versus balloon-occluded retrograde transvenous obliteration (BRTO) for the management of gastric varices. Semin Intervent Radiol 2011;28:339–49.

102. Saad WE, Sabri SS. Balloon-occluded retrograde transvenous obliteration (BRTO): technical results and outcomes. Semin Intervent Radiol 2011;28: 333–8.

103. Saad WE. The history and evolution of balloon-occluded retrograde transvenous obliteration (BRTO): from the United States to Japan and back. Semin Intervent Radiol 2011;28:283–7.

104. Al-Osaimi AM, Sabri SS, Caldwell SH. Balloon-occluded retrograde transvenous obliteration (BRTO): preprocedural evaluation and imaging. Semin Intervent Radiol 2011;28:288–95.

105. Garcia-Tsao G, Bosch J. Management of varices and variceal hemorrhage in cirrhosis. N Engl J Med 2010;362(9):823–32.

106. Kitamoto M, Imamura M, Kamada K, et al. Balloon-occluded retrograde transvenous obliteration of gastric fundal varices with hemorrhage. AJR Am J Roentgenol 2002;178:1167–74.
107. Akahoshi T, Hashizume M, Tomikawa M, et al. Long-term results of balloon-occluded retrograde transvenous obliteration for gastric variceal bleeding and risky gastric varices: a 10-year experience. J Gastroenterol Hepatol 2008;23: 1702–9.
108. Cho SK, Shin SW, Lee IH, et al. Balloon-occluded retrograde transvenous obliteration of gastric varices: outcomes and complications in 49 patients. AJR Am J Roentgenol 2007;189:W365–72.
109. Belghiti J, Grenier P, Nouel O, et al. Long-term loss of Warren's shunt selectivity. Angiographic demonstration. Arch Surg 1981;116:1121–4.
110. Jalan R, John TG, Redhead DN, et al. A comparative study of emergency transjugular intrahepatic portosystemic stent-shunt and esophageal transection in the management of uncontrolled variceal hemorrhage. Am J Gastroenterol 1995;90:1932–7.
111. Sarfeh IJ, Rypins EB. Partial versus total portocaval shunt in alcoholic cirrhosis. Results of a prospective, randomized clinical trial. Ann Surg 1994;219:353–61.

Approach to the Management of Portal Hypertensive Gastropathy and Gastric Antral Vascular Ectasia

 CrossMark

Kamran Qureshi, MD[a], Abdullah M.S. Al-Osaimi, MD[b],*

KEYWORDS

- Liver cirrhosis • Portal hypertension • GI bleeding
- Transjugular intrahepatic portosystemic shunt (TIPS)

KEY POINTS

- Gastric antral vascular ectasia (GAVE) and portal hypertensive gastropathy (PHG) are 2 distinct causes of chronic gastrointestinal bleeding.
- In patients with cirrhosis, often these mucosal lesions can be relatively easy to distinguish on upper endoscopy based on their appearance: as "watermelon stomach" (red stripes pattern) in the case of GAVE, or "snake skin" (mosaic pattern) in the case of PHG, or location: gastric antrum for GAVE and fundus or upper body in PHG.
- Diffuse red spots or nodular pattern on gastric mucosa is occasionally encountered in cirrhotics, which is seen with both GAVE and severe PHG.
- When the diagnosis is unclear, biopsy and histologic evaluation (and use of GAVE score) help in differentiating GAVE from PHG.

INTRODUCTION

Portal hypertensive gastropathy (PHG) and gastric antral vascular ectasia (GAVE) are 2 important causes of gastrointestinal bleeding (GIB). Overall, both are gastric mucosal lesions that are uncommon causes of overt GIB but are frequently associated with chronic blood loss and iron deficiency anemia.[1] GAVE and PHG are typically seen in distinct patient populations; however, both conditions are encountered in patients with liver cirrhosis and portal hypertension and can cause nonvariceal GIB. The clinical

Disclosures: None.
[a] Division of Hepatology, Department of Medicine, Temple University Health System, Temple University School of Medicine, 3440 North Broad Street, Kresge West, Room 209, Philadelphia, PA 19140, USA; [b] Division of Hepatology, Department of Medicine, Temple University Health System, Temple University School of Medicine, 3440 North Broad Street, Kresge West, Room 216, Philadelphia, PA 19140, USA
* Corresponding author.
E-mail addresses: Abdullah.Al-Osaimi@tuhs.temple.edu; abdullah_alosaim@hotmail.com

Gastroenterol Clin N Am 43 (2014) 835–847
http://dx.doi.org/10.1016/j.gtc.2014.08.012
0889-8553/14/$ – see front matter © 2014 Elsevier Inc. All rights reserved.
gastro.theclinics.com

presentation and morphologic appearance of these lesions can be relatively similar, yet the management is clearly different. Thus, it is imperative to make an accurate diagnosis and differentiation between GAVE and PHG to formulate suitable treatment decisions.

In this article, the pathogenesis, diagnosis, and recent advancements in the management of both GAVE and PHG are briefly reviewed, with an emphasis on the treatment options in the presence of advanced liver disease.

GASTRIC ANTRAL VASCULAR ECTASIA
Epidemiology

The exact prevalence of GAVE is unknown because of its relatively silent presentation and its association with a wide variety of systemic diseases.[2] In addition, GAVE was not described reliably in the past, and it was not until 1995 that the distinction was made between GAVE and PHG in patients with cirrhosis.[3] During the evaluation of chronic anemia, GAVE is typically found to be the cause in elderly women and is also is associated with several chronic systemic diseases (chronic renal failure, autoimmune diseases, systemic sclerosis, cardiac diseases, and bone marrow transplantation).[2,4] On routine upper endoscopy, GAVE is seen in 3% and 2% of patients with advanced liver disease and those undergoing liver transplantation, respectively.[5] GAVE is considered to be responsible for 4% of nonvariceal upper GIB in patients with and without portal hypertension.[6]

Diagnosis

GAVE is described as a vascular lesion consisting of abnormally dilated and tortuous gastric mucosal capillaries (ectasia) with mural spindle cell proliferation (smooth muscle cells and myofibroblasts), focal thrombosis, and fibrohyalonosis.[7] These histologic findings are incorporated into the "GAVE score" (**Table 1**), which can be used to make a diagnosis of GAVE with high accuracy (70%–85%) on a gastric biopsy to differentiate it from PHG.[3] Biopsy, however, is often not needed to diagnose GAVE because of its characteristic morphologic appearance. Conventionally, upper endoscopy has been used to diagnose GAVE based on the finding of reddish spots either organized in stripes radially projecting proximally from the pylorus (watermelon stomach) or arranged in a diffuse (honeycomb stomach) or nodular pattern (nodular antral gastropathy) (**Fig. 1**).[2,8] These lesions are seen in the form of erythematous and at times raised

Table 1 GAVE score			
	0	1	2
Fibrin thrombi and/or ectasia in mucosal vessels	Absent	Only one feature present	Both present
Spindle cell proliferation (smooth muscle cell and myofibroblasts hyperplasia) in superficial mucosal vessels	Absent	Increased	Markedly increased
Fibrohyalonosis around the ectatic capillaries of the lamina propria	Absent	Present	—

Score ranges from 0 to 5. GAVE score greater than 3 is considered highly diagnostic for the presence of GAVE.

Adapted from Payen JL, Calès P, Voigt JJ, et al. Severe portal hypertensive gastropathy and antral vascular ectasia are distinct entities in patients with cirrhosis. Gastroenterology 1995;108(1):138–44; with permission.

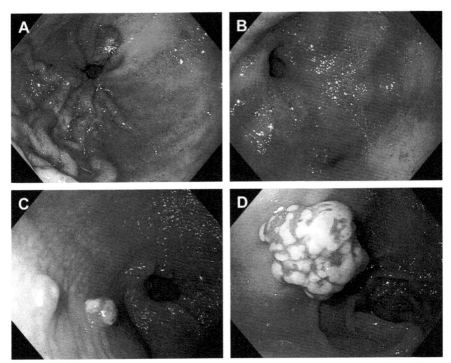

Fig. 1. Mild GAVE with stripes (*A*); moderate GAVE with mild active GIB (*B*); mild/small nodular GAVE or nodular antral gastropathy (NAG) (*C*); large NAG (*D*).

mucosa with visible underlying ectatic vessels, which are located mainly in the antrum of the stomach.[9] In cirrhotics, a clear distinction from PHG, especially in a diffuse or nodular type pattern, is difficult to make on endoscopic inspection and a biopsy is often needed. Among other endoscopic modalities, capsule endoscopy has been recently used to evaluate GAVE. In addition, endoscopic ultrasound (EUS) is also used, and the EUS appearance of GAVE is described as spongiform mucosa and submucosa with well-preserved muscularis propria and hypertrophied gastric antrum.[10] Red blood cell scan and CT scan findings of GAVE have also been described in a few case reports.[11] Platelet marker CD61 immunostain identifies microthrombi within the vessels and increases the diagnostic accuracy of biopsy specimen evaluation.[12]

Pathogenesis

GAVE is considered to be an acquired abnormality, resulting in ectasia of mucosal microvasculature, which results from mechanical stress or neuroendocrine abnormalities. Hemodynamic and autoimmune factors have also been implicated in the pathogenesis of GAVE and its exact cause remains to be further elucidated. The finding of antropyloric dysfunction and abnormal antral motor response to meals in some patients with GAVE relate to the hypothesis that repeated forceful peristalsis induces prolapse and trauma to the antral mucosa, which leads to microvascular abnormalities found in GAVE.[13] Several neuroendocrine hormones (gastrin, vasoactive intestinal polypeptide [VIP], 5-hydroxytryptamine, prostaglandin E2, nitric oxide, and/or glucagon) have also been suggested to play a role in the development of GAVE.[14,15] Their levels are found to be elevated in some cirrhotics with GAVE. It is postulated that the accumulation of vasoactive substances that are poorly metabolized by the cirrhotic liver results in mucosal microvascular damage and ectasia. It is actually the loss of hepatic function rather than the portal hypertension in liver cirrhosis that is associated with GAVE, in contrast to PHG.[16] GAVE has been reported to have completely resolved after liver transplantation, and portal decompressive techniques have been reported to not improve GAVE and its associated GIB.[17] Up to 60% of GAVE patients have concurrent autoimmune disease (eg, Raynaud disease, systemic sclerosis, Sjogren syndrome) and several auto-antibodies have been detected in patients with GAVE.[18–20] The association of several other chronic diseases (eg, renal, cardiac, and/or hematologic) with GAVE also needs further investigation.[2,21]

Management

Similar to any patient with GIB, initial management of these patients consists of adequate resuscitation and hemodynamic stabilization. In patients with GAVE, GIB is most often chronic, with patients presenting with symptoms of anemia, occult blood in their stool, with or without iron deficiency anemia. GAVE is mostly identified as a part of the workup of GIB on upper endoscopy or during screening endoscopies. It is reasonable not to treat GAVE lesions, which are found incidentally or are not the source of bleeding (primary prophylaxis). For symptomatic/bleeding lesions, endoscopic ablative techniques are usually first-line treatment. Thermoablative procedures are used more commonly in clinical practice, while the use of cryotherapy, radiofrequency, or mechanical ablation is less frequent because, generally, they require more expertise.

Major thermoablative techniques include argon plasma coagulation (APC) and neodymium:yettrium-aluminum garnet (YAG) laser therapies, which have been investigated extensively to control GAVE-related GIB. Both techniques are equally effective with up to 80% to 100% eradication of lesions and abolishment of need of blood transfusion in up to 50% to 80% of patients after 2 to 3 sessions on average.[22,23] There are no head-to-head trials comparing these techniques; they do differ in their safety profile. APC is a reasonably newer (**Fig. 2**), noncontact technique with lesser depth of coagulation and thus carries a lesser risk of gastric perforation as compared with YAG.[24] YAG therapy is often complicated with gastric ulceration. In addition, cases of pyloric stenosis with gastric outflow obstruction, and hyperplastic gastric polyps forming after repeated sessions of YAG procedure, have been reported.[25] A case of multifocal gastric cancer 5 years after multiple sessions of YAG laser therapy has also been reported.[26] The technical details of these endoscopic procedures are not the focus of this article. The choice of procedure is mainly determined by the availability of expertise and technologies in any center. APC ablation is being used more prevalently these days because of better availability, lower cost, and good safety profile.

Endoscopic band ligation (EBL) for GAVE showed a significantly higher rate of bleeding cessation with fewer treatments sessions and reduced need for blood transfusions because of a greater increase in hemoglobin levels after treatment, as compared with endoscopic thermal therapy in a study by Wells and colleagues.[27] This mechanical ablative procedure (EBL) has been reported in a few case reports[28]; however, its utility requires expertise, has not yet become popular in many centers, and requires further controlled trials before it can be recommended. In addition, several other endoscopic techniques including cryoablation (needs specialized equipment), bipolar coagulation probe (greater depth of energy delivery), endoscopic mucosectomy, and radiofrequency ablation have been attempted with encouraging results for refractory GAVE cases.[29] These techniques also need larger, prospective studies before their general use, to establish their efficacy and safety.

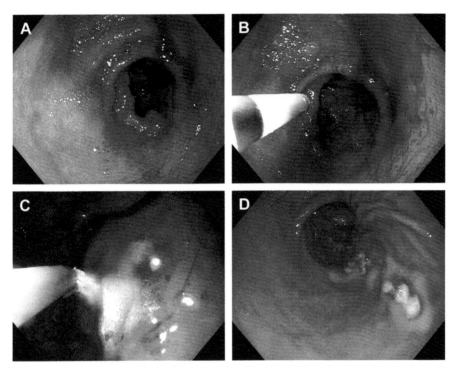

Fig. 2. Moderate GAVE with significant active GIB (*A*); APC probe introduced via endoscope (*B*); APC deploying argon gas for coagulation to control bleeding (*C*); post-APC hemostasis (*D*).

Several classes of drugs have been used to control GAVE-related GIB in case reports and clinical studies. Generally, if endoscopic therapy is not effective or not feasible, medical options are possible. Hormonal therapy with estrogen-progesterone combination pills demonstrated cessation of GIB from GAVE.[30] The GAVE lesions were not eradicated and patients required higher doses, as bleeding recurred with dose reduction during the follow-up period.[31] Maintenance with higher-dose estrogen-progesterone might contribute to untoward side effects of hormonal therapy, including increased risk of endometrial and breast cancer. Octreotide is a somatostatin analogue and has multiple local neuroendocrine effects, including decreasing gastrin levels (growth factor for gastric mucosa), suppression of serotonin, VIP, secretin, motilin, and pancreatic polypeptide.[32] These factors have all been implicated in the pathogenesis of GAVE. In addition, octreotide has been shown to decrease splanchnic circulation and has local anti-angiogenic effects. In addition, it has been shown clinically to effectively reduce the chronic bleeding from gastric vascular abnormalities. Its utility in GAVE still remains of unclear benefit.[33] Other agents, like thalidomide, serotonin antagonists, tranexamic acid, and corticosteroids, have shown some clinical efficacy in separate case reports. Immunosuppressive therapies, methyl prednisone, and cyclophosphamide were used in a patient with systemic sclerosis and resulted in complete resolution of GAVE-related GIB, suggesting the importance of control of the underlying disease as definitive therapy for GAVE.[34]

Surgical resection of the gastric antrum with Billroth-I anastomosis provides definitive cure and has been used in difficult-to-treat cases after endoscopic and medical failures.[35] The analysis of several case reports revealed that a surgical approach (mainly antrectomy) carries up to a 6.6% 30-day mortality.[35]

Gastric Antral Vascular Ectasia in the Presence of Liver Cirrhosis

Liver cirrhosis is found in up to 30% of cases of GAVE.[36] It often presents with chronic, persistent GIB leading to iron deficiency anemia. Overall, cirrhotic patients with GAVE-related GIB carry a higher mortality risk. It is often present with underlying portal hypertension and PHG. Diffuse/nodular pattern is more frequently seen along with PHG in cirrhotics, and clear distinction is sometimes difficult on endoscopic evaluation and, in such cases, careful biopsy and histologic evaluation are preferred. As mentioned above, the use of the GAVE score on histology has high diagnostic accuracy in distinguishing GAVE from PHG.[3] This distinction is of clinical importance because management options are uniquely different for the definitive treatment of GIB from either of these gastric lesions. Treatment of portal hypertension (eg, β-blockers, or portosystemic shunts including transjugular intrahepatic portosystemic shunt [TIPS]) does not have a significant effect on GAVE-related GIB. Endoscopic treatment is mostly the preferred option,[6] APC therapy was found to be effective in 88% of patients with cirrhosis and it required fewer treatment sessions to completely control the GIB related to GAVE, as compared with those without cirrhosis. However, high mortality (53%) was observed in a study among cirrhotics during a 20-month follow-up period and was mostly related to hepatic decompensation. EBL has not been well studied in patients with liver cirrhosis and safety and efficacy of medical therapy has been well defined in this population. Abdominal surgery (antrectomy) carries a high risk of morbidity and mortality in cirrhotics, especially in patients with portal hypertension. Careful selection of patients, accurate diagnosis, and prompt treatment are prudent in cirrhotic patients with GIB related to GAVE. Liver transplantation resulted in complete resolution of GAVE in a patient despite persistent portal hypertension, possibly because of the cure of their underlying liver failure.[17]

In summary, asymptomatic, nonbleeding GAVE lesions do not require any therapy. GIB should be managed with transfusions as needed with a hemoglobin target of 7 to 8 g/dL (cirrhotics) and iron replacements for iron deficiency anemia. Endoscopic therapy (APC) should be attempted first, followed by medical management if endotherapy fails. Surgery can be used in refractory cases of GIB, as a rescue therapy.

PORTAL HYPERTENSIVE GASTROPATHY
Epidemiology

As its name indicates, PHG is found in patients with portal hypertension. It is seen in patients with cirrhosis and also in cases of noncirrhotic portal hypertension. The prevalence of PHG, as mentioned in the literature, varies from 20% to more than 80%, with higher prevalence in decompensated cirrhosis as compared with patients with chronic hepatitis C and milder liver disease or those without cirrhosis.[37,38] In addition, some report that PHG develops less frequently in patients who also have concomitant gastroesophageal varices[39]; however, some reports suggest that endoscopic ligation and sclerotherapy of varices increase the risk of developing PHG, albeit the risk is found to be temporary.[40] Based on the diagnoses used, PHG is indicated to be the cause of 3% to 5% of chronic GIB[41] and 2% to 12% of acute GIB in cirrhosis.[37] Interestingly, from a large prospective study of nonresponder chronic hepatitis C patients with advanced fibrosis, the incidence of PHG is 12.9% per year and worsening PHG develops at a rate of 6.7% per year.[38]

Diagnosis

PHG is usually an incidental or a related finding on an upper endoscopy performed on cirrhotic patients for either variceal screening or acute GIB. It appears as a snake-skin-like mosaic pattern of the mucosa in milder forms and flat or raised red-brown spots in severe cases (**Fig. 3**).[42] Interobserver variability has been reported in the literature for the endoscopic diagnosis of PHG based on these morphologic patterns.[43] If these mucosal lesions are biopsied, PHG usually demonstrates mucosal/submucosal ectatic vessels without thrombin clots or fibrinohyalonosis. As mentioned above, the absence of these findings and GAVE score will differentiate PHG from GAVE in difficult-to-diagnose cases.[3] The distribution of PHG lesions is usually in the fundus and upper body of the stomach (see **Fig. 3**) and similar mucosal abnormalities are often found in the small (duodenopathy) or large (colopathy) intestine in patients with severe portal hypertension and/or liver cirrhosis. Capsule endoscopy has been used to help diagnose PHG and portal hypertensive lesions in distant parts of gastrointestinal tract.[44] Recently, a few case reports have suggested indirect assessment of PHG either by blood testing or ultrasound examination.[45] Moreover, transient elastography combined with platelet count is found useful for predicting the absence of esophageal varices and PHG in HIV patients with liver cirrhosis in a recent study.[46]

Pathogenesis

Most studies have proposed portal hypertension as the essential underlying factor leading to PHG. Some investigators found mucosal friability and increased levels of local mediators leading to gastric mucosal injury, oxidative stress, and impaired healing.[47] Typically, inflammation and vascular mural changes are not seen in the abnormally dilated vasculature seen in PHG lesions.[48,49] Portal hypertension, when estimated by measuring the hepatic venous pressure gradient, has not demonstrated consistent correlation with the presence of PHG.[50,51] Portal and systemic vascular hemodynamic alterations in patients with liver cirrhosis are found to be worse in patients who also have PHG as compared with those who do not have PHG.[52] In addition, gastric mucosal blood flow abnormalities are also observed in PHG lesions independent of portal hypertension.[53] There is no reliable indicator of severity of PHG, except that it is frequently persistent and progressive in patients with portal hypertension associated with liver cirrhosis, as compared with those with noncirrhotic portal hypertension.

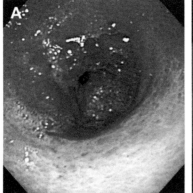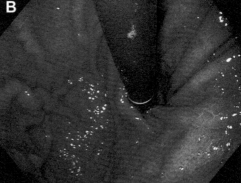

Fig. 3. Mosaic pattern of portal hypertensive gastropathy.

Management

PHG is mostly asymptomatic, and the primary prophylaxis of GIB from nonbleeding PHG should be advised based on the presence and grading of gastroesophageal varices. In a study of patients with isolated nonbleeding PHG, 160 mg of long-acting propranolol per day for 6 weeks showed significant improvement in the endoscopic grading of PHG.[54] Any patient with asymptomatic PHG should be followed with surveillance endoscopies per protocol, because PHG is found to worsen over time in up to 30% of patients.[42] In patients with associated esophageal varices that require medical prophylaxis, the use of nonselective β-blockers could further potentially benefit those same patients with PHG. If PHG is identified in the setting of variceal bleeding and endoscopic therapy is applied for secondary prophylaxis of GIB, some studies have suggested that there is a transient worsening of PHG.[55] In such cases, the introduction of β-blocker therapy could be of benefit to prevent worsening of PHG.

The most common presentation of PHG is chronic gastrointestinal blood loss and iron deficiency anemia (incidence around 10%–15% at 3 years).[56] Adequate iron replacement and, as needed, blood transfusions are used to correct the anemia. Nonselective β-blockers have been shown to decrease recurrent bleeding episodes secondary to PHG. As secondary prophylaxis of bleeding from PHG, one study showed that propranolol is effective in the prevention of rebleeding during 30 months of follow-up.[57] The dose of β-blocker should be titrated to the maximally tolerated dose for adequate heart rate control and minimal side effects. Although several studies have shown benefit of nonselective β-blockers (eg, propranolol, nadolol) in reducing portal hypertension, carvedilol, a nonselective β-blocker and α-1 receptor-blocker, has been shown to be superior to propranolol for reducing portal hypertension and associated GIB.[58]

Acute GIB is an uncommon presentation of PHG (incidence <3% at 3 years)[2]; however, if it occurs, such bleeding episodes can be severe and difficult to manage. Initial management with appropriate resuscitation and antibiotic coverage should be individualized and promptly instituted. Systemic therapy with intravenous somatostatin, octreotide, terlipressin, and/or vasopressin has been shown to reduce portal hypertension and gastric blood flow and control bleeding in patients with PHG.[59] Propranolol has been investigated for the acute management of bleeding from severe PHG and was shown to effectively control the GIB within 3 days.[60] Use of β-blockers can be challenging in the acute setting because of systemic hypotensive and antisympathomimetic effects. Endoscopic therapy for acute bleeding from PHG may provide temporary control of GIB and remains investigational. APC application is proven successful in controlling bleeding from PHG and reducing transfusion requirements in a small study.[61] Hemospray, a nanopowder hemostatic agent licensed for endoscopic hemostasis of nonvariceal UGIB in Europe and Canada, has been shown in preliminary data to be effective in stopping acute bleeding from portal hypertensive mucosal diseases.[62] Hemospray has no effect on portal pressure or the underlying natural disease.

In cases of failure of medical or local therapies for acute or chronic GIB, patients that require frequent transfusions or are clinically worsening, portosystemic shunt therapies should be considered, either through surgery or through the placement of a TIPS. These shunts effectively decompress the portal system to terminate bleeding from PHG.[63] A surgical shunt is preferred in patients with noncirrhotic portal hypertension. Patients who undergo shunt surgery have an improvement in the endoscopic appearance of the PHG lesions and a reduction in the number of transfusions required.[64,65] Patients with liver cirrhosis and portal hypertension who receive TIPS show an improvement of PHG lesions on endoscopy (in as short as 6 weeks after

Table 2
Comparison of treatment modalities for GAVE and PHG

Treatment Modality	GAVE	PHG
Primary prophylaxis	Not indicated	Not indicated (unless associated with large varices)
APC	Primary therapy[22]	For temporary hemostasis[61]
YAG laser therapy	Primary therapy[23]	—
EBL	Can be used in primary therapy for larger lesions[27]	May transiently worsen when done for associated varices[40]
RFA (radiofrequency ablation)	For large refractory lesions[29]	—
Hemospray	—	Local hemostasis[62]
β-blockers (propranolol, Carvedilol)	No benefit[16]	Primary therapy for acute or chronic bleeding[57]
OCP (oral contraceptive pills)	Temporary control of bleeding[30]	—
Octreotide	Possible benefit[33]	Primary therapy in acute bleeding[59]
Liver transplantation	Improves/resolves[17]	Improves with resolution of portal hypertension
TIPS	No benefit[16]	For refractory cases or emergency[65]
Surgical portosystemic shunts	No benefit	For refractory cases
Surgical resection (antrectomy)	For refractory cases[35]	—

shunt placement and in up to 3 months) in cases with more severe PHG.[66] Consideration of TIPS placement should be a team approach with the gastroenterologist, hepatologist, surgeon, and interventional radiologist involved in the decision-making process. TIPS placement carries a potential risk of rapid deterioration of hepatic function leading to liver failure and need for liver transplantation.

SUMMARY

In conclusion, GAVE and PHG are 2 distinct causes of chronic GIB. In patients with cirrhosis, often these mucosal lesions can be relatively easy to distinguish on upper endoscopy based on their appearance: as "watermelon stomach" (red stripes pattern) in the case of GAVE, or "snake skin" (mosaic pattern) in the case of PHG, or location: gastric antrum for GAVE and fundus or upper body in PHG. However, diffuse red spots or nodular pattern on gastric mucosa is occasionally encountered in cirrhotics, which is seen with both GAVE and severe PHG. When the diagnosis is unclear, biopsy and histologic evaluation (and use of GAVE score) help in differentiating GAVE from PHG. The exact diagnosis of the cause of GIB is crucial and the treatment modalities are distinctly different and are summarized in **Table 2**.

REFERENCES

1. Mathurin SA, Agüero AP, Dascani NA, et al. Anemia in hospitalized patients with cirrhosis: prevalence, clinical relevance and predictive factors. Acta Gastroenterol Latinoam 2009;39(2):103–11 [in Spanish].

2. Gostout CJ, Viggiano TR, Ahlquist DA, et al. The clinical and endoscopic spectrum of the watermelon stomach. J Clin Gastroenterol 1992;15(3):256–63.
3. Payen JL, Calès P, Voigt JJ, et al. Severe portal hypertensive gastropathy and antral vascular ectasia are distinct entities in patients with cirrhosis. Gastroenterology 1995;108(1):138–44.
4. Tobin RW, Hackman RC, Kimmey MB, et al. Bleeding from gastric antral vascular ectasia in marrow transplant patients. Gastrointest Endosc 1996;44(3):223–9.
5. Ward EM, Raimondo M, Rosser BG, et al. Prevalence and natural history of gastric antral vascular ectasia in patients undergoing orthotopic liver transplantation. J Clin Gastroenterol 2004;38(10):898–900.
6. Dulai GS, Jensen DM, Kovacs TO, et al. Endoscopic treatment outcomes in watermelon stomach patients with and without portal hypertension. Endoscopy 2004;36(1):68–72.
7. Suit PF, Petras RE, Bauer TW, et al. Gastric antral vascular ectasia. A histologic and morphometric study of "the watermelon stomach". Am J Surg Pathol 1987; 11(10):750–7.
8. Ito M, Uchida Y, Kamano S, et al. Clinical comparisons between two subsets of gastric antral vascular ectasia. Gastrointest Endosc 2001;53(7):764–70.
9. Burak KW, Lee SS, Beck PL. Portal hypertensive gastropathy and gastric antral vascular ectasia (GAVE) syndrome. Gut 2001;49(6):866–72.
10. Parente F, Petrillo M, Vago L, et al. The watermelon stomach: clinical, endoscopic, endosonographic, and therapeutic aspects in three cases. Endoscopy 1995;27(2):203–6.
11. Herman BE, Vargo JJ, Baum S, et al. Gastric antral vascular ectasia: a case report and review of the literature. J Nucl Med 1996;37(5):854–6.
12. Westerhoff M, Tretiakova M, Hovan L, et al. CD61, CD31, and CD34 improve diagnostic accuracy in gastric antral vascular ectasia and portal hypertensive gastropathy: an immunohistochemical and digital morphometric study. Am J Surg Pathol 2010;34(4):494–501.
13. Charneau J, Petit R, Calès P, et al. Antral motility in patients with cirrhosis with or without gastric antral vascular ectasia. Gut 1995;37(4):488–92.
14. Quintero E, Pique JM, Bombi JA, et al. Gastric mucosal vascular ectasias causing bleeding in cirrhosis. A distinct entity associated with hypergastrinemia and low serum levels of pepsinogen I. Gastroenterology 1987;93(5):1054–61.
15. Saperas E, Perez Ayuso RM, Poca E, et al. Increased gastric PGE2 biosynthesis in cirrhotic patients with gastric vascular ectasia. Am J Gastroenterol 1990; 85(2):138–44.
16. Spahr L, Villeneuve JP, Dufresne MP, et al. Gastric antral vascular ectasia in cirrhotic patients: absence of relation with portal hypertension. Gut 1999; 44(5):739–42.
17. Vincent C, Pomier-Layrargues G, Dagenais M, et al. Cure of gastric antral vascular ectasia by liver transplantation despite persistent portal hypertension: a clue for pathogenesis. Liver Transpl 2002;8(8):717–20.
18. Watson M, Hally RJ, McCue PA, et al. Gastric antral vascular ectasia (watermelon stomach) in patients with systemic sclerosis. Arthritis Rheum 1996; 39(2):341–6.
19. Goel A, Christian CL. Gastric antral vascular ectasia (watermelon stomach) in a patient with Sjögren's syndrome. J Rheumatol 2003;30(5):1090–2.
20. Valdez BC, Henning D, Busch RK, et al. A nucleolar RNA helicase recognized by autoimmune antibodies from a patient with watermelon stomach disease. Nucleic Acids Res 1996;24(7):1220–4.

21. Arendt T, Barten M, Lakner V, et al. Diffuse gastric antral vascular ectasia: cause of chronic gastrointestinal blood loss. Endoscopy 1987;19(5):218–20.

22. Probst A, Scheubel R, Wienbeck M. Treatment of watermelon stomach (GAVE syndrome) by means of endoscopic argon plasma coagulation (APC): long-term outcome. Z Gastroenterol 2001;39(6):447–52.

23. Ng I, Lai KC, Ng M. Clinical and histological features of gastric antral vascular ectasia: successful treatment with endoscopic laser therapy. J Gastroenterol Hepatol 1996;11(3):270–4.

24. Liberski SM, McGarrity TJ, Hartle RJ, et al. The watermelon stomach: long-term outcome in patients treated with Nd:YAG laser therapy. Gastrointest Endosc 1994;40(5):584–7.

25. Geller A, Gostout CJ, Balm RK. Development of hyperplastic polyps following laser therapy for watermelon stomach. Gastrointest Endosc 1996; 43(1):54–6.

26. Bernstein CN, Pettigrew N, Wang KK, et al. Multifocal gastric neoplasia after recurrent laser therapy for the watermelon stomach. Can J Gastroenterol 1997;11(5):403–6.

27. Wells CD, Harrison ME, Gurudu SR, et al. Treatment of gastric antral vascular ectasia (watermelon stomach) with endoscopic band ligation. Gastrointest Endosc 2008;68(2):231–6.

28. Chong VH. Snare coagulation for gastric antral vascular ectasia ablation. Gastrointest Endosc 2009;69(6):1195.

29. McGorisk T, Krishnan K, Keefer L, et al. Radiofrequency ablation for refractory gastric antral vascular ectasia (with video). Gastrointest Endosc 2013;78(4): 584–8.

30. Tran A, Villeneuve JP, Bilodeau M, et al. Treatment of chronic bleeding from gastric antral vascular ectasia (GAVE) with estrogen-progesterone in cirrhotic patients: an open pilot study. Am J Gastroenterol 1999;94(10):2909–11.

31. Moss SF, Ghosh P, Thomas DM, et al. Gastric antral vascular ectasia: maintenance treatment with oestrogen-progesterone. Gut 1992;33(5):715–7.

32. Nardone G, Rocco A, Balzano T, et al. The efficacy of octreotide therapy in chronic bleeding due to vascular abnormalities of the gastrointestinal tract. Aliment Pharmacol Ther 1999;13(11):1429–36.

33. Barbara G, De Giorgio R, Salvioli B, et al. Unsuccessful octreotide treatment of the watermelon stomach. J Clin Gastroenterol 1998;26(4):345–6.

34. Lorenzi AR, Johnson AH, Davies G, et al. Gastric antral vascular ectasia in systemic sclerosis: complete resolution with methylprednisolone and cyclophosphamide. Ann Rheum Dis 2001;60(8):796–8.

35. Novitsky YW, Kercher KW, Czerniach DR, et al. Watermelon stomach: pathophysiology, diagnosis, and management. J Gastrointest Surg 2003;7(5): 652–61.

36. Jabbari M, Cherry R, Lough JO, et al. Gastric antral vascular ectasia: the watermelon stomach. Gastroenterology 1984;87(5):1165–70.

37. Merli M, Nicolini G, Angeloni S, et al. The natural history of portal hypertensive gastropathy in patients with liver cirrhosis and mild portal hypertension. Am J Gastroenterol 2004;99(10):1959–65.

38. Fontana RJ, Sanyal AJ, Mehta S, et al. Portal hypertensive gastropathy in chronic hepatitis C patients with bridging fibrosis and compensated cirrhosis: results from the HALT-C trial. Am J Gastroenterol 2006;101(5):983–92.

39. Iwao T, Toyonaga A, Oho K, et al. Portal-hypertensive gastropathy develops less in patients with cirrhosis and fundal varices. J Hepatol 1997;26(6):1235–41.

40. D'Amico G, Montalbano L, Traina M, et al. Natural history of congestive gastropathy in cirrhosis. The Liver Study Group of V. Cervello Hospital. Gastroenterology 1990;99(6):1558–64.

41. Primignani M, Carpinelli L, Preatoni P, et al. Natural history of portal hypertensive gastropathy in patients with liver cirrhosis. The New Italian Endoscopic Club for the study and treatment of esophageal varices (NIEC). Gastroenterology 2000; 119(1):181–7.

42. Sarin SK, Sreenivas DV, Lahoti D, et al. Factors influencing development of portal hypertensive gastropathy in patients with portal hypertension. Gastroenterology 1992;102(3):994–9.

43. de Franchis R, Faculty BV. Revising consensus in portal hypertension: report of the Baveno V consensus workshop on methodology of diagnosis and therapy in portal hypertension. J Hepatol 2010;53(4):762–8.

44. Canlas KR, Dobozi BM, Lin S, et al. Using capsule endoscopy to identify GI tract lesions in cirrhotic patients with portal hypertension and chronic anemia. J Clin Gastroenterol 2008;42(7):844–8.

45. Burak KW, Beck PL. Diagnosis of portal hypertensive gastropathy. Curr Opin Gastroenterol 2003;19(5):477–82.

46. Montes Ramirez ML, Pascual-Pareja JF, Sánchez-Conde M, et al. Transient elastography to rule out esophageal varices and portal hypertensive gastropathy in HIV-infected individuals with liver cirrhosis. AIDS 2012;26(14):1807–12.

47. Drăghia AC. Histochemical and histopathological study of the gastric mucosa in the portal hypertensive gastropathy. Rom J Morphol Embryol 2006;47(3): 259–62.

48. Sarfeh IJ, Tarnawski A. Gastric mucosal vasculopathy in portal hypertension. Gastroenterology 1987;93(5):1129–31.

49. Lan C, Sun X, Dong L, et al. The role of endotoxin in the pathogenesis of gastric mucosal damage in cirrhotic rats with portal hypertensive gastropathy. Asian Pac J Trop Med 2011;4(3):212–4.

50. Kim MY, Choi H, Baik SK, et al. Portal hypertensive gastropathy: correlation with portal hypertension and prognosis in cirrhosis. Dig Dis Sci 2010;55(12): 3561–7.

51. Bellis L, Nicodemo S, Galossi A, et al. Hepatic venous pressure gradient does not correlate with the presence and the severity of portal hypertensive gastropathy in patients with liver cirrhosis. J Gastrointestin Liver Dis 2007;16(3):273–7.

52. Kumar A, Mishra SR, Sharma P, et al. Clinical, laboratory, and hemodynamic parameters in portal hypertensive gastropathy: a study of 254 cirrhotics. J Clin Gastroenterol 2010;44(4):294–300.

53. Ohta M, Hashizume M, Higashi H, et al. Portal and gastric mucosal hemodynamics in cirrhotic patients with portal-hypertensive gastropathy. Hepatology 1994;20(6):1432–6.

54. Hosking SW. Congestive gastropathy in portal hypertension: variations in prevalence. Hepatology 1989;10(2):257–8.

55. de la Peña J, Rivero M, Sanchez E, et al. Variceal ligation compared with endoscopic sclerotherapy for variceal hemorrhage: prospective randomized trial. Gastrointest Endosc 1999;49(4 Pt 1):417–23.

56. Iwao T, Toyonaga A, Sumino M, et al. Portal hypertensive gastropathy in patients with cirrhosis. Gastroenterology 1992;102(6):2060–5.

57. Pérez-Ayuso RM, Piqué JM, Bosch J, et al. Propranolol in prevention of recurrent bleeding from severe portal hypertensive gastropathy in cirrhosis. Lancet 1991; 337(8755):1431–4.

58. Bañares R, Moitinho E, Matilla A, et al. Randomized comparison of long-term carvedilol and propranolol administration in the treatment of portal hypertension in cirrhosis. Hepatology 2002;36(6):1367–73.
59. Zhou Y, Qiao L, Wu J, et al. Comparison of the efficacy of octreotide, vasopressin, and omeprazole in the control of acute bleeding in patients with portal hypertensive gastropathy: a controlled study. J Gastroenterol Hepatol 2002; 17(9):973–9.
60. Hosking SW, Kennedy HJ, Seddon I, et al. The role of propranolol in congestive gastropathy of portal hypertension. Hepatology 1987;7(3):437–41.
61. Herrera S, Bordas JM, Llach J, et al. The beneficial effects of argon plasma coagulation in the management of different types of gastric vascular ectasia lesions in patients admitted for GI hemorrhage. Gastrointest Endosc 2008;68(3): 440–6.
62. Smith LA, Morris AJ, Stanley AJ. The use of hemospray in portal hypertensive bleeding; a case series. J Hepatol 2014;60(2):457–60.
63. Mezawa S, Homma H, Ohta H, et al. Effect of transjugular intrahepatic portosystemic shunt formation on portal hypertensive gastropathy and gastric circulation. Am J Gastroenterol 2001;96(4):1155–9.
64. Urata J, Yamashita Y, Tsuchigame T, et al. The effects of transjugular intrahepatic portosystemic shunt on portal hypertensive gastropathy. J Gastroenterol Hepatol 1998;13(10):1061–7.
65. Kamath PS, Lacerda M, Ahlquist DA, et al. Gastric mucosal responses to intrahepatic portosystemic shunting in patients with cirrhosis. Gastroenterology 2000;118(5):905–11.
66. Ripoll C, Garcia-Tsao G. The management of portal hypertensive gastropathy and gastric antral vascular ectasia. Dig Liver Dis 2011;43(5):345–51.

Index

Note: Page numbers of article titles are in **boldface** type.

A

Acid injury, 711–712
Acid suppression, for erosive lesions, 708
Adenocarcinoma, gastric, 710–711
American Association for Study of Liver Diseases recommendations, 787, 791, 808
Angiodysplasia, 708–710
Angiography, catheter, 746–750
Angiotherapy, ultrasound-guided, 732–734
Ankaferd Blood Stopper, 685–686, 726–728
Antibiotics, for variceal bleeding, 670, 772–773, 797–798, 821
Anticoagulants, peptic ulcer bleeding and, 689–693
Antiplatelet therapy
    as bleeding risk, 646–648
    peptic ulcer bleeding and, 689–691
Antrectomy, for peptic ulcer, 757–759
Apixaban, peptic ulcer bleeding and, 692–693
Argon plasma coagulation, for peptic ulcer bleeding, 683–684
Aspartate aminotransferase, in variceal bleeding, 767
Aspiration precautions, in variceal bleeding, 821
Aspirin
    as bleeding risk, 646–648
    peptic ulcer bleeding and, 689–690

B

Balloon catheters, for radiofrequency ablation, 729–731
Balloon retrograde transvenous obliteration, 776–777, 813–814, 825–826
Balloon tamponade, 775, 801, 822–823
Band ligation
    for GAVE, 838
    for variceal bleeding, 799–800
Batteries, ingestion of, 712
Baveno guidelines, 787, 791
Beta blockers
    for portal hypertension gastropathy, 842
    for varices, 786–791
Biliary tract, bleeding from, 712–713
Billroth-1 anastomosis, for GAVE, 839–840
Bipolar electrocautery, for peptic ulcer bleeding, 682–683
Bisphosphonates, as bleeding risk, 647–648
Blakemore tube, 671, 801

Gastroenterol Clin N Am 43 (2014) 849–856
http://dx.doi.org/10.1016/S0889-8553(14)00118-6
0889-8553/14/$ – see front matter © 2014 Elsevier Inc. All rights reserved.

gastro.theclinics.com

Blood transfusions, 671, 772
Boerhaave syndrome, 711–712

C

Cameron lesions, 708
Cancer, 710–711
Capsule endoscopy, for portal hypertension gastropathy, 841
Carbon dioxide cryotherapy, 728
Carvedilol, for varices, 788–790
Catheter angiography, 746–750
Caustic injury, 711–712
Cephalosporins, for variceal bleeding, 773
Chemoradiotherapy, for neoplastic lesions, 710–711
Child-Turcotte-Pugh score, 767–768, 784
Cirrhosis
    as bleeding risk, 649
    GAVE with, 840
    treatment of, 786
    variceal bleeding in. *See* Variceal gastrointestinal bleeding.
Clinical Rockall Score, 668
Clips, 712, 722–725
Clopidogrel, peptic ulcer bleeding and, 690–691
Clots, removal of, in peptic ulcer, 686–687
COGENT trial, 690–691
Coil therapy, 743, 810–812
Computed tomography, for variceal bleeding, 770, 785
Computed tomography angiography, 746
Contact electrocoagulation, for peptic ulcer bleeding, 682–683
Contact heater probe, for peptic ulcer bleeding, 683
Corticosteroids, for vasculitis, 713–714
Cryotherapy, 728
Cyanoacrylate
    for gastric varices, 808–810
    for variceal bleeding prophylaxis, 792
    for variceal bleeding treatment, 801–802, 808–811

D

Dabigatran, peptic ulcer bleeding and, 692–693
Definitive surgery, for peptic ulcer, 757
Dieulafoy lesions, 645, 708–710
Drugs, erosive lesions due to, 708
Duodenitis, erosive esophago-gastric, 708

E

Echoendoscope, forward-view, 814–815
Edoxaban, peptic ulcer bleeding and, 692–693
Electrocoagulation, for peptic ulcer bleeding, 682–683
Embolization
    agents for, 740, 742

for neoplastic lesions, 710–711
for variceal bleeding, 810–811
in transcatheter angiography, 746–750
Encephalopathy, hepatic, 772, 821–822
Endoclips, for peptic ulcer bleeding, 684–685
EndoClot, for peptic ulcer bleeding, 685–686
Endoscopic management
    failure of
        interventional radiology alternative for, **739–752**
        surgical alternatives for, **753–761**
    for nonvariceal bleeding, emerging therapies for, **721–737**
    for nonvariceal nonulcer bleeding, **707–719**
    for peptic ulcer bleeding, **677–705,** 755–756
    for variceal bleeding, 773–774
        esophageal, **795–806**
        gastric, **807–818**
Endoscopy, diagnostic
    benefits of, 650–654
    emergency, 656–657
    for peptic ulcer bleeding, 678–680
    procedure for, 654–656
    prognostic value of, 650–655
    quality of, 655–656
    timing of, 656–657
Endotracheal intubation, for variceal bleeding, 770, 797
Epinephrine injection, for peptic ulcer bleeding, 681–682
Erosive causes, of UBIB, 708
Esophagogastric bleeding. *See* Variceal gastrointestinal bleeding.
Esophago-gastric-duodenitis, erosive, 708
Esophagogastroduodenosccopy, for variceal screening, 784–786
Esophagus
    Boerhaave syndrome of, 711–712
    Mallory-Weiss tears of, 711–712
    resection of, for variceal bleeding, 775–776
    trauma to, 711–712
Estrogen-progesterone therapy, for GAVE, 839
Ethanolamine oleate, for variceal bleeding, 799

F

Fibrin glue, for variceal bleeding, 810
FibroTest, in variceal bleeding, 770
Fluid therapy, for variceal bleeding, 770–772, 797, 820–821
Focal catheters, for radiofrequency ablation, 729–730
Foreign body ingestion, 711–712
Forrest classification, for peptic ulcer bleeding, 650–654
Forward-view echoendoscope, 814–815

G

Gastrectomy, for peptic ulcer, 757–759
Gastric adenocarcinoma, 710–711

Gastric antral vascular ectasia, 708–710, 836–840
    cirrhosis with, 840
    cryotherapy for, 728
    diagnosis of, 836–837
    epidemiology of, 836
    hemostatic sprays for, 727
    pathogenesis of, 837–838
    radiofrequency ablation for, 729–731
    treatment of, 838–840
Gastric ischemia, bleeding from, 713–714
Gastric varices, bleeding from, **807–818**
Gastropathy. *See also* Gastric antral vascular ectasia.
    portal hypertension, 709–710, 840–843
GAVE. *See* Gastric antral vascular ectasia.
Glasgow-Blatchford Score, 668
Gold probe, for peptic ulcer bleeding, 683

H

Helicobacter pylori infections, 645–646, 688
Hemobilia, 712–713
Hemospray powder, 726–728
    for erosive lesions, 708
    for neoplastic lesions, 710–711
    for portal hypertension gastropathy, 842
    for variceal bleeding, 801–802
Hemostasis, endoscopic therapies for. *See* Endoscopic management.
Hemostatic powders and sprays, 685–686, 725–728
Hemosuccus pancreaticus, 712–713
Hepatic encephalopathy, 772, 821–822
Hepatic venous pressure gradient, in variceal bleeding, 767–769, 784
Hepatopancreaticobiliary tract, bleeding from, 712–713
Hiatal hernia, Cameron lesions due to, 708
Hormone therapy, for GAVE, 839

I

Immunosuppressive therapy, for vasculitis, 713–714
Infections, in variceal bleeding, 772–773
Injection therapy, for peptic ulcer bleeding, 681–682
Interventional radiology, **739–752**
    adverse events in, 747, 750
    evolution of, 740
    for variceal bleeding, 813, 824–826
    materials and methods for, 740–749
    results of, 747

K

Kidney failure and dysfunction
    as bleeding risk, 649
    in variceal bleeding, 772, 822

L

Laser therapy, for GAVE, 838
Ligation, of varices, 789–791
Linton-Nicholas tube, for variceal bleeding, 822–823
Liquid nitrogen cryotherapy, 728
Liver, stiffness of, in variceal bleeding, 769–770

M

Magnets, ingestion of, 712
Malignancy, 710–711
Mallory-Weiss tears, 711–712
MELD (Model for End-Stage Liver Disease) Score, in variceal bleeding, 767–768
Microcatheters, 740–741
Microcoils, 743
Minimal surgical approach, for peptic ulcer, 757
Model for End-Stage Liver Disease (MELD) Score, in variceal bleeding, 767–768
Monopolar electrocautery, for peptic ulcer bleeding, 682–683
Mortality
    from nonvariceal UGIB, 648–650
    in peptic ulcer bleeding, 754
    in variceal bleeding, 766–769

N

Nadolol, for varices, 787–788
Nasogastric aspiration, as diagnostic tool, 668–669
Neoplastic lesions, 710–711
Noncontact thermal therapy, for peptic ulcer bleeding, 683–684
Nonsteroidal anti-inflammatory drugs
    as bleeding risk, 646–648
    erosive lesions due to, 708
    peptic ulcer bleeding and, 688–689
Nonvariceal gastrointestinal bleeding, **707–719**. *See also* Peptic ulcers, bleeding from.
    causes of, 644–645
    diagnosis of, 650–657
    epidemiology of, 643–650
    erosive causes of, 708
    from hepatopancreaticobiliary tract, 712–713
    in neoplastic lesions, 710–711
    in vascular anomalies, 708–710
    mortality from, 648–650
    nonulcer, endoscopic treatment of, **707–719**
    risk factors for, 645–648
    traumatic, 711–712
    treatment of, **707–719, 721–737**
Norfloxacin, for variceal bleeding, 797–798

O

Octreotide
    for GAVE, 839
    for variceal bleeding, 798, 824

Overstitch device, 730–732
Over-the-scope clips, 712, 722–725

P

Padock clips, 722–725
Pancreas, bleeding from, 712–713
Partial gastrectomy, for peptic ulcer, 757–759
Peptic ulcers, bleeding from, **677–705**
    endoscopic treatment of, 680–693, 755–756
    Forrest classification for, 650–654
    incidence of, 644–645
    mortality in, 754
    preendoscopic prokinetics for, 678
    rebleeding after endoscopy, 754–755
    risk factors for, 645–648
    surgery for, **753–763**
Peritonitis, 772–773
Platelet count, for variceal bleeding, 770, 785–786
Portal decompressive surgery, 826
Portal hypertension
    decompressive surgery for, for variceal bleeding, 775–776
    variceal bleeding prophylaxis in, **784–794**
Portal hypertension gastropathy, 709–710, 840–843
Portal vein thrombosis, 826
Propranolol
    for portal hypertension gastropathy, 842
    for varices, 787–788
Proton pump inhibitors
    postendoscopic, 687
    preendoscopic, 670

R

Radiofrequency ablation, 729–731
Rivaroxaban, peptic ulcer bleeding and, 692–693

S

Saeed Multiple Ligator, for variceal bleeding, 799–800
Salvage surgery, for peptic ulcer, 759
Scintigraphy, 746
Sclerotherapy
    for peptic ulcer bleeding, 682
    for variceal bleeding, 798–799
Selective cyclooxygenase inhibitors
    as bleeding risk, 647
    peptic ulcer bleeding and, 688–689
Selective vagotomy, for peptic ulcer, 757–759
Sengstaken-Blakemore tube, for variceal bleeding, 801
Sodium morrhuate, for variceal bleeding, 799

Somatostatin
    for variceal bleeding, 773, 798, 823
    preendoscopy, 670
Speedband, for variceal bleeding, 799–800
Spleen, stiffness of, in variceal bleeding, 769–770
Sprays, hemostatic, 725–728
Stents, 712, 734, 775, 801
Surgery
    for endoscopic failure, **753–763,** 826
        alternatives to, 760
        definitive approach to, 757
        early versus delayed, 755–757
        endoscopic retreatment after, 760
        minimal approach to, 757
        selection of technique for, 757–760
    for GAVE, 839–840
    for variceal bleeding, 775–777
Suturing, endoscopic, 730–732

T

TC-325, 685–686, 726–728
Terlipressin, for variceal bleeding, 798, 823
Thermal therapy, for peptic ulcer bleeding, 682–684
Thermoablation, for GAVE, 838
Thrombin, for variceal bleeding, 810
Tissue adhesives, 734
    for peptic ulcer bleeding, 682
    for variceal bleeding, 801–802
Transarterial embolization, for neoplastic lesions, 710–711
Transcatheter angiography, 746–750
Transjugular intrahepatic portosystemic shunt, 813, 824–825
    for portal hypertension gastropathy, 842
    for variceal bleeding, 774–776
Traumatic lesions, 711–712
Truncal vagotomy, for peptic ulcer, 757–759

U

UGIB. *See* Upper gastrointestinal bleeding.
Ultrasonography, in variceal bleeding, 770
Ultrasound-guided angiotherapy, 732–734
Upper gastrointestinal bleeding, **665–675**
    causes of, 744
    definition of, 744
    diagnosis of, 745
    imaging for, 745–746
    in peptic ulcer. *See* Peptic ulcer.
    in portal hypertension, **835–847**
    incidence of, 665–666
    initial management of, 666–667

Upper (*continued*)
  nonvariceal. *See* Nonvariceal gastrointestinal bleeding.
  presentation of, 666
  risk stratification for, 667–669
  treatment of. *See also specific disorders and techniques.*
    interventional radiology for, **739–752**
    options for, 744–745
  variceal. *See* Variceal gastrointestinal bleeding.
  vascular supply in, 744

V

Vagotomy, for peptic ulcer, 757–759
Vapreotide, for variceal bleeding, 798
Variceal gastrointestinal bleeding, **765–782**
  assessment of, 821–826
  diagnosis of, 769–770, 796–797
  epidemiology of, 765
  esophageal, **795–806**
  gastric, **807–818**
  mortality in, 766
  natural history of, 796–797
  predictive models for, 767–769
  prophylaxis for, **783–794**
  surveillance for, 791
  treatment of, 770–776, 797–802
    endoscopic, **795–818**
    esophageal, **795–806**
    gastric, **807–818**
    nonendoscopic, **819–833**
Vascular anomalies, 708–710
Vasculitis, bleeding from, 713–714
Vasoactive medications
  for variceal bleeding, 773, 798
  preendoscopy, 670
Vasopressin
  for portal hypertension gastropathy, 842
  for variceal bleeding, 773, 798, 823
  preendoscopy, 670
Video capsule endoscopy, 669, 785

W

Warfarin
  as bleeding risk, 647
  peptic ulcer bleeding and, 689–691

Z

Zoom endoscopy, 654

United States Postal Service

Statement of Ownership, Management, and Circulation
(All Periodicals Publications Except Requestor Publications)

1. Publication Title	2. Publication Number	3. Filing Date
Gastroenterology Clinics of North America	0 0 0 - 2 7 9	9/14/14

4. Issue Frequency	5. Number of Issues Published Annually	6. Annual Subscription Price
Mar, Jun, Sep, Dec	4	$320.00

7. Complete Mailing Address of Known Office of Publication (Not printer) (Street, city, county, state, and ZIP+4®)

Elsevier Inc.
360 Park Avenue South
New York, NY 10010-1710

Contact Person
Stephen R. Bushing
Telephone (Include area code)
215-239-3688

8. Complete Mailing Address of Headquarters or General Business Office of Publisher (Not printer)

Elsevier Inc., 360 Park Avenue South, New York, NY 10010-1710

9. Full Names and Complete Mailing Addresses of Publisher, Editor, and Managing Editor (Do not leave blank)

Publisher (Name and complete mailing address)

Linda Belfus, Elsevier Inc., 1600 John F. Kennedy Blvd., Suite 1800, Philadelphia, PA 19103-2899

Editor (Name and complete mailing address)

Kerry Holland, Elsevier Inc., 1600 John F. Kennedy Blvd., Suite 1800, Philadelphia, PA 19103-2899

Managing Editor (Name and complete mailing address)

Adrianne Brigido, Elsevier Inc., 1600 John F. Kennedy Blvd., Suite 1800, Philadelphia, PA 19103-2899

10. Owner (Do not leave blank. If the publication is owned by a corporation, give the name and address of the corporation immediately followed by the names and addresses of all stockholders owning or holding 1 percent or more of the total amount of stock. If not owned by a corporation, give the names and addresses of the individual owners. If owned by a partnership or other unincorporated firm, give its name and address as well as those of each individual owner. If the publication is published by a nonprofit organization, give its name and address.)

Full Name	Complete Mailing Address
Wholly owned subsidiary of	1600 John F. Kennedy Blvd, Ste. 1800
Reed/Elsevier, US holdings	Philadelphia, PA 19103-2899

11. Known Bondholders, Mortgagees, and Other Security Holders Owning or Holding 1 Percent or More of Total Amount of Bonds, Mortgages, or Other Securities. If none, check box ☐ None

Full Name	Complete Mailing Address
N/A	

12. Tax Status (For completion by nonprofit organizations authorized to mail at nonprofit rates) (Check one)
The purpose, function, and nonprofit status of this organization and the exempt status for federal income tax purposes:
☐ Has Not Changed During Preceding 12 Months
☐ Has Changed During Preceding 12 Months (Publisher must submit explanation of change with this statement)

PS Form 3526, August 2012 (Page 1 of 3 (Instructions Page 3)) PSN 7530-01-000-9931 PRIVACY NOTICE: See our Privacy policy in www.usps.com

---

13. Publication Title	14. Issue Date for Circulation Data Below
Gastroenterology Clinics of North America	September 2014

15. Extent and Nature of Circulation			Average No. Copies Each Issue During Preceding 12 Months	No. Copies of Single Issue Published Nearest to Filing Date
a. Total Number of Copies (Net press run)			854	894
b. Paid Circulation (By Mail and Outside the Mail)	(1)	Mailed Outside-County Paid Subscriptions Stated on PS Form 3541. (Include paid distribution above nominal rate, advertiser's proof copies, and exchange copies)	349	359
	(2)	Mailed In-County Paid Subscriptions Stated on PS Form 3541 (Include paid distribution above nominal rate, advertiser's proof copies, and exchange copies)		
	(3)	Paid Distribution Outside the Mails Including Sales Through Dealers and Carriers, Street Vendors, Counter Sales, and Other Paid Distribution Outside USPS®	194	206
	(4)	Paid Distribution by Other Classes Mailed Through the USPS (e.g. First-Class Mail®)		
c. Total Paid Distribution (Sum of 15b (1), (2), (3), and (4))		▶	543	565
d. Free or Nominal Rate Distribution (By Mail and Outside the Mail)	(1)	Free or Nominal Rate Outside-County Copies Included on PS Form 3541	99	114
	(2)	Free or Nominal Rate In-County Copies Included on PS Form 3541		
	(3)	Free or Nominal Rate Copies Mailed at Other Classes Through the USPS (e.g. First-Class Mail)		
	(4)	Free or Nominal Rate Distribution Outside the Mail (Carriers or other means)		
e. Total Free or Nominal Rate Distribution (Sum of 15d (1), (2), (3) and (4)		▶	99	114
f. Total Distribution (Sum of 15c and 15e)		▶	642	679
g. Copies not Distributed (See instructions to publishers #4 (page #3))		▶	212	215
h. Total (Sum of 15f and g)		▶	854	894
i. Percent Paid (15c divided by 15f times 100)		▶	84.58%	83.21%

16. Total circulation includes electronic copies. Report circulation on PS Form 3526-X worksheet.

17. Publication of Statement of Ownership
If the publication is a general publication, publication of this statement is required. Will be printed in the December 2014 issue of this publication.

18. Signature and Title of Editor, Publisher, Business Manager, or Owner	Date
Stephen R. Bushing — Inventory Distribution Coordinator	September 14, 2014

I certify that all information furnished on this form is true and complete. I understand that anyone who furnishes false or misleading information on this form or who omits material or information requested on the form may be subject to criminal sanctions (including fines and imprisonment) and/or civil sanctions (including civil penalties).

PS Form 3526, August 2012 (Page 2 of 3)

Printed and bound by CPI Group (UK) Ltd, Croydon, CR0 4YY

03/10/2024

01040496-0002